Everything you
always wanted to know about sex*

*BUT WERE AFRAID TO ASK™

ALL NEW EDITION

Everything you
always wanted to know about sex*

*BUT WERE AFRAID TO ASK™

ALL NEW EDITION

David Reuben, M.D.

HarperCollins*Publishers*

HarperCollins books may be purchased for educational, business, or sales promotional use. For information please write: Special Markets Department, HarperCollins Publishers, Inc., 10 East 53rd Street, New York, NY 10022.

FIRST EDITION

Designed by Jonathan Nathan

Library of Congress Cataloging-in-Publication Data
Reuben, David R.
    Everything you always wanted to know about sex* *but were afraid to ask: all new edition / David Reuben.—1st ed.
       p. cm.
    Includes index.
    ISBN 0-06-019267-4
    1. Sex. 2. I. Title
    HQ31.R436 1999
    306.7—dc21   98-43025

99 00 01 02 03 ❖/RRD 10 9 8 7 6 5 4 3 2 1

To my wife, Barbara,
who has given me 13,780 days of happiness . . .
and still counting . . .

And to all the MUNCHKINS . . .
For their Loyalty, their Courage, and their Devotion

CONTENTS

ACKNOWLEDGMENTS

To Ben Camardi, my Agent (he deserves upper case), who displayed those rarest of qualities these days. He was loyal, tenacious, and unflinching every step of the way.

To the 100 million men and women around the world who read the Original Edition and gave me the encouragement and the mission to give them the All New Edition—with the fervent wish that it will bring them the satisfaction and fulfillment that they so richly deserve.

DAVID REUBEN, M.D.
New York, NY

An Open Letter to My Fellow Physicians

David Reuben, M.D.
Harold Matson Co.
276 Fifth Avenue
New York, NY 10001

Tel: 212-679-4490
Fax: 212-545-1224

E-mail: mydoctor@everysex.com

My Dear Colleagues,

It has been some time since I've had the pleasure of writing to you.

All of us have noted the dramatic changes in the medical aspects of Human Sexuality over the past few decades. It has been challenging and at the same time exciting—it has made our daily practice even more compelling than in the past.

I hope you will find this book useful in counseling and orienting your patients. Today more than ever, the field of Human Sexuality is cluttered with self-styled experts of dubious credentials who may do actual harm to your patients while eroding your professional status with them.

I am happy to assure you that every fact and every detail in this book is reinforced by reference to the authoritative scientific literature. You will also note that I have taken every opportunity to refer readers to the one person who is most qualified to give them information and advice regarding their personal sexual problems. That person is you, their personal physician.

If you have any questions or suggestions, I will be very happy to hear from you.

With very best wishes for your continued success,

Fraternally yours,

David Reuben, M.D.
David Reuben, M.D.
U. of Illinois College of Medicine '57

DR/cg

AN OPEN LETTER TO MY READERS

David Reuben, M.D.
Harold Matson Co.
276 Fifth Avenue
New York, NY 10001

Tel: 212-679-4490
Fax: 212-545-1224

E-mail: mydoctor@everysex.com

My Dear Friends,

I'm happy to have the pleasure of greeting you once again. I want to take this opportunity to thank you for the warm acceptance that you have given to my books over the past years—all eight volumes. At the same time, I am keenly aware of the responsibility on my part that goes along with the confidence you have placed in me.

In the All New Edition of *Everything you always wanted to know about sex* *But were afraid to ask*, I have been meticulous in presenting the most authoritative medical and scientific findings in a way that will be useful to you and your family. At the same time I have taken care to alert you to some of the real hazards and pitfalls of sex in the twenty-first century.

My goal, as always, is to do everything I possibly can to assure your good health, your unrestricted happiness, and your personal triumph. I hope that this New Edition contributes to those goals.

As always, if you have any questions or suggestions, I'd be delighted to hear from you.

With very best wishes for your continued success and happiness,

Sincerely,

David Reuben, M.D.
David Reuben, M.D.
U. of Illinois College of Medicine '57

Please read this!

I'm confident that you already know this but I would like to emphasize it again.

NOTHING IN THIS BOOK IS MEDICAL ADVICE.

It is educational and informative. I hope it will encourage you to discuss any medical problem you might have with your trusted personal physician.

He can give you medical advice and treatment because he can see you and examine you. Since I can't see you or examine you through the pages of this book, I couldn't begin to give you the tiniest bit of medical diagnosis, advice, or treatment.

As they say on those ads on TV where a race driver runs off a mountain at 100 miles an hour and then the caption reads:

"Don't try this at home!"

That's really what I'm saying to you . . .

Don't try *anything* in this book without getting the advice of a doctor you know and trust. Neither I nor my publisher assume any responsibility for anything that may result from your failure to do so.

Now that we've cleared that up . . . I hope you enjoy every word on every page. And I hope this book brings you a better life in every way . . . every day.

DAVID REUBEN, M.D.
New York, NY

Chapter 1
BEYOND THE BIRDS AND BEES

It has been thirty years almost to the day since the original publication of *Everything you always wanted to know about sex* *But were afraid to ask*. In that interval a lot has changed. Men go to Outer Space almost the way they used to go from New York to London. Even the jet pilot I mentioned in the Introduction to the Original Edition has now become a Space Voyager and steered his Craft into the vast darkness of Space. But he still can't propel his penis those seven inches into the vast darkness of the vagina.

The woman physicist who explored the mysteries of nuclear particles in the original edition has discovered an entirely new form of attraction between sub-nuclear particles—but she still hasn't discovered why her own sexuality drives her to an attraction for women instead of men.

As I pointed out then, the control of our sexual knowledge and information has been in the hands of those least qualified scientifically and emotionally to lead us. It has been in the hands of people who've tried to suppress and deny the most human of all human feelings—our sexual instincts. It has been in the hands of people who didn't know a hormone from an enzyme and yet told us in agonizing detail how to regulate the most intimate aspect of our personal lives.

But now that we are on the verge of the twenty-first century, all that has changed. . . .

Or has it?

Not quite. Now the self-appointed gurus of human sexuality are the "Touchy-Feely," "Whatever-Does-It-For-You," folks. Most of them are self-styled "experts" with credentials not even remotely related to the slightest knowledge of human sexuality. Some of them have the impressive title "Dr." in front of their names. But if you probe a little deeper, you will see that it's rarely a doctorate in medicine. More often it's for studies in an area not even remotely related to human sexuality. Sometimes that "Dr." is even farther removed from years of study.

Their message usually amounts to something like "If it feels good, do it!" Their advice is amateur, improvised, and often scientifically disastrous. And their primary appeal is a glib self-assurance and the unconditional approval of any and every form of sexual behavior. And there's something very strange about it.

When the average person has the flu, they go to the most competent medical doctor they can find, follow the doctor's advice carefully, and make sure the flu is cured.

But when they have to deal with the sexual challenges that face everyone day after day, they suddenly lose their way. They turn to a book or a lecture by someone who may have gotten their full store of knowledge about human sexuality by selling real estate or teaching aerobics. Here's the problem:

Human sexuality involves the most detailed knowledge of anatomy, biochemistry, physiology, pathology, internal medicine, surgery, obstetrics, and gynecology—to mention only a few of the studies involved. After years of study, to be competent in that area, you must read at least a dozen medical journals each month, and treat patients for years.

How can someone imagine that a hairdresser who took a few courses in psychology can lead them through the often perilous twists and turns of sex? In a real sense, they would almost be better off going to the self-styled "sex guru" for treatment of their flu— and to their doctor for help in their sexual challenges.

Instant sex experts are also experts in seduction. They give their followers strength and self-confidence by giving them permission to do anything and everything sexual. There's only one little problem:

Why do we need their permission to do anything?

Just because they say something is "good" for us, that doesn't make it good. And because they something is "bad" for us, that doesn't make it bad.

And besides, there are a few other important questions to ask. If they know so much about sex, how come most of them:

- Have been married—and divorced—so many times?
- Have had so many affairs?
- Look so obviously depressed and disappointed?
- Give advice that doesn't work for us no matter how hard we try?

Before we take the advice of anyone about sexual matters it's worthwhile to remember one vital—and wonderful—fact: Sex should be the simplest and most straightforward thing we do.

That is, if we make the right sexual decisions with the right people, we feel good. Right away. Without any doubt. And not just good. We feel wonderful!

If we make a bad sexual decision with bad people, we feel bad. Really bad.

Sometimes we feel bad for an hour. Sometimes we feel bad for a week. And sometimes we feel bad for a lifetime. And if we make a really bad choice, sometimes that "lifetime" won't be very long.

Even if the self-styled "sex gurus" tell us our bad choice is "good," we still feel bad.

But that brings up a very big and very important question:

If those dozens of self-styled "sex experts" don't know what's "good" for us sexually and what's bad, who does know?"

Who is smart enough to tell us what is best in each and every situation that we face from the age of five (when sex really starts to involve us seriously) to the age of ninety?

Who has the intelligence and insight and unerring instinct to point us in the right direction every time?

I'm going to tell you who has that ability and I'm going to tell you where to find them.

If you want to know who it is and where they are, just look in the mirror!

It's *you*! All you need to find sexual satisfaction and sexual happiness throughout your life is the honest, straightforward facts about human sexuality.

You're smart enough and cool enough to make the right sexual decisions every time—if you only know exactly what you're dealing with. You can make the best choices, for example:

- If you know the real truth about condoms—which may be quite different from what you've been seeing every day on TV . . .
- If you know the real truth about abortion pills—which may be quite different from what you've been seeing every day on TV . . .
- If you know the real truth about the sexual perversions in your own town and neighborhood—which may be quite different from what you've been seeing every day on TV . . .
- If you know the real truth about how a woman has an orgasm—which may be quite different from what you've been seeing every day on TV . . .
- If you know the real truth about homosexuality—which is quite different from what you've been seeing every day on TV . . .

Then, and only then, can you make the right decisions for yourself and your husband or wife, for your partner, for your children and your family. Knowledge is power, and sexual knowledge is Super-Power.

That's what the first edition of *Everything you always wanted to know about sex* *But were afraid to ask* was all about. It gave more than 100 million people around the world the honest, scientifically sound information they needed to make sex as exciting and enjoyable as it should be. They learned how to make sex fun, fulfilling, and fascinating. They learned how to avoid the traps and potholes and bottomless pits of human sexuality—and there are plenty of them.

I know they learned that because they told me. Tens of thousands of letters from dozens of countries around the world confirm that anyone who knows "Everything They Always Wanted to Know about Sex*" can enjoy sex more than they ever imagined—far beyond their wildest dreams!

But thirty years is a long time in any area of *medical science*—and sex is medical and it is science. In that period of time a lot of new and totally unpredictable events have occurred:

- An epidemic of sexual diseases never seen before in the history of the world. The number one bacterial disease in the United States these days isn't pneumonia or strep throat. It is a vaginal infection known as "chlamydia!"
- Untold millions of people around the world have died from an incurable almost always fatal sexual disease that was unknown (or even nonexistent) thirty years ago.

- Abortion is legal almost everywhere in the United States and there are pills you can take that provoke an abortion and machines you can make in your garage that produce an abortion.

- There are drugs that can give a man a hard erection fifteen minutes after taking them. And maybe they can do the same kind of thing for women.

- There are surgical operations on the sexual organs that can change them in ways we never imagined—and perhaps never expected.

- Thirty years later the birth control pill is everywhere, and still most women haven't been told that it is the only prescription drug proven to increase life expectancy in women.

That's why more than ever, sexual satisfaction, sexual safety, and sexual sanity are among life's greatest challenges. As I said in the original edition: "The purpose of this book is to tell the reader what he *wants* to know and what he *needs* to know to achieve the greatest possible degree of sexual satisfaction."

The only thing that has changed is that the new *Everything you always wanted to know about sex* *But were afraid to ask* covers everything that has happened sexually in the past thirty years.

But that's not all. There's one more aspect of sex that's vital to really getting the most out of sex. That most essential element is: humor. Sex is fun—there's no doubt about that. It's really the most fun anyone can have. But sex is also funny. Human beings are the only animals that can laugh about sex—and that's what makes our sex so uniquely human. Just like the original edition, the new edition of *Everything you always wanted to know about sex* *But were afraid to ask* has plenty of good humor within its pages.

When I wrote the original version thirty years ago, I had one idea in mind: The more you know about sex, the more you can enjoy it.

That concept has been confirmed by more than 100 million readers in fifty-two countries around the world.

As I also said in the original edition:

An active and rewarding sexual life, at mature level, is indispensable if one is to achieve his full potential as a member of the human race. Those whose sexual behavior is shrouded in ignorance and circumscribed with fear have *little chance of finding happiness in their short years on this planet. The goal of this book is to replace ignorance with knowledge and replace fear with confidence by telling honestly and directly: EVERYTHING YOU ALWAYS WANTED TO KNOW ABOUT SEX* *BUT WERE AFRAID TO ASK.*

Every word of that is as true today as it was on the original day of publication.

With that in mind, in the pages that follow, it is my sincere hope that all the new and exciting things you find here will help you to enjoy sex and sexuality much more than ever before.

Chapter 2
MALE SEXUAL ORGANS

How big is the normal penis?

That's the question of the century. And it's the wrong question. Every male, virtually from the very moment he is aware of his marvelous organ, is plagued by doubt. Is his penis big enough? Is it long enough? Is it wide enough?

Whenever and wherever a man has the chance to catch a glimpse of another man's penis, he immediately takes a mental snapshot of it and puts it alongside the permanent image of his own penis. At the Country Club, in the high school locker room, in military barracks, in public washrooms, you can see every man cast a lightning-fast sideways glance at another man's organ as his mental micrometer calculates the length of the stranger's phallus.

Unfortunately the Penile Olympics are a no-win proposition—in more ways than one. What if you find a penis longer and wider than yours? It ruins your day, right? And then the next day you spy a puny penis that makes yours look like it belongs on a raging bull? You feel good until the afternoon break when you go to the washroom and stand next to a fellow whose organ looks like it belongs on a bull elephant. That trashes your afternoon but good. And for most men, it goes on that way for a lifetime. They suffer—and they don't have to suffer.

Why don't they have to suffer?

Because they are asking the wrong question. Instead of "How long is the normal penis?" they should be asking "How long is the normal vagina?"

Because that's what it's really all about. The penis isn't there for decoration. It isn't a trendy little appendage to fill out tight jeans and clinging bathing trunks. It isn't there to fascinate the ladies by swinging gaily to and fro every time you take your pants off. The penis is really just an amazing, exciting, superbly designed tool to deliver a teaspoon or two of warm fluid into the waiting vagina. The useful length of the penis is determined by the working length of the vagina.

How long is that?

The average adult vagina ranges from about 3½ inches to about 5 inches in length. The average penis is about 4 inches long in its normal non-erect state. That's "average"—a penis can be only 2 inches long in the "resting" stage and still be quite normal. That means that virtually every adult male has a penis that can reach and vigorously massage every square inch of almost any vagina.

Since penile length is a hereditary characteristic, transmitted through genes, any man whose penis is too short to even enter the vagina will have trouble reproducing. A short-penised race would have died out half a million years ago.

But doesn't the length of the penis change with an erection?

It certainly does—and that's another reason not to get involved in the "Penile Olympics." The organ that hangs there all shriveled up may suddenly grow 20 percent or more when it gets down—or up—to business. But really big penises are few and far between. A very long—and very rare—penis might reach 12 inches in the erect state.

What about the men who star in porno films? They seem to have very big penises.

The key phrase there is "seem to have." Even male porno stars generally have a real-world penis length up to 30 percent shorter than advertised. For example, here's a list of stars—with names disguised to protect their careers—with their real measurements and their advertised penis length.

Star	Advertised Size (Inches)	Real-Life Size (Inches)
A	10	7½
B	9	7
C	12	9
D	10	8
E	11	9
F	12	8

As we see, even these penile superstars are just a little longer in the phallus than the average man. And besides that, they know some tricks that we don't know.

For example?

Well, they often closely clip or shave their pubic hair. That makes their penis look bigger. Then, most of them are relatively short and thin—almost emaciated. That makes their organ look even larger.

And what makes female actresses shed bitter tears makes male porn stars smile with satisfaction.

What's that?

The normal camera lens is a magnifying lens. That's why the leading ladies always complain, "I have to starve myself to death! That camera adds 10 pounds to my weight!"

And of course, a lens that can add 10 pounds to a thin lady can easily add a couple of inches to a normal penis.

Male stars sometimes also pop their penises into a vacuum pump (see Chapter 6 for details on those devices) and pump them up before big scenes.

But there's a fool proof way to bring porno-penises into line with reality.

What's that?

Just look at the actor's hands. He can pump up his penis, but he can't pump up his hands. A man's hands (not his feet) are usually sized in proportion to his penis. Compare the size of the porno star's hands with the size of his penis and then compare your hands and your penis. You'll be amazed, delighted—and relieved.

The truth is that almost all adult penises are more alike than they are different. They all fit into more or less the same size range. And they do what they are designed to do—deliver semen into the vagina. And of course, that's the way it should be. If a man's penis is long enough to reach from his body into the vagina, that's all it takes. It's a waste of time to fret about an inch more or less. Or to put it another way, worrying about an inch or two of penis size is "a lot of issue about a little tissue."

How can a man really tell if his penis is normal size?

The easiest way is to measure it. Just stand comfortably and measure from the pubic bone to the tip of your penis. (No cheating!) That's the "resting size." (Note: It's not a good idea to ask your wife or lady friend to help you in this process—because of the manipulation involved, you may never get an accurate measurement.) Then very gently (if you can comfortably, don't strain) pull your penis as far as it stretches. Don't go for that extra half inch, please!

That measurement is the "stretched length." The next time you have an erection, stand up and gently move your penis downward until it is parallel to the floor. Again measure from the pubic bone to the tip. That's the "erect length."

Interestingly enough, the stretched length of your penis will be almost the same as the erect length. Of course, if you think about it, it has to be that way. Your organ can only get as long as it is, no longer. Pumping in blood under pressure can add about 5 percent to the length.

And speaking of pressure, men shouldn't be under any pressure when it comes to the size of their penis. If your penis is more than 3 inches long when it is erect, you're still in the normal range. And even if it's shorter, remember Dr. Reuben's First Law of Sexual Satisfaction: "If It Works, Don't Fix It—You Can't Get a New One if You Break It!"

But can a man have his penis made bigger if he really wants to?

With modern plastic surgery almost anything is possible. But think of it this way. Most men feel uncomfortable if they even stand too close to the kitchen counter when their wife is slicing a salami. A fellow has to be pretty well motivated to let someone take a gleaming knife to his privates. Yet some of them do.

There are a number of ways a doctor can cut into and around a penis to make it "bigger"—and the result is not always what the patient expects.

How does it work?

Well, the "quick-and-easy" method just takes a couple of snips. The penis is really suspended from the pubic bone by a kind of cord called a "ligament." If you cut that ligament, since the penis is a heavy fleshy tube, it drops down, hangs lower, and suddenly "looks" longer. It might look as if it's an extra inch or so longer, but the actual length hasn't been changed one millimeter. It's just that the organ has been cut loose from its moorings and it hangs lower. It's like cutting the elastic on your socks. Your socks get droopier but they haven't gotten any longer. Unfortunately the man has to pay for that extra "overhang." When he has an erection, his reworked penis won't stand up at such a nice angle as before. It's almost as if it's getting revenge on him for being taken down a peg or two.

Cutting that vital ligament also makes the penis unstable during sex. It flops around and can't be controlled nearly as well. It also increases the risk of a fractured penis.

A fractured penis? Can a penis get broken?

Although it sounds like a bad dream, it can happen. An erect penis is hard—almost like a bone—because it is full of blood under pressure. Imagine a 6-inch length of very lightweight but rigid plastic pipe closed off at both ends and full of water. If you grab it hard in both hands and bend it sharply, it will fracture.

The stiff penis is similar to that plastic pipe. It's full of blood, and just under the skin it is encased in a tight canvaslike circular ligament—almost like a bandage. If, during sex, the gentleman bends his penis too hard against the woman's pubic bone, he can tear that ligament-bandage and break his rigid penis like a wooden matchstick.

How do you fix a fractured penis?

Not in the usual way. You don't put it in a plaster cast—although that permanent erection might seem attractive to some. And you don't put it in a sling—that's not socially smooth. Actually it's a surgical problem.

The actual procedure is a little scary. First, the skin of the penis is "de-gloved." That means it's loosened up and then slipped back over the organ like you take a glove off your finger. Then the torn ligament is sewn up and the skin put back in place. With luck, in about two weeks the patient is back doing what he did before—but this time, very carefully. The experience is so unsettling that few men are careless enough to fracture their penis twice in a lifetime.

Besides making it longer, is there any way to make a penis fatter—wider in diameter?

As they used to say, "What the mind of man can conceive, the hand of man can achieve." Well, in this case it's not exactly the hand . . .

That kind of operation on the penis gets a little complicated. It involves a sort of reverse liposuction. The surgeon sucks fat from somewhere else in the body and then injects it into the shaft of the penis. So the penis doesn't really get bigger, it just gets fatter! And that's when the problem begins.

What problem?

Think of it this way. Normally, people want to get thin—they want to lose fat. When their fat decreases—by dieting or liposuction—they struggle to keep it from coming back. In penis restructuring, it's exactly the opposite. You are desperately trying to make something fatter and to keep that fat where you put it! But Mother Nature is against you. No matter what the patient does, the fat that was grafted onto the penis is usually absorbed and the organ eventually goes back to its original size. Unfortunately the patient's bank account does not go back to its original size.

The operation has several known complications, including poor cosmetic appearance such as knobby fat nodules along the shaft plus skin deformity and scarring. Sometimes the penis doesn't even work as well as it did before the remodeling.

But is that kind of surgery a good idea?

Like all plastic surgery, it's an individual decision. But maybe there's truth in the old saying: "It's not how long you make it, it's how you make it long."

And besides, none of these procedures makes the penis function even the tiniest bit better.

What will make a penis work better?

That depends on what the problem is in the first place. Most of the time, the real problem with a penis that won't work right has nothing to do with the penis. Almost always—with rare exceptions—the glitch is in the brain.

The proof is in the postage stamps.

In the postage stamps?

That's right. As most men know—and many wives and girlfriends have discovered—men frequently have erections on awakening in the morning. Most men explain them away as reflex erections because of a full bladder. It may sound plausible, but that's not the correct explanation. Although few men are aware of it, almost every night almost every man has several erections while he is asleep.

Those erections are caused by dreams and unconscious sexual fantasies and are perfectly normal. Not only are they normal, they are tremendously useful in diagnosing and treating erectile problems. Here's how it functions:

Suppose your TV set doesn't work. Before you take it to the repair shop and start to have it repaired, you should always check to see if it is plugged in.

Now if a man has trouble getting erections, before we send him to the doctor, it's worthwhile seeing if the problem is in the equipment or in the connection. That's where the postage stamps come in.

How does that work?

Logically. If a man can't produce an erection during sexual intercourse, there are two possibilities. It could that his physical equipment—spinal nerves, blood reservoirs of the penis, blood vessels to and from the penis, and all the rest—isn't working. Or it could be that something is happening in his brain that short-circuits the whole erection process.

The obvious solution is to see if he ever gets an erection. All you have to do is check him into the hospital, attach an expensive and complicated electronic instrument to his penis that measures the diameter of the shaft, let him go to sleep, and see if the instrument detects and records any erections during the night. That will cost about five hundred dollars if the poor fellow ever manages to fall asleep with all those wires clamped onto his sensitive organ.

There's an easier way. On the way home from work, he just picks up a roll of postage stamps from the Post Office. At bedtime, he unrolls a few, wraps them gently around the shaft of his penis just below the head, and glues them together to make a little collar of stamps. It's not exactly a fashion statement, but it's a lot cheaper and easier than a stay in the hospital.

Then what?

Then he goes to sleep and waits. If he wakes up in the morning with those nice commemorative pictures of Mount Rushmore hanging around his testicles, he can whistle all the way to breakfast. It's unmistakable proof that his physical equipment is working fine and any problem he might have is almost surely emotional. Total cost for the test, depending on the kind of stamps and the size of the penis, could be $2.50. Of course, those stamps might just be reusable—depending on individual tastes.

Is there any risk to this test?

The only one I know of is what happened to Roger. Let Rhonda, his wife, tell it:

> *"Well, Roger had really been worried about his sexual problem for the past six months. He'd been having trouble getting hard and he was like, obsessed with it. He was get-ting desperate and I was kind of worried about him. He kept talking about this strange specialist in Hong Kong who might be able to help him. He kept saying he only wished he had enough money to go there and how he knew he could never afford it.*
>
> *"Well, one night last week at bedtime, I was putting on some face cream in the bathroom and when I walked into the bedroom I saw Roger sitting up in bed. He was tremen-dously red in the face and sweating and he was sticking all these air mail stamps on his organ.*
>
> *"I thought, 'My God, he's lost his mind! He thinks he can send his penis away to Hong Kong to that Chinese doctor!'*

"Well, it turned out OK because when he woke up in the morning all the stamps were torn and we finally got to the bottom of his problem, but he really had me worried there for a moment!"

Roger's case may have been extreme, but men do worry a lot about erections.

What do they worry about?

Well, besides whether or not they are going to have an erection, they worry about the angle of their penis during an erection and which way it points. But they shouldn't worry because as far as erections go, almost everything is normal. For example, about 25 percent of all normal erections are lower than horizontal. And about 15 percent of normal erections are distinctly curved downward.

Although that may not fit the stereotype of the "perfect male," it has its distinct advantages. No more wives or girlfriends with stiff necks in the morning—oral sex with a downward slanted penis is a whole lot easier. (That's why they make drinking straws that bend downward in the middle.) And remember, nearly half of all normal erections are under 5¾ inches long.

When you think about it, the way an erection happens is really amazing.

What makes an erection happen?

The interesting thing is that after all these years, no one knows the whole story. But this is what we do know:

The penis itself is constructed like one of those inflatable rubber air mattresses. Along the shaft, from the pubic bone to the tip of the organ, there are two long thin balloons that are normally collapsed. These are wrapped in a covering like a thick canvas. In the center of the shaft, there is a tube called the urethra—it carries urine and sperm to the outside.

There is a set of valves that controls blood flow to these balloons. When the valves are opened, blood surges under pressure into these balloons, literally blowing up the penis like an air mattress. If everything is working right, the valves then snap shut and the blood is trapped in the now-inflated organ. Interestingly, it doesn't take very much blood to pop up the penis.

How much blood does it take?

Actually about two tablespoonsful, or about enough to fill a small shot glass. But getting the blood into the penis isn't that easy, because the arteries that supply the penis are little ones. They're only about the size of the arteries that supply your index finger. It would be nice to have slightly better blood delivery service considering that the average man worries a lot more about his penis than his index finger. But that's the way things are and we have to do the best we can.

But what exactly brings on an erection?

That's a good question. If we knew that, we could make a lot of men—and a lot of women—a whole lot happier. But we know this much. As soon as something happens to trigger an erection, a tremendous barrage of chemicals is released all over the body. They include adrenaline, norepinephrine, acetylcholine, and prostaglandins. And for some unknown reason, in the process of building an erection the substance known as "laughing gas," or nitrous oxide, is released. Could that be the reason why most men with erections have that same cheerful grin on their face? (Or could it be something else?)

But the amazing—and so far unexplained—aspect of erection is the number of things that can make the penis pop up. A beautiful naked woman stretching out in bed alongside a man will trigger an erection. That's to be expected. But a picture of the same naked woman can have the same effect. Even the memory of the woman can unleash the chain of events that makes the penis pound with the pulsating pressure of that critical 1 ounce of blood.

There's another strange quality about an erection that's hard to explain precisely. A man with an erection cannot sit down, cannot lie down, cannot walk around in comfort. Perhaps the Spanish proverb tells it best:

"Cuando cabeza chica se calienta, cabeza grande ya no piensa!"
(When the Little Head gets hot, the Big Head stops thinking!)

A hard hot penis screams for ejaculation!

What happens during ejaculation?

Ejaculation is a complex sequence of events executed with split-second timing. It is reminiscent of a missile launching into Outer

Space. Actually it is a missile launched into "Inner Space." By comparison it makes the most complicated man-made launch look like a game of marbles.

Once erection has taken place (a minor miracle in itself), and the penis is in place in the vagina, the circuits begin to hum. Sensory receptors within the skin of the penis lock into the body's electrical system. They measure the heat of the vagina, friction against the penis, pressure of the vaginal wall against the penile shaft, amount of vaginal lubrication present, etc. These "situation reports" are constantly relayed to the sexual centers in the spinal cord and brain. In response, these centers direct more blood to the penis, increase the sensitivity of the touch receptors in the organ, and build up nervous energy in the lower segment of the spinal cord.

As intercourse progresses, a constant flow of nerve impulses races between the sexual organs and the central nervous system, building up and reinforcing themselves. At the same time, all other stimulation is integrated into the system. Looking at the sexual partner, touching her, being touched by her—they all contribute to the rapidly building tension. It is comparable, in one sense, to blowing up a balloon. The pressure gets greater and greater and greater until finally there is a sudden and dramatic explosion—ejaculation! Then things start to happen fast.

The urethra is sealed off so urine will not be expelled accidentally. Secretions from the prostate gland, seminal vesicles, and testicles are mixed on the spot. Simultaneously, involuntary arching of the back muscles drives the entire body forward as the man's pelvic muscles contract to hurl the penis deeper into the vagina. At this point consciousness is obliterated and the man loses all contact with the world—except for those few cubic inches of vagina surrounding his penis.

A powerful internal pump swings into action squirting a quarter-ounce or so of seminal fluid into the vagina in about six consecutive jets. The semen speeds through the air at eleven miles per hour and ten seconds later it's all over—until the next time.

How many sperm are in each ejaculation?

On the average there are about 500 million sperm swimming in each quarter-ounce of semen, or about twice the population of the United States. The average man propels about 18 quarts of seminal fluid in his lifetime, or nearly 1.5 trillion sperm. Therefore he is able, theoretically, to father about two hundred times the number of people now living on this planet. Fortunately on the average only 3 out of 288 acts of intercourse results in impregnation.

What does the ejaculate consist of?

Strangely enough, the list of ingredients in semen looks a lot like the label on a bottle of vitamin pills. Semen contains at least two vitamins: vitamin C and vitamin B12. It also contains important minerals, including calcium, potassium, magnesium, phosphorus, and zinc. It contains two sugarlike substances: fructose and sorbitol. It is also very high in protein. That makes it, in addition to its other obvious qualities, an excellent nutritional supplement. But it won't replace a balanced diet. It's important to note that semen is also high in cholesterol and sodium, and for those who should avoid these substances, caution is indicated.

Is oral sex OK for vegetarians?

One of my patients, Jenny, a professional nutritionist, came face-to-face with the problem and worked it out this way:

> *"I'm a strict vegetarian, Doctor, and I'm really serious about it. I don't eat any animal products and I don't even buy clothes made from leather. But I love oral sex. And then all of a sudden one day, I realized that what I was doing wasn't exactly vegetarian!"*
>
> *"What did you do?"*
>
> *"Well, when I told my husband, Bill, about it he was like in shock. I mean, both of us love it, but if it goes against my principles, what could I do? I finally worked it out. I still do it and I still love it—but I don't swallow! Not even one drop!"*

But that's not the only hazard of oral sex.

What other danger is there?

It's not exactly a danger, but the average ejaculate is a little over a teaspoonful and contains about 15 calories. For those who count calories, it has to be taken into consideration. Calorie counting may get in the way of oral sex for women but there's something that can get in the way of regular sex for men.

What's that?

The "Bent-Nail Syndrome," otherwise known as "Peyronie's Disease." It's a strange name for an unfortunate problem, and if you have it, your penis can look exactly like that: a "bent-nail." Having sex with a Peyronie's penis is a unique and absolutely unforgettable experience. As the years go by, a woman may forget the face and the name of her Peyronie's partner, but she will never forget his penis. Although it's a relatively rare disease, its sexual effects are so spectacular that it's worth knowing about.

What causes it?

No one knows. Fortunately it only affects about 1 percent of all men but it is certainly spectacular in appearance. No one knows for sure but there is a possibility that hitting or excessive bending of the penis can bring it on years later. Theoretically violent sex or too-vigorous masturbation can trigger the condition. When erection occurs, the shaft of the penis may point northwest while the head of the organ looks southeast. It doesn't exactly look like a corkscrew but it's getting there.

Peyronie's Disease is caused by hardening of certain areas of the fibrous layers of the penis at random spots. One hardened area pulls in one direction while the other pulls in a different direction, giving the penis an odd twist. That makes normal sex complicated and sometimes even confusing—for both the man and the woman.

What's the treatment?

Sometimes it doesn't need any treatment. Sometimes it goes away by itself in six months to a year. That means it could be worthwhile to postpone treatment for at least a year to see if the penis straightens out by itself. In the meantime regular and frequent—and gentle—sex just might help.

In really serious cases, surgery can be done, but there are two possible complications: loss of erection capacity or shortening of the penis. As one of my patients said when he heard those two alternatives: "Shortened penis or loss of erection capacity? Don't you have something in Column C?"

Are there any other problems that affect erection?

There's one that might be called the "King Midas Disease." Remember the story about King Midas, who wished that everything he touched would be turned into gold? And when he got his wish, it became very complicated—his food and drink all turned to gold along with everything else he touched.

Well, there's a sexual equivalent called "Priapism" after "Priapos," the Greek god of the penis and male sexuality. It's a case of "You want an erection? I'll give you a real erection!"

But when they get it, no one with priapism likes it very much.

Why not?

For a man, an erection is a problem to be solved. You can't live with it—it's like all the blood in your body has been pumped into your penis and is bursting to get out. You need an ejaculation and fast! But with priapism, that doesn't help. A man with priapism can have sex three times in a row and masturbate five times in succession, and the penis still stays hard as a rock and as tender as a toothache.

What causes priapism?

Usually it's caused by some serious underlying disease like leukemia or an infection of the urinary tract. And it has become much more common recently with the new medications that can be injected directly into the penis to produce an instant erection (see Chapter 6). A little carelessness with the technique and you can get an erection that just won't go away.

As any man who has had it will testify, priapism is an emergency condition. That means emergency treatment. The doctor sticks a fairly thick needle into the shaft of the penis—carefully—and sucks the blood out of those two tubes, the corpora cavernosa. (Ouch!) That usually solves the problem.

What role do the testicles play in male sexuality?

If the penis is the star of the show, the testicles write the script. They produce testosterone, a truly magic hormone. Without testosterone, there would not be a single man in the entire world.

How is that?

It works like this. In the uterus, according to current concepts, every fetus is destined to be a female, and that's the way it will develop—unless it secretes testosterone. Once testosterone is produced, instead of female sexual organs, male organs develop and the fetus becomes a male. During the development of a male baby, there's still a lot of testosterone around that causes temporary enlargement of the penis and testicles. A newborn male baby has equipment that you wouldn't expect him to have for many years to come. That can be a big surprise for some new mothers!

Over the next few weeks the sexual organs shrink to baby-size as the level of testosterone declines, but about eleven years later those same testicles start to pump out that hormone again. That makes the penis grow dramatically and triggers many other male characteristics like a beard, big muscles, and a deep voice. It also gives men their very special male outlook on life—like their interest in football.

Is testosterone really why men like football?

Strange as it seems, it could be. Testosterone is produced by the testicles and to a lesser extent by the adrenal glands (that's why women also have some testosterone circulating in their bloodstream). The hormone has an effect on almost every structure in the body, but it has a very special effect on the brain. It makes men aggressive, willing to threaten other men, and eager for contact sports. It motivates them to seek sexual contact with women and influences their sexuality in important ways.

Research into the real effects of testosterone is still in its infancy, although even a century ago Sigmund Freud seemed to have had an understanding of the situation. Once, during a discussion with some of his advanced students, one of them stood up and asked, "Isn't it true, Dr. Freud, that the way a man acts in life is determined by the size of his penis?"

Freud smiled and replied, "Not exactly. I rather think that the size of a man's penis is determined by the way he acts in life!"

Strange as it may seem, there is now clear scientific evidence that a man can raise his testosterone level and if not the size of his penis at least the way it functions, by positive thinking.

Really? How does it work?

It turns out that tennis players who are up for a big match can secrete a lot more testosterone than opponents who are less assertive. But that's only the beginning. If they win, their testosterone zooms up another few notches. And as you would expect, when players lose a match, their testosterone slumps.

And it goes on and on. Players who win produce more testosterone, which makes them more confident and able to win, and that in turn pumps out more testosterone.

Freud was right, and even more important, you can apply these findings to your own sexual experiences. The more confident you are about your next sexual event, the more testosterone you will produce and the better you should perform. That in turn should carry over to each successive copulation. It's really a win-win situation.

Is there anything else that pushes up testosterone levels in men?

Not as much. On the other hand stress, as every man can testify, lowers testosterone levels. Army recruits in basic training and soldiers in combat can lose about 40 percent of their testosterone. That's bad news for the Army because a man with 40 percent less testosterone is less eager to fight. But armies traditionally have found ways to raise their soldiers' testosterone before battle.

What do they do?

For centuries, armies have provided prostitutes for soldiers to pump them up sexually and raise their testosterone before combat. In recent years military officials in certain countries show videotapes of pornography and violence to the troops before sending them into action. The generals may not be physicians or psychiatrists, but over the centuries they have found out what works.

Do high testosterone levels cause any problems?

Unfortunately, yes. The testicles have to work hard to produce all that testosterone plus the sperm they have to constantly supply. That's why they are sometimes two little time bombs hanging there in the scrotum.

Time bombs?

Unfortunately, yes. Organs that have a lot of metabolic activity are very vulnerable to malignant tumors, and the testicles are no exception. Cancer of the testicle is the most common form of cancer in men between the ages of twenty and thirty-four. About two out of every thousand white males will get cancer of the testicles sometime in their lives. That's bad news—but there's good news to compensate for it.

What's the good news?

It's more than 95-percent curable—if it's detected in time. And that's not too hard. A lot of women worry about breast cancer, and that encourages them to perform the self-examination. Well, men worry a lot about their testicles—they don't call them "The Crown Jewels" for nothing. And fortunately there is an equivalent self-exam for men. The next time you're in the shower and your testicles are well descended from the heat and humidity of the shower, take a moment to write yourself an insurance policy on those "jewels."

Encircle each testicle carefully with your thumb and finger and feel the outline. You should feel something like an egg (that's why they call them "huevos"—eggs—in Spanish). The "egg" hangs from a stalk and has what feels like a worm on its back side. That's all you should feel. If you feel a lump or a hard mass or anything that doesn't seem right, see your doctor promptly. You want to be in that 95 percent of the statistics.

But if you're lucky you won't even have to do that self-examination.

Why not?

Maybe you have a lady who will do it for you. The testicles are not particularly sensitive sexually because they are too tender to the touch. Really they shouldn't be out there where they can be bumped around. At least when our ancestors ran around on all fours, they were back there out of harm's way, not right there in front the way they are now. But the testicles don't make sperm well unless they're cooler than body temperature. That's why they have to swing in the wind.

But even if the testicles aren't sexually responsive, the scrotum is. The skin of that wrinkly sac is almost as sensitive sexually as the penis. The woman who really wants to excite her man to peak performance knows how to take advantage of the sexual sensitivity of the scrotum. And in the process, she can't help getting a feel for the condition of the testicles. Just as many lives have been saved by a husband finding a lump in his wife's breast, a woman can save her man by detecting a lump in his testicle. It's worth it.

Is circumcision a good idea?

That depends on a lot of factors. First and foremost, if it's part of your religious belief, that's not a topic to discuss here. You should make your own decision based on personal considerations.

But if it's a medical question, here goes:

Male circumcision (for the details of female circumcision, see Chapter 3) consists of cutting off the foreskin of the penis. At birth, the loose skin of the shaft of the penis extends down over the head of the organ and forms a loose covering—sort of like a knitted wool cap pulled down over your head. There is an opening at the end, of course, for urine and semen to get out. That foreskin slides back and forth and can be retracted or pulled backward to expose the "glans" or head of the penis. By making a circular incision just behind the head of the organ (that's what "circumcision" really means—a "circular cut") you can cut off that foreskin and expose the head of the penis permanently.

But if you think about it, circumcision is really a strangely contradictory kind of operation.

Contradictory? Why contradictory?

Well, in spite of the obsession with penis length and the wish of so many men for the longest possible penis, circumcision actually takes length from that organ. Although it doesn't cut away anything from the penis itself—except in those tragic cases where the surgeon makes a mistake—circumcision does shorten the total length of the penis by a fraction of an inch.

Why do they perform circumcision?

The answer to that question delves deeply into controversy and differences of opinion. (But remember, nothing in this section refers to religious circumcision. That's a very personal matter and totally beyond the scope of this book.)

Although we don't usually think of it that way, the most commonly performed sexual plastic surgery procedure is circumcision of the penis.

Circumcision originated long before the birth of Christ, who was himself circumcised along with the Twelve Disciples. The operation was performed as far back as the Stone Age and was regularly done in ancient Egypt. It was even common among the Aztecs. Today it is performed by such diverse groups as the Australian aborigines, the Tacuna Indians of Brazil, Abyssinian Christians, and of course modern Jews, Moslems, and Ethiopians.

In the Bible, the first reference to circumcision is in Genesis 17:11:

"And ye shall circumcise the flesh of your foreskin; it shall be a token of the covenant betwixt me and you."

In those times the penis was remodeled with a sharp stone as prescribed in Exodus 4:25:

"Then Zipporah took a sharp stone, and cut off the foreskin of her son, and cast it at his feet, and said, Surely a bloody husband art thou to me."

The same implement, a sharp stone, is used today by some primitive tribes; those who are slightly more advanced use a broken piece of glass. Among the Jews, a ceremonial steel knife is wielded by a ritual surgeon, called a *mohel,* who restricts his practice to circumcisions. He operates on the squirming eight-day-old infant freehand—something few modern surgeons would attempt. The idea of the *mohel* has always caused anxiety—understandably—and one of the best defenses against anxiety is humor. That explains the dozens of jokes about the *mohel.*

For example?

An American is visiting France and stays overnight in a small town. He awakens in the morning to find that his watch has stopped. Searching through the narrow streets, he finally comes across a small shop with a big sign showing a watch hanging over the entrance. He goes in to find a middle-aged man with a beard behind the counter.

Relieved, he plops his wristwatch on the counter.

"When I woke up this morning, this watch had stopped."

The pudgy gentleman shakes his head and hands the watch back to him. "I don't know anything about watches. I'm a mohel. I do circumcisions."

"You do circumcisions? Then why do you have that big watch hanging over your door?"

The fellow shrugs his shoulders.

"What do you want me to hang up there?"

Modern medical circumcision is standardized and nearly automatic. The infant is strapped to a rack—usually plastic—and a bell-shaped device, also plastic, is slipped between penis and foreskin. A loop of nylon thread is knotted around a groove at the base of the bell, constricting the prepuce. The surgeon runs the scalpel blade once around the penis and it's all over. The bell is left in place a day or two, the infant meanwhile urinating through an opening in the top of the bell.

Aside from religious beliefs, the origin of this operation is unknown. Until recently virtually every doctor in the United States was taught that circumcision was essential and should be performed on every male infant before he went home from the hospital.

You said "until recently." Has anything changed?

Yes, it has. Like a lot of other things in medicine, circumcision has come under close scrutiny in recent years and now there are two separate and distinct schools of thought. One believes that circumcision is still the right way to go. The other group, as well organized and as vociferous, believes that circumcision is unnecessary, mutilating, and even dangerous.

What do they say?

The people who are in favor of circumcision point out that cancer of the penis only occurs in uncircumcised men—with rare exceptions. They also say that urinary infections are more common in males who are uncircumcised. Another point advocates of circumcision mention is that men who are circumcised are less likely to get AIDS and other sexually transmitted diseases.

The group against circumcision—and both groups have physicians among them—insists that circumcision is a bad idea. They say that the risk of cancer of the penis for uncircumcised men is very small—1 in 100,000. They also point out that most of the medical risks can be avoided by "good personal hygiene" (translation: pulling back the foreskin and washing the head of the penis regularly and carefully).

They say that there is some risk to the operation. That's true. They also say that getting rid of the foreskin takes some of the feeling out of sex. And there are some other interesting points. Circumcision is usually done without anesthesia and it hurts the baby. There's also a very complicated philosophical question: Do the parents have the right to decide that the penis of the newborn infant should be modified—without consulting the baby?

Who's right?

Maybe that's not what decides the issue. In the United States, about 85 percent of all male babies are circumcised. (The exact figures are hard to get at since not all these operations are recorded.) But in Europe, barely 10 percent of all male babies lose their foreskins. And worldwide, the figure is about 20 percent. And that may bring us to the real explanation.

What's that?

Think about it. Who makes the decision to circumcise the newborn baby? Unless it's a religious decision—made long before birth— it's almost always the Mother! I've seen it personally a thousand times. The woman comes to the hospital in labor, the nurse takes down the routine information, and says, almost casually:

> *"And if it's a boy, you want him circumcised, don't you?"*

Nine times out of ten, the mother nods, and that's that!

But why do mothers choose circumcision so often?

That was a puzzle for a long time. Obviously they don't weigh all the statistics and medical complications. They just know what they want for their sons. They want their boys to have circumcised penises—and here's the surprising reason:

Most American women prefer circumcised organs in their own sexual partners—and by a big margin. In various surveys most women believe that a circumcised penis is cleaner, looks sexier, and is nicer to handle.

But then it gets strange.

Why strange?

Because in one survey almost 80 percent of the women said that a circumcised penis "seems more natural"! Whatever a circumcised phallus may be, it isn't natural. But like everything else in the world of sex, it just depends on what you're used to.

But that's not the whole story. There are less than 200 million American females compared with almost 3.5 billion females in the rest of the world. In Europe, 90 percent of the men are not circumcised and it's a good bet that European women believe an uncircumcised organ is cleaner, looks sexier, and is nicer to handle. And you can be sure they think it's more natural!

What if a man is circumcised and wants to undo it?

You mean, can he get his foreskin back? Unfortunately that bit of tissue is gone forever, but thanks to the magic of modern medicine, he can get something back.

There are several procedures in plastic surgery to construct something like a foreskin. The operation is expensive and carries the usual risks of surgery. A man has to be well motivated to undergo it. But there's something else he can do that doesn't cost as much and gives an interesting result.

What's that?

He can make a new foreskin himself. This is probably the ultimate do-it-yourself project. But before we go into the details, let me say:

Don't try this at home!

I don't recommend it. Repeat: *I don't recommend it.*
The explanation that follows is only for educational purposes.
You'll see why in a moment.
The skin on the shaft of the penis is loose—it has to be or an erection would literally skin the organ. Someone figured out—probably in desperation—that you can stretch that skin if you really put your

mind to it. So it's possible to fasten weights to the skin of the penis, behind the head of the organ, and pull some of that loose skin forward until it covers the head of the phallus and looks like a foreskin.

Is it easy to do?

That depends on what you consider easy. It takes about a year of walking around with a weight taped to the end of your most delicate appendage. From time to time that weight is bound to fall off—usually during a critical job interview or when you're meeting your fiancée's parents for the first time. All you have to do is bend down to pick up that kinky little leather harness with the lead balls that fell down your pants leg and explain to your future employer or prospective in-laws what your problem is. Good luck.

However, if you persist, you just might get something that looks like a foreskin eventually.

But then is circumcision a good idea?

Yes, no, and maybe. It depends on what you want for yourself and your son. It's a very personal decision and the American Academy of Pediatrics sums it up very well:

> *"Newborn circumcision has potential medical benefits and advantages as well as disadvantages and risks. When circumcision is being considered, the benefits and risks should be explained to the parents and informed consent obtained."*

The rest is up to you.

Chapter 3
FEMALE SEXUAL ORGANS

Is it really true that the clitoris is simply a miniature penis?

Many experts consider the clitoris to be a penis that just didn't grow. They describe the entire female genitalia as male organs that never matured. Understandably, all the scholars who feel this way are men. Women experts look at it another way. According to them, the penis is nothing more than an overgrown clitoris. They consider the male organ a primitive version of the more "refined" female sexual apparatus.

Who's right?

As usual, everybody is about half right. At an early stage in development, the human embryo has both male and female sexual organs. They exist in the form of "anlage," a German word for primitive tissue that later differentiates into a specialized organ.

The embryo has a bisexual phallus; in those destined to be male it differentiates into a penis. Future girls will end up with a clitoris. According to the chromosomal decision made at the microsecond of conception, the tiny being may evolve one day into either a top-less dancer or a well-muscled lifeguard. For the moment, however, the future female charmer is as well equipped as the men who will,

30

twenty years from now, stuff bills into her G-string in appreciation of her feminine charms. Likewise, the future lifeguard has, potentially, all the pelvic endowments of the bikini-clad lovelies who will one day swarm around him.

Fortunately for those concerned, long before birth the sexual structures of the suppressed sex atrophy and almost disappear. At the time of delivery the normal infant has clear-cut and distinctive sexual features. The obstetrician has no trouble telling the excited parents whether it's a boy or girl. But if he were completely honest, he would say: "Congratulations, you are the proud parents of a six-pound-two-ounce-98-percent-girl!"

Why only 98 percent?

Because at least 2 percent of the sexual organs of the male and female really belong in the other sex. In their sexual organs, boys are 2-percent girls and girls are 2-percent boys. This is the proportion in normal people—in abnormal cases the percentage can be a lot higher. For example, the testicles can be thought of as female ovaries that have found a new home in the scrotum. (Some experts prefer to consider the ovaries as merely testicles that did not descend. The point of view usually depends on whether the expert has testicles or ovaries.)

If the embryo is going to be a boy, the future testicles will drop through the pelvic cavity into what would have been the labia majora and expand them into a scrotum. The undifferentiated phallus increases dramatically in size and in the process is pierced by the urethra to become the penis.

If the embryo is to follow the female path, there are fewer changes required. The ovaries stay where they are. The labia majora also remain essentially unchanged. Only a few minor alterations are required to produce uncomplicated structures like the vagina and labia minora.

Does that mean that if the original sexual organs don't develop, the embryo will be female?

Not exactly. At the earliest stages, the embryo has little more than gonads—future ovaries or testicles and genital swellings—future labia majora or scrotum and phallus—future penis or clitoris. If the child is going to be sexually distinctive as male or female, development must occur in one direction or the other. In the male this development is fairly complicated. The female has a much shorter distance to travel.

This has led some researchers, most of them women, to suggest that every embryo is originally female. About half of them (the unlucky ones according to these ladies) develop into males.

Is that true?

Maybe. There is, however, one element of female superiority that is undeniable.

In relatively primitive animals such as chickens, urination, defecation, and reproduction are all conducted at one common orifice known as the cloaca. (Literal-minded scholars coined the term—in Latin *cloaca* means "sewer.")

On moving up the evolutionary scale, the functions of the various openings become increasingly specialized. At what we like to consider the top of the tree, human beings, the male has progressed to the point of developing a separate orifice for defecation. He is still committed however to time-sharing for urination and reproduction; the urethra serves both purposes.

The female, meanwhile, has reached the top. She is a deluxe model, anatomically speaking, with complete segregation of structure and function: three jobs, three orifices. Male superiority? Well, men like to think so anyway.

Do all the female sexual organs have a counterpart in the male?

Yes, they have to. Since the genitalia were originally identical, there must be at least a remnant of each female organ in the male and of each male organ in the female.

Then do men have a vagina?

Every man carries with him a little souvenir of the time when his masculinity was not so obvious. In the anatomy books it is called vagina masculina, or male vagina. Once upon a time it was destined to become a real vagina, but that never worked out. It is simply a tiny tag of tissue tacked onto the edge of the bladder. Men even have an equivalent of the hymen. Virgin or not, this tiny memento remains permanently intact in every adult male. It is called the "seminal colliculus"—*colliculus* is Latin for "little hill." Not nearly as informative as the female hymen, it is simply a little hill of tissue next to the prostate gland, another leftover of the woman that he might have been.

If there is a hymen in men, is there a prostate gland in women?

Yes, there is, or at least the equivalent. In women the prostate gland turns out to be Skene's glands, two tiny openings on either side of the urethra. Aside from becoming badly infected in ladies with gonorrhea, they seem to have long ago lost any function.

Bartholin's glands, which get the credit (without doing the work) for supplying vaginal lubrication during intercourse, have developed into structures known as the bulbourethral glands in the male.

The bulbourethrals don't do much but what they do, is crucial. They rarely supply more than one tiny drop of secretion during intercourse, but it is a mighty important drop.

Important?

Yes. This is the way it can happen. The scene is a doctor's office. An attractive twenty-two-year-old girl, Lois, sits across from the doctor who has just finished examining her. She is very upset.

> *"But Doctor, I couldn't be! I mean, there's no way! I just don't see how!"*
>
> *The mascara begins to flow down her cheeks, propelled by a gush of tears.*
>
> *"I'm sorry, but there just isn't any question about it—you are six weeks pregnant."*
>
> *"But I never did anything. He wanted to but I wouldn't let him because I didn't want to get—"*
>
> *Another flood of tears.*
>
> *"Why don't you tell me exactly what you did let him do, so we can figure out what happened?"*
>
> *Quickly Lois touches up her makeup.*
>
> *"Well, we were over at my place and we got to, you know, fooling around, and so he wanted to put it in me but I was afraid. So I said, 'No, you can just rub it around the outside but you can't, you know, put it in . . .'"*
>
> *"Then what happened?"*

"Well, then he did. I mean, you know by then I had my panties off and he started rubbing me with his thing. But he started getting excited and I thought he was going to uhm, you know, spurt out all over me, so I pushed him away."

That first treacherous drop claimed another victim. The initial secretion originating at the bulbourethral glands appears shortly after erection. No more than an expectant drop at the end of the penis, it can contain as many as 50,000 sperm. If these are wiped against the vulva by an aggressive penis, only one of the kicking, squirming swimmers needs to snake its way up the vagina into the cervix. Then we have a case like Lois: all the consequences without any of the compensations.

What are the chances of something like that really happening?

Because of the long distance involved—from the labia to the cervix—the chances are against being impregnated this way. On the other hand, some girls are more likely to play this game instead of full-fledged intercourse because of the false sense of security it gives them. Since the odds are directly proportional to the number of exposures, it gets riskier each time. A bigger gamble is the common practice of inserting the penis, starting pelvic thrusts, and whipping it out just before ejaculation. A bad way to have sex and a good way to get pregnant.

What about the breasts?

This is another example of rudimentary organs present in both sexes. In this case they remain undeveloped until needed. In the male this means they never develop (under normal conditions); in the female they are quiescent until puberty.

The only exception is the first few days of life. Then both male and female breasts are active. They produce a clear secretion called colostrum, or "witches milk." The milk-producing glands in the breasts of both sexes are triggered to secrete by the large amount of sex hormones present in the infant's body at birth. In a few days the hormones subside and the "milk" disappears.

It's interesting that the breasts themselves are actually sweat glands that have increased in size and become specialized in function. That means the milk is a specialized form of sweat, enriched with proteins from the mother's blood. Fortunately this unromantic fact is buried deep in the textbooks of Embryology. Imagine the effect on the millions of red-blooded American men lusting after big sexy breasts if they realized they were romantically involved with oversized sweat glands.

Why do women have only two breasts?

This is the type of question that no mere human being can answer with authority. It obviously was decided that way by some Higher Power. However, we can guess at some possible reasons: since humans usually have only one offspring at a time, two breasts still leave one in reserve. In the Animal Kingdom, only human beings, primates, and elephants have a single set of breasts at the nipple line. Other species are more amply endowed, with six or more pairs of mammary glands.

But there are exceptions. About 1 out of every 200 women has extra nipples. They usually extend in a line downward over the abdomen from the regular nipples to the pubic area. Sometimes a woman notices a dark spot or two on each side of her chest below and right in line with her nipples. These may be vestiges of extra nipples. In rare cases a woman may have an extra set of breasts located just below the original pair. In a culture with such admiration for breasts, it is a wonder that these ladies are not in greater demand.

What about the hymen?

The hymen is a structure that gets attention all out of proportion to its function, which is—nothing. For centuries it has been regarded as the Barometer of Chastity—Guardian of Purity—Sentinel at the Gates of Venus. Nothing could be further from the truth.

It is possible for a woman to have sexual intercourse twenty times a day, give birth to a dozen children, and still have that Flag of Virtue, the hymen, waving at the vaginal portal. It all depends on the kind of hymen she is born with.

How does it work?

To understand the hymen's relative position in the genital area, it helps to have a model. If you hold your hand up and make a circle with the thumb and first finger, the enclosed space represents the vaginal opening. The webbing between the thumb and finger is the hymen in its usual position. Ordinarily, during the first sexual act, the penis pushes through the hymen, tearing it in several places. Repeated intercourse continues to erode the membrane, leaving only a few shreds to mark its former position of glory. In some cases the hymen is flexible, and instead of breaking before the penile assault, it merely bends. It is forced down toward the vaginal floor and allows the penis to glide over it. At childbirth the same thing can happen in reverse. Very rarely, the child's head can push the hymen outward without tearing it.

In many parts of the world, the hymen is a big deal. It is considered the symbol of virginity, and for some yet unexplained reason every full-fledged American man wants to make it with a virgin. A young-looking prostitute with a stretchable hymen, if she plays her cards right, can make a fortune by surrendering her maiden state over and over again at premium prices.

Certain of the more swinging establishments in European cities make the ceremony into quite a production. It requires a gent (not a regular customer) with a penchant for virgins. The lady of the house chooses her specialist—the one with the flexible hymen—and arranges for the two to meet—at triple the going rate. The lucky couple occupies a room fitted with a dozen peepholes—admission is charged. (Nowadays closed-circuit TV in color is becoming more popular for viewing.)

The performance is always a sell-out to the men (and ladies) who enjoy this kind of thing. Accompanied by appropriate shrieks and squeals, the ravisher has his way. Virginity loses again. Thirty minutes later, after a hot bath and a little massage, the hymen is back in position ready to do its bit keeping its mistress in the upper brackets.

Isn't there always bleeding when the hymen is really broken?

Usually, but professional virgins also bleed. Careful analysis might reveal that an hour earlier the blood flowed in the veins of a chicken, but then most customers are not interested in probing that deeply.

Then an intact hymen is not a reliable indicator of virginity?

Correct. And a tattered or absent hymen doesn't mean the young lady has dispensed her favors freely. Some women just don't have much of a hymen. Others lose what they had by vigorous exercise. Sliding down poles and climbing trees are not exactly designed to keep a tiny tab of delicate tissue in place. Another old enemy of the vaginal gatekeeper is masturbation. Introducing a finger or two into the vagina can be tough on a virgin's hymen.

A relatively recent innovation, the vaginal tampon to absorb menstrual flow, is also an easy way to say good-bye to this fragile membrane. The only reliable sign of a virgin vagina is what doctors call an imperforate hymen, and they are rarely seen by anyone but doctors.

How come?

This type of hymen closes off the vaginal entrance completely. It is rarely noticed until menstruation begins—or more precisely, does not begin.

Usually if a girl does not start to menstruate by the age of sixteen or so, her mother becomes anxious and takes her to the doctor. After a quick check of the vaginal orifice he makes the diagnosis. The opening is completely sealed off by a bulging hymen. Actual menstruation may have begun six months ago, but instead of draining to the outside, the fluid has backed up into the vagina. A few nicks with the scalpel and the problem disappears. So does the hymen.

At what age does menstruation normally start?

It varies. Every girl has her own biological timetable, so there is no normal age for the onset of menstruation. The range is from six to eighteen years, with most girls beginning between ten and fourteen years of age.

It's interesting that the average age when the menses begin has changed in the past fifty years in the United States. Back in the 1870s the average age for menstruation to begin was fourteen years and eight months. Nowadays it's about 12 years and 8 months for white girls and 12 years and 1 month for Afro-American youngsters. But something has changed—and no one knows what it is.

What's that?

According to a recent medical survey covering more than 17,000 girls, by the age of eight, fifty percent of Afro-American girls had pubic hair or breast development. At the same age, only about 15 percent of white girls had similar sexual characteristics. That can be a big problem, because few eight-year-old tots are able to deal with the problems of sexual development.

What causes it?

As usual when something so unexpected occurs, no one knows the cause. There are a couple of interesting theories, however. Some people think that the estrogen-like substances and placental extracts in black hair care products and hormone-containing cosmetics may be involved. And of course, there are a lot more estrogen-like substances in our environment than in the past. But how does it work and why? Stay tuned.

What actually is menstruation?

Menstruation is the final event in a long series of complex maneuvers executed by the body with split-second timing. The whole process unfolds according to a detailed script prepared by an internal computer. The plan is reviewed constantly, moment by moment, and updated monthly. In spite of the advances of science, our knowledge in this area is still rudimentary.

Controlling the menstrual cycle is roughly equivalent to launching a space vehicle, the egg, at the same time the launching pad is being built. Simultaneously, a gigantic landing facility, the uterus, must be prepared in case the little traveler through inner space should come back in a new form—fertilized. Concurrently, preparations must be made to tear down everything that has been built up in order to start again from scratch each month. It is like demolishing Cape Canaveral on the first of every month and rebuilding it by the thirtieth.

As the menstrual period finishes, the ovaries begin pouring one of the primary female sex hormones, estrogen, into the bloodstream. The presence of estrogen is reported to the Central Control Area, the pituitary gland at the base of the brain. In response, Central Control directs the release of a supporting hormone, FSH or Follicle Stimulating Hormone. FSH stimulates increased production of estrogen. While estrogen acts on every reproductive organ, it specifically triggers rapid growth of the inner lining of the uterus.

At the surface of the ovary, the egg scheduled for launch that month is already straining at its moorings. Now secretion of the other female sex hormone, progesterone, begins. When the presence of progesterone is detected by the pituitary, it responds with a counter-hormone, LH or Luteinizing Hormone.

Most of the progesterone is funneled to the uterus where it intensifies the preparations already under way. Central Control is constantly monitoring hormone levels in all areas of the body. When the ratio of FSH to LH reaches the critical point, a rapid countdown begins, and the ovum is hurled into the abdominal cavity.

Into the abdominal cavity? Doesn't it go into the Fallopian tubes?

With any luck, eventually. But it goes into the abdomen first. As the egg bursts from the surface of the ovary it travels freely into the vast emptiness of the pelvis. At the upper end of the Fallopian tubes, two enormous funnels with grasping fingers grab eagerly at the tiny egg. Most eggs slide willingly into the friendly grasp.

Then what?

Meanwhile, back at the uterus, big things are happening. The lining has enlarged dramatically. Each individual cell is swelling up until it is bursting at the seams. The blood vessels have become immense and are pulsating rhythmically. Day after day the build up continues as the detection systems remain constantly alert for information about the fate of the recently launched egg.

If the egg is not fertilized, Central Control reluctantly pushes the red button marked "DESTRUCT" and everything comes crashing down. Ruthlessly the blood supply to the uterine lining is choked off. Cells on the surface are left to starve and die. They will soon slough off by the millions. Menstruation is under way.

For the next three to seven days, all that remains of the ambitious undertaking of the past three weeks goes down the drain. Appropriately, menstruation has been called "The Weeping of a Disappointed Uterus." But all is not lost: the human body is perpetually optimistic. The entire project will begin again next month.

What does the menstrual flow consist of?

Not what most people think. Although it may seem like much more, only about a cupful or so of thin red fluid trickles out of the vagina during each menstrual period. And menstrual fluid is not all blood. It's only about half blood mixed with varying amounts of mucus and "clots." These so-called "clots" are actually pieces of the uterine lining that have broken away. Menstrual blood itself does not clot.

Why not?

The reason eluded researchers for years: they finally discovered that menstrual blood cannot clot because it has already clotted. As blood pours out of the uterine wall, it coagulates quickly. As always, a short time after coagulating, the blood liquefies and once again flows freely.

Is that all there is to menstruation?

Not quite. Some unanswered questions remain:

- Why does the menstrual tide, like the ocean tide, ebb and flow with the cycle of the moon? (That gives rise to the quaint Spanish reference to menstruation. A woman who is menstruating is said to be "*cornuda por la luna*" or "gored by the moon," like a bullfighter is gored by the bull.)
- Why do nosebleeds sometimes accompany the menstrual flow?
- Why do many women feel inexplicably depressed during menstruation? (Most crimes of violence committed by women occur during menstrual periods.)
- Why do women who live together—as in college dormitories— eventually begin to have synchronized menstrual periods?

Anything else?

One more thing. Why is it that women go to such great lengths to conceal the fact that they are menstruating? Why do they refer to it as "The Curse" or "sick" or "A Visitor from Down South"? Why do ads for tampons and menstrual pads insist that their products are invisible and undetectable?

Rhonda is thirty-one and a successful trial lawyer. She has her own explanation:

"Doctor, haven't you ever asked yourself why we women have to hide everything about menstruation as if we were

committing some crime? I mean, we have gotten so sensitive about it that we even call it 'Being Sick.' But really, menstruating is 'Being Well.' Only healthy women menstruate. As you say in your book, it's really only some clotted blood, some tissue fluid, and some dead cells that we get rid of. It's not as if we were dangerous or something like that!

"Did you ever ask yourself how it would be if men menstruated? First of all they'd have menstrual pads with National Football League colors. The government would invest billions in a Research Foundation to find a cure for PMS. Sports would take on a different look. Like this headline, for example:

"SUPER BOWL CANCELED! BOTH TEAMS SIDELINED BY MENSTRUAL CRAMPS!

or

MAN ROBS BANK, BLAMES PMS!"

Are men really frightened by menstruation?

Everybody is frightened by menstruation—at least at first. After all, it is pretty scary to have what looks like fresh blood suddenly dribbling from one of your body openings. Even experienced women, when they have extra-heavy flows, sometimes wonder "Will it ever stop?"

And when a young boy sees his mother and sisters "bleeding" every month, it can worry him. Maybe that's the reason men don't want to know that a woman is menstruating—or why they don't even want to say the word "menstruation." "Having her period" sounds so much safer—even if it sounds more like giving birth to a punctuation mark. Here's some advice from one of my female patients: "It would be a wonderful idea for every man to pick a nice quiet corner and say, 'MENSTRUATION!' one hundred times out loud. Then they wouldn't get so red in the face when they hear the word."

Is that attitude about menstruation something new?

Not at all. The whole subject of menstruation has fascinated mankind for thousands of years. Even the earlier portions of the Bible refer to it. In Leviticus 15:19:

> *"And if a woman have an issue, and her issue in her flesh be blood, she shall be put apart seven days: and whosoever toucheth her shall be unclean until the even."*

What does that mean?

Like any Bible quotation, it is open to an unlimited number of interpretations. However, a few rapid calculations are revealing.

Let us assume the start of menstruation is considered the first day. The flow continues, say, seven days. If the woman is "unclean," that is, not approachable for sexual intercourse, for the next seven days, the first available moment after the onset of the menstrual period will be fourteen days later. Interestingly enough, that corresponds to the most likely day of ovulation. Intercourse on that day has an excellent chance of returning a fertilized ovum to the waiting uterus.

What guarantee is there that a woman will have intercourse on that specific day?

There is no guarantee, of course. However, if she has been waiting impatiently for two weeks and her husband has likewise been counting the hours until his wife is available again, they will probably take advantage of the first opportunity. Synchronizing the lowering of the monthly sexual barriers with the day of greatest fertility was a stroke of genius on the part of the ancient Hebrews. Maybe that is the real meaning of I Chronicles 27:23:

> *"the Lord had said he would increase Israel like to the stars of the heavens."*

Why does menstruation stop during pregnancy?

It doesn't always. In a small number of cases monthly bleeding continues throughout pregnancy. Not quite so rare is a menstrual flow during the first month or two. Usually the increase in maternal hormone levels during pregnancy, bolstered by the hormones from the newly formed placenta, is adequate to keep the uterine lining from decomposing. Lactation may further delay the return of the period.

How come?

Another hard question. Lactation itself is not well understood. At birth both breasts are generally prepared to supply abundant milk. If the child begins to nurse, nervous impulses go from the nipples to Central Control in the pituitary gland. This produces still another hormone, Lactogenic Hormone, which starts the milk flowing and keeps it available until nursing stops. At the same time, menstruation is suppressed. Almost like magic, when the sucking stops, the milk stops.

Then the woman can't become pregnant if she isn't menstruating?

Not exactly. Pregnancy is less likely during lactation (reason unknown), but in reproduction anything is possible. Fertilization can occur before, after, or during menstruation. Lots of unmarried chaps who pay child support will testify to that.

How do the female genitalia change in preparation for intercourse?

Erection of the penis is relatively simple compared with what must take place before girls are ready for copulation. Let's begin at the bottom and work up.

First, the blood vessels supplying the vulva dilate and bring on the feminine equivalent of a penile erection. The spongy tissues around the labia minora as well as the labia themselves swell and grow turgid. The clitoris becomes erect and may peep from under its diminutive foreskin. The labia majora increase in size, and Bartholin's glands, the two sentinels located astride the vaginal opening, do—nothing. Once considered the prime source of lubrication—"lover's liniment"—they have been demoted as medical research has discovered a new and fascinating source of these essential juices. The walls of the vagina themselves ooze a super-slippery substance that smoothes the way for eager couples. In the research lab, by means of a special camera in the form of a transparent, optically correct plastic penis, the glistening drops can be observed gently forming on the vaginal wall.

In the meantime, engorgement of the vulva has formed a sort of sexual anteroom in front of the vagina. This increases the effective length of the vaginal canal and thus increases the size of the penis it can accommodate. More important, it brings the sexually sensitive structures—clitoris and labia minora—closer to the penis.

The vagina is also changing. In cross section the relaxed vagina looks like the letter H; the roof is in contact with the floor. During sexual excitement it swiftly assumes the shape of a cylinder to receive an energetic piston, the penis.

What is the function of the clitoris?

The clitoris is the center of sexual sensation in women. Though it is tiny in comparison with the penis, it has at least the same number of nerve cells and nerve fibers as the penis, crowded into a much smaller space. It is a sexual time bomb with a short fuse. Actually, a pair of fuses. The labia minora, looking like twin rooster's combs, are attached to the hood or prepuce of the clitoris. Pulling on them applies a gentle tug on the clitoris itself. As the labia are alternately pulled and released, the prepuce slides back and forth over the head of the clitoris. As the gentle friction continues, the clitoris swells even more, making each tug even more exquisite.

How do the labia get pulled?

If the vagina can be considered a cylinder and the penis a piston, the labia minora are a crankshaft. With each stroke of the penis into the vagina, the ends of the labia are pulled toward the vagina, drawing down on the prepuce and clitoris. As the penis is withdrawn, the labia are released and the prepuce slides back over the clitoris. At the same time, the penis is massaging the labia, the vagina, and the related structures. If everything goes right the result is orgasm.

What happens during orgasm?

Everything. All the transmission lines and circuits of the entire body are suddenly and deliciously overloaded. The wires get red-hot, the fuses blow, the bells chime—and then it's all over until the next time.

As a woman approaches orgasm the whole pace of her body accelerates. The heart rate zooms up to 160 or more. Respiration gives way to panting and groaning. Blood pressure can double. In the meantime, the pelvis is going wild. All the veins of the pelvic area are at the point of bursting. The vulva is throbbing rhythmically almost to the point of grabbing at the surging penis. The sensory nerves are at their peak, soaking up each tiny drop of sensation. So much current is drawn by the sexual structures that the lights in the cerebrum begin to dim. The woman loses track of her surroundings, and all attention is focused on that vital 5 percent of her body.

Suddenly the master switch is flipped and it happens! Indescribable sensations race from the vulva, vagina, and clitoris throughout the nervous system. The primitive areas of the brain seize control. The back arches, the pelvis lunges forward, the muscles surrounding the vulva expand and contract and send waves of feeling racing over the entire body. The pelvic veins empty rapidly, droplets of sweat burst out on the skin, and a sense of relaxation flows through the entire body.

How many orgasms can a woman have?

Nobody really knows. Recent investigators stopped the experiments after fifty or so consecutive climaxes. The experimental technique itself was rather ingenious. Under carefully controlled conditions, with trained observers, movie lights, tape recorders, and a video camera grinding away, a female volunteer engaged in sexual intercourse with a male volunteer. They copulated until she reached orgasm, duly recorded by electrodes taped to various parts of her body, as well as by the camera and tape recorders. The gentleman immediately withdrew from the scene and was replaced by another more or less eager volunteer. This process continued until two score and ten intrepid spirits had given their best for science. The lady was still more or less willing, but the experimenters were hungry for dinner, the recorders were running out of tape, the video cameras were running out of videotape, and anxious wives were beginning to telephone their husbands at the laboratory.

Wasn't the female subject tired?

The official records describe her as "tired but happy." One wonders how many orgasms she might have had without the lights, video cameras, recorders, and eager observers.

Actually there are several varieties of orgasm in the female. Male orgasms tend to be of the all-or-nothing variety—a tremendous buildup of tension followed by an explosive release. Woman have this type of orgasm too, but they are also capable of "skimming."

This is a series of sexual climaxes that consist of a rapid increase in tension with an equally rapid release, rising immediately to another peak. The effect is something like a flat pebble skimming over the surface of the waves. The peaks are never as high and the valleys are never as deep as a full-scale orgasm, but it is said to be an exquisitely gratifying experience just the same. Most of the female multiple orgasms are of this variety.

How can a woman continue to reach climax after climax when a man is finished after the first time around?

The answer depends on their different sexual structure and functioning. Erection in the male is dependent on engorgement of the veins of the penis. When sexual tension subsides after the first orgasm, the erection droops as the blood begins to drain from the organ. Even if sexual stimulation continues, once the erection fades the organ must go through the full cycle of relaxation, rest, and re-erection. Sometimes this cycle can be speeded up, but the stages must proceed in that order.

The female has no such limitation. Large veins deep in the pelvic area as well as those in the sexual organs themselves never need to empty completely after orgasm. The blood can ebb and flow according to the degree of sexual excitement.

Immediately after orgasm, sexual stimulation usually diminishes and the message goes out from the brain and spinal cord to open the drainage valves. If sexual activity should resume, the order is countermanded and the internal and external genitalia become engorged with blood once again.

Then orgasm is caused by blood flowing in the sexual organs?

Not exactly. There are three components to the orgasmic experience; if any of them are missing, orgasm does not take place.

First and most important is the nervous element. Sensations are fed to a cluster of nerves in the spinal cord, sort of an Orgasm Central Control, from every part of the body. Before intercourse, as her partner caresses the woman's breasts, the sensations are fed into the spinal nerve plexus. When she places her hand on his penis, those sensations are routed via the brain to Orgasm Central. Any sexually stimulating sounds or words are also picked up and relayed to the spinal centers. As the man mounts her and begins to slide his penis into her vagina, the number of nervous messages increases a hundred times. The sensation of his skin rubbing against hers, the odor of his body, the pressure of his chest upon her breasts, the throbbing of his penis against her labia minora and vaginal entrance—these are all picked up by the appropriate sensing mechanisms and raced to Orgasm Central.

At about that stage the mechanism becomes self-feeding. Nervous impulses are now going in both directions, to the spinal center and from it. This is what builds up to orgasm. It's like an old-fashioned baseball pitcher winding up—around and around and around, building up momentum all the time, until finally the stored energy is released explosively.

The impulses from the vagina, clitoris, labia, and even the internal pelvic structures increase a thousandfold as the penis thrusts in and out. Finally the critical stage is reached, no more sensations can be tolerated, and Orgasm Central gives the command.

Then the second component of orgasm enters the picture. Nerve impulses from the spinal centers cause vigorous muscular contraction. The network of muscles that form a circular tunnel around the vagina clamp down, let go, and clamp down, again and again. Even the uterus contracts under the intense nervous stimulation. Some people have suggested that at orgasm the uterus can even suck up the sperm that are squirted into the vagina. An experiment performed some years ago indicated that at orgasm the uterus of a female horse could suck up an impressive amount of liquid in less than six seconds. It still has to be confirmed in human subjects.

Then there is the third element in orgasm—vascular. The vigorous muscular contractions pump all the blood out of the veins, the resulting vacuum drains the tissues of the vulva, and sexual tension swiftly declines. That, for the moment, is that.

What part does the uterus play in sexual intercourse?

Sexual feeling is confined primarily to the clitoris, the labia minora, and the anterior wall of the vagina. The rest of the vagina has much less sensation, and the cervix, or lower end of the uterus, can hardly feel anything at all. During medical exams the cervix is often held with a sharp-toothed instrument; the patient is rarely aware that anything is happening. This is notable since most men put a lot of emphasis on the length of the penis (women know better) as an indicator of sexual prowess. Most of the real accomplishments occur in the first 3 inches of the female reproductive apparatus—it is a rare man who cannot stand up to that.

There is one exception. A certain number of women react sexually to deep pelvic pressure. It is more common among those who have had several children; they may have developed an awareness of the uterus and cervix during pregnancy and labor. These women experience an intensification of pleasure during intercourse and specifically during orgasm if the penis penetrates deeply into the vagina and presses against the cervix. But even here a long penis is not required. By shifting her body and flexing her legs, the woman can effectively shorten the length of her vagina and get the result she wants.

If a woman can have so many more orgasms than a man, how come some women can't have any orgasms at all?

There is a big difference between having the potential to achieve an orgasm and achieving it. The only thing that stands between any woman and an unlimited number of orgasmic experiences is about 2 pounds of tissue—the brain. The decision to have a sexual climax is not made in the vagina—it occurs in the brain at the other end of the body. Nature does not require sexual enjoyment for reproduction. Once the sperm make it to the vagina, She makes no further demands. According to the Laws of Nature enjoyment of sexual intercourse is optional and left to the discretion of the participants.

Is there any way a man can tell if a woman has really had an orgasm?

Since most women know what men want to hear, especially in the department of sex, they are always willing to acknowledge an orgasm, even if they haven't had one. It doesn't cost them anything and goes a long way toward inflating the male ego. A great number of men in our society feel their manhood enhanced if their partners experience orgasm. Rarely do they inquire too deeply—if she says "yes," that's that. It makes it easier—at least for the moment. However if he really wants to know, there are two approximate indicators.

Immediately after orgasm a certain number of women experience what is called a sexual flush. This is a measles-like rash over the entire chest. It comes on suddenly, lasts a few minutes, and then gradually fades away. Not every woman experiences this, and the same holds true for erection of the nipples. At orgasm some women's nipples stand smartly at attention—and some don't.

The important thing to remember is that in sexual intercourse, orgasm happens in the brain—not the vagina or clitoris or in the penis. The penis may give the vagina the best workout in the world, but if the brain isn't plugged in, it's like nothing ever happened.

What's the difference between a vaginal orgasm and a clitoral orgasm?

Nothing. Absolutely nothing. Many years ago Sigmund Freud theorized that women experienced two distinct types of orgasm, vaginal and clitoral. The clitoral orgasm was presumably based on masturbation in childhood and was considered childish and immature. Vaginal orgasm was related to "adult" sexual organs, and Dr. Freud considered it "mature." The vaginal variety was said to be a more intense, more fulfilling experience. Based on this theory, which was essentially a philosophical concept, psychiatric thinking hardened like so much psychic cement. Few psychiatrists thought to ask the women what they really felt, although they were the ones who were having the clitoral or vaginal orgasms in the first place.

If direct experiments and observations had been possible in Freud's time, he probably would have been a pioneer in that area too. But since a truly scientific look at human sexuality has had to wait until recently, Freud's ideas must be revised accordingly. They must make way for an Orgasmic Bill of Rights.

Orgasmic Bill of Rights?

Yes. "All Orgasms Are Created Equal." Years of careful observation and analysis involving thousands of men and women who copulated, masturbated, and engaged in nearly every variation thereof right in the scientific laboratory have yielded some important answers about female orgasm.

Unless the clitoris participates in some way, orgasm does not take place. Remember, the clitoris is attached to the vagina and the vagina is attached to the labia minora—and the labia minora are attached to the clitoris. All of them are interconnected by a vast network of nerves. The whole collection of sexual organs is connected directly to the spinal cord and thus to the brain. That makes it impossible to say that orgasm is entirely dependent on one structure or another.

What difference does it make, vaginal or clitoral orgasm?

None at all. Once again, the guiding principle should be The Orgasmic Bill of Rights. And that's good news to women because they can stop worrying about it. An orgasm is an orgasm. Orgasms may vary in frequency and intensity but they all begin and end at the same place—the vaginal-labial-clitoral axis. Just as the planets revolve around the sun, vagina-labia-clitoris revolve around orgasm. Feelings of guilt instilled by well-meaning psychiatrists can be cast aside. Every orgasm resulting from penis-vagina intercourse is, by definition, mature.

What if the vagina is stimulated without exciting the clitoris?

It's very hard. Any object large enough to stimulate the vagina also stimulates the clitoris by pulling down on the labia. Furthermore, nerves from the clitoris extend downward over the entire vulva into the walls of the vagina itself. When the penis is in the vagina pressing against the vaginal walls, it is still titillating the clitoris. Even this tiny detail has been scientifically measured.

What did it show?

In carefully performed experiments, increasing the pressure in the lower one-third of the vagina—where all the action occurs—caused a tremendous increase in blood flow to the clitoris. After about a second or so of pressure in the lower part of the vagina, blood flow to the clitoris increases up to 1,000 percent. The same kind of powerful blood flow happens when the head of the penis is stimulated. So when the head of the penis presses hard against the vagina, the clitoris comes to attention and even more blood rushes into the penis. As the head of the penis swells, it triggers more blood flow to the clitoris. A perfect example of teamwork in action.

If a woman were to lose her clitoris, say in an operation, could she still have orgasms?

Certainly. Some women have had that kind of surgery, because of cancer, for example. But nerves and blood vessels from the clitoris extend to every part of the vulva. Even if the organ itself is removed, the remaining nervous connections are more than adequate for orgasm.

However, some women have the clitoris removed for non-medical reasons.

Remove the clitoris for "Non-medical reasons"? Why should anyone want to do that?

It's a complicated problem. Among certain religious groups "female circumcision" is a religious rite comparable to male circumcision. Everyone's religious convictions must be respected, so it's not entirely a medical decision.

There are many forms of the operation—one technique involves removing just the tip of the clitoris and/or its tiny foreskin. Another more drastic procedure is the "clitoridectomy" where the entire clitoris, including the foreskin, is removed. The operation is usually done by people who are not medically qualified and without any anesthesia whatsoever. It is painful—to say the least. Currently in the United States and some European countries, there is a tremendous wave of protest against it.

How come?

Many people—especially in the United States—feel outraged that young girls are having their clitoris operated on and even removed. They refer to the procedure as "FGM" or "Female Genital Mutilation" and are horrified by it. The problem is complicated by the fact that many families come to the United States from other countries where total or partial removal of the clitoris is common; when they arrive, they insist on doing the operation here. To many Americans, it seems cruel and irrational. But they have short memories.

Short memories? How come?

It wasn't so long ago that removal of the clitoris was done every day in the United States. And hardly anyone even noticed. It happened like this:

Influenced by European specialists, about 1890 American doctors decided that female masturbation was a serious problem that produced many other diseases. Since most women masturbate by rubbing the clitoris, the doctors' solution was simple: Cut it off! And that's what they proceeded to do.

For a quarter of a century, thousands of grown women had that most exquisitely sensitive organ sliced off in a hospital by a doctor. Amputation of the clitoris was a medically approved and recommended treatment. FGM was alive and well in America not too many years ago.

Does that mean that female circumcision is OK?

Not at all. It simply means that the sexual organs are so powerfully entwined with the innermost feelings and attitudes of society that strange things can happen. And it can lead to some strange contradictions.

Like what?

Like piercing, for example. While there is a tremendous outcry in the United States against female circumcision as distorting and deforming the female genitals, no one seems to be distraught about piercing. And it can come pretty close to some of the techniques of "Female Genital Mutilation."

For example?

Let's take a look at it. The operation is usually done by people who are not medically qualified and generally without any anesthesia whatsoever. It's usually done in piercing establishments by "piercers." These are business men or women who sell the "piercing jewelry" and "pierce" customers who buy their products.

It is painful—to say the least. Female piercing looks more like torture than anything else. Usually a sharp rod something like an ice pick is shoved through part of the female sexual equipment. Sometimes the operator shoves the sharp instrument through the foreskin of the clitoris above or below that very sensitive little organ either up-and-down or from side-to-side. Then they might insert—into the raw and bleeding genital tissues—a ring with a steel ball at each end. In piercing lingo, it's called a "CBR," or "Captive Bead Ring." When it's all over, the lady jumps off the table and waddles away.

That sounds gruesome. Is that all there is?

No, there's more. Some women also have their labia minora pierced and rings put into the labia. Many women have three or four rings on each side of the opening to the vagina. Putting a ring through the foreskin that covers the clitoris or through the labia is pretty scary to most people. If the woman were strapped to the table against her will and holes were poked in her delicate sexual organs and rings clamped into them, you'd be able to hear her screaming in the next county. The sheriff would be there in ten minutes and we'd have a human rights, sexual harassment, and sexual torture case on our hands.

But strangely enough, that's what women all over the United States and Europe pay big money for every day. And for some women, that's not nearly enough. Provided she qualifies, a woman can step up to the "big time" in the world of piercing.

How does she qualify?

She has to have a clitoris that is at least one-quarter inch wide and moves freely within its foreskin. If Nature has given her that much she can go on to the ultimate piercing. That means she has someone punch a hole right though the shaft of the clitoris itself. Then they clamp a Captive Bead Ring or some other kind of "jewelry" right through it and she limps home.

Is there anything wrong with that?

Not necessarily. It's a personal decision and if that's what a woman wants, she can do it. But there is an interesting paradox:

While people today are protesting against the involuntary muti-lation of females by operations on the clitoris, less than 100 years ago, medical doctors were recommending and performing precisely that procedure. And right now today, as you read this, women are paying to have their own labia pierced with metal rings and their delicate and ultra-sensitive clitoris drilled and ringed.

Why do women have themselves pierced?

Two reasons, both of them fascinating. First, a correctly placed ring or ball constantly tickles and bumps the clitoris as the woman moves. If it's done right it can trigger erection and titillation of the organ. At work, walking to lunch, watching TV, even crossing her legs and tapping her toe, she can engage in secret and exciting mas-turbation. If it sounds strange, listen to what one patient, Jenny, a 23-year-old professional dancer, explained:

"Why do I have a steel ball bouncing off my clit every time I move? Is that your question, Doctor? Well, all I can say is, if you haven't tried it, don't knock it!"

What's the other reason?

S&M. A steel ring through the clitoris or labia works perfectly for Sado-Masochistic games. To that group of people who like their sex mixed with pain, it's fun to have someone pull on those rings or hook little chains to them and drag you around. Every time they jerk on those rings, pain surges through all your most delicate sex-ual equipment.

You say it's not your idea of fun? Well, it isn't mine either, but when it comes to sex, as Shakespeare observed in Hamlet:

There are more things in heaven and earth, Horatio,
Than are dreamt of . . .

We'll see some more things that were never dreamt of in the chapters that follow.

Chapter 4
SEXUAL INTERCOURSE

What is sexual intercourse?

Magic, pure magic. If we stand back a little bit and look at sexual intercourse—as if we had never seen it before—"magic" would be the only word for it.

Imagine this. One night, in a burst of blue light, a couple of Martians suddenly appear in your bedroom. They are tall and thin, dressed in silver jumpsuits. They are a male and a female and they are curious. They ask:

"How do you Earthlings have sex?"

You're eager to help and you answer them.

"Well, it's like this. A man and a woman get together somewhere and they look at each other. Then they talk to each other and touch each other. Then all of a sudden their sexual organs start to swell up. The man's penis gets big and hard and hot—and very uncomfortable. The woman's clitoris gets hard, her labia swell, and the entrance to her vagina gets wet and slippery. They can't stop any of this from happening—it's almost completely out of their control."

The Martians are listening intently and they are puzzled. "Then what happens?"

"Then the man can't hold back any longer. He has to plunge his penis into the woman's opening, the vagina, and the woman really wants that hard stiff penis inside her."

"Very interesting," say the Martians. "Why is that?"

"No one knows. They just have to do it that way. They can't resist it. It's like a drug!"

"Then what?" they ask.

"Then the man pushes his penis into the vagina and almost takes it out and then pushes it in again and they rub those two swollen organs together, slowly at first, then faster and faster and faster. All of a sudden the friction makes the penis start to pulsate uncontrollably and squirt out a teaspoon of whitish liquid."

"Then what?"

"Then the couple have something like an epileptic seizure! They sort of lose consciousness while they have these wild muscle spasms."

The Martians look at each other in disbelief. "But why do people do that?"

"Because they love it! Because it's the most exciting and enjoyable thing they ever do! That's the one thing in the world they like the best!"

"They like that?"

The Martians look at each other, shake their heads in amazement, and disappear in another flash of blue light.

That is pretty much what sexual intercourse looks like—and yet it is truly the most amazing and wonderful and enjoyable thing that human beings ever do.

But is sex that important?

Yes, it is. Aside from the fact that if it weren't for sex you wouldn't be here reading this page, sex can be the most constructive, the most positive, the most rewarding aspect of human existence. But sex is like a hammer.

Like a hammer?

That's right. You can use it to build a beautiful Temple to Love—or you can smash your thumb with it. You can use it to reinforce the love that bonds you to your mate—or you can conk someone on the head with it. Rape, child abuse, and the deliberate spread of STDs (Sexually Transmitted Diseases)—those are the criminal misuses of sex. But the penis and vagina aren't to blame—just as the hammer isn't to blame when it zaps your thumb. It's the person who wields the hammer—or the penis or vagina—who is responsible. But to get the most out of sex—and to use it in the best possible way, you have to understand the different kinds of sexual intercourse.

How many kinds of sexual intercourse are there?

Sexual intercourse actually involves three distinct experiences masquerading as one. Sometimes the three events occur simultaneously, sometimes in succession, and very often they happen separately.

What do they consist of?

The first type of sexual intercourse is reproductive sex or "ReproSex." It's simple, straightforward, easily understood, and relatively speaking, unpopular. Every year people spend billions of dollars on birth control items to avoid ReproSex. In the average person's lifetime, ReproSex occurs on about five occasions or less. All the requirements of this form of sexuality can be managed nicely in three or four minutes and probably could be performed more efficiently by a disinterested third party—as it is occasionally in artificial insemination. ReproSex is merely a means of introducing Mr. Sperm to Miss Egg—what they do after that is up to them.

ReproSex has the approval and endorsement of Ministers of the Gospel, moral leaders, and maiden aunts. Though they may not engage in it themselves, for obvious reasons they recommend it for the masses.

ReproSex is uniformly unpopular with teenagers, unmarried lovers, carefree young bachelors, single girls, and ladies with ten or more children. Major world governments endorse or discourage this variety of sexual intercourse depending on the population supply at the moment.

What's the second form of sex?

Sex can also be a means of expressing love. When all the words have been said, the deep emotional bond that flows from the dramatic fusion of two bodies and two spirits can be the most profound way of saying "I love you." It can exist among men and women at any stage of their lives, tends to be perishable if not carefully preserved, and those who have experienced it say it tends to grow stronger with the passage of time. Marriage is not a prerequisite, and some cynics even say that marriage takes the love out of sex. Everybody is in favor of LoveSex, especially writers of popular songs and vendors of greeting cards, though not everyone has the chance to experience it.

How about the third form of sex?

The third kind of sexual intercourse has acquired a bad name over the years. Many Western religions are against it, Moral Educators unanimously condemn it, parents are (apparently) against it—and everyone wants to get as much of it as they can. This is sex for fun, for the sheer physical and emotional exhilaration of feeling all the good feelings that come from a complete sexual experience. This is FunSex at its best. Almost everyone under the age of twenty-five is openly for it, and nearly everyone else wishes for it actively, if secretly. There is nothing wrong with FunSex. Human beings—and for that matter, all mammals—are provided with a penis or vagina and an overwhelming compulsion to use them. There is no reason why they shouldn't, and specifically in a way that will bring them the maximum pleasure—without getting them into trouble.

Whole libraries have been devoted to amassing arguments against the sensible enjoyment of sex. Even after centuries of this insidious form of brainwashing, most human beings remain basically unconvinced. But there is a major obstacle to getting the full pleasure from sex.

What's that?

Obtaining the maximum enjoyment from sexual intercourse requires knowledge. Our modern society is careful to teach people how to run their automobiles but deliberately avoids teaching them how to run their sexual organs. What passes for sex education is like the French joke:

> "What is flirtation?
> "It's when the hand is in the you-know-what and the you-know-what is in the hand, but the you-know-what is never in the you-know-what."

After the usual course in sex education, the high school senior emerges with the amazing knowledge that two you-know-whats somehow fit together. That, too, is a joke, but a grimmer one. If the schools wasted less time on the physiology of reproduction with all the beautiful diagrams of frantically swimming sperm (which nobody cares about anyhow) and spent more time on the physiology of orgasm (which everybody cares about), this would be a happier world.

And of course, nowadays there's another big problem in sex education.

What's that?

Disease. Because of the out-of-control epidemics of STDs—including the old ones as well as the new ones—most of what should be useful education in sexuality is devoted to how to prevent, diagnose, and treat the deadly diseases that sex can bring. At the same time, the current educational system devotes a lot of time to training students in the installation, operation, and maintenance of rubber one-finger gloves—condoms—to be worn by the male organ. Obviously that's important, but it misses one vital point. If you're going to have sex with a penis or a vagina, you run a big risk of getting a disease—especially these days. But if you have sexual intercourse—and emotional intercourse—with another human being, you reduce your chance of infection significantly. If you are part of their life and they are part of your life, neither of you wants to expose the other to any unhappiness—much less a fatal disease.

What can a person do to increase his enjoyment of sex?

The answer to that question is a five-letter word: L-E-A-R-N. The key to sexual enjoyment is to learn what sex is all about, how it works, and what to do to make it work for you. But you won't find it in a Handy-Dandy-Do-It-Yourself-Sex-Manual written by an overweight ex-chorus girl or an unemployed saxophone player. Titles like *99 Ways to Turn Your Dentist into a Love-Slave* or *How to Make All the Women in Your Car Pool Lust After You in Only 7 Days* aren't for real. If you think about it, anyone who is going to help you understand human sexuality has to have an extensive knowledge of anatomy, physiology, biochemistry, pathology, bacteriology, internal medicine, psychiatry, and a dozen or so other areas of advanced study. It also helps if they have diagnosed and treated a few thousand people with sexual problems. (Dancing naked on the tables in a bar or having sex with a thousand men does not precisely meet the definition of "diagnosis and treatment.")

So before you put your faith in any tome on sex, ask the author where he or she acquired their knowledge of the most complex medical-scientific part of human existence—sex.

Why is it so important to know so much about sex to enjoy it? Can't you just do it?

Sure. A lot of people do. And a lot of people drive automobiles without knowing what they are doing. They crash. They hurt other people. They get in jail. They end up hating cars and people.

A lot of people drive their sexual organs without knowing what they are doing. They crash. They hurt other people. They get in jail. They end up hating sex and people.

Taking the time to learn about sex and understand sex is probably the most rewarding thing anyone can do in their entire lifetime. Sex is nice. But it's more than just nice. While you are having fun you are accomplishing something useful. You are showing affection, cementing human relationships, and significantly improving your health and increasing your life expectancy (see Chapter 16, "September Sex" for the details on how sex actually can actually improve your health). Of course, having sex accomplishes one other little task: it preserves the human race.

But you can't accomplish any of those things well unless you understand sex. And the more you understand it, the better you will be able to enjoy it.

Where do you start?

Right here. The first step is to visualize human beings from a sexual point of view as medical scientists see them. Think of a person as having two Sexual Poles just as the Earth has two Poles—a North Pole and a South Pole. For people, the North Pole is the Head—composed of the Brain and those little-known but vitally important direct extensions of the brain called the "Cranial Nerves." (That's the part that most books on sex completely ignore.) The South Pole is composed of the sexual organs themselves. In men it's the penis and testicles. In women it's the clitoris, vagina, labia, and associated structures. But there's more. In women the Lower Pole covers the same area that would be covered by a pair of short shorts. In back, that includes the area from the waist to the buttocks extending to the perineum (the area between the anus and the vagina). In front, from the waist past the vagina around to the perineum. The whole Lower Pole is really a gradient—the sensitivity and the sensation is weakest around the waist and intensifies rapidly as one approaches the actual sexual organs. There is also a V-shaped area on the chest that takes in the nipples and the breasts. If the head and Cranial Nerves are the North Pole, then the breasts are in Canada.

The Sexual Map for men is about the same but with less sensitivity than women over the abdomen and buttocks—most of the nerve supply for men is concentrated in that Primary Ballistic Missile, the penis. Some men have sexual sensitivity around the breasts and nipples, but this is less intense than in women.

One of the great problems in sexual intercourse is that the Upper Pole—the Head—is constantly at war with the Lower Pole— the Sexual Organs.

Why should they be at war?

Marlene knows how it is. She's seventeen and a freshman in college:

> *"It's really hard to deal with sometimes, Doctor. Like I'm going out with this boy. We start in—you know, kissing and fooling around. At first, I'm completely in control. But then I get hotter and he starts touching my breasts and I start to get wet down there. Then he gets more excited and kind of climbs on top of me and starts rubbing up against me and I feel my clitoris starting to get hard. And it's like my brain begins to melt and it's all happening between my legs . . ."*

That's when the Lower Pole starts to win the War.

It can happen the other way too. Nancy tells how it feels. She is twenty-nine and has been married six years:

> *"I don't understand it. When Bill and I start to have sex, everything is OK at first. The kissing and all that is nice and I start to get really excited. But when he starts playing with me down there . . ."*

She paused and glanced furtively in the general direction of some indefinite space between her navel and her knees.

*"Then I start to freeze up and I let him do it but it's like I
don't feel anything. I mean, I start to think about whether
it's right and if I'm going to get pregnant or something."*

Nancy's North Pole wins the War and Nancy and Bill lose
every battle.

What's the solution?

Make Peace. Teach the Upper Pole and the Lower Pole to work
together so that you and your partner can enjoy sex to the fullest.
Start with the Head.

The truth is that the sexual organs—in men and women both—
are nothing more than receptors. They feel things just like you feel
things with the tips of your fingers. Of course the tip of a penis is
somewhat more sensitive than the tip of a finger, and the tip of a clitoris is thousands of times more sensitive than a fingertip. But the
principle is the same. All the tremendously powerful sensations that
the sexual organs/receptors gather are sent to the brain. At any
moment, as it is being bombarded with all these dynamite sexual
sensations, the brain can scream "NO!" and pull the plug on sex.

And the brain will do it.

It's Midnight. Husband and wife are just getting into some wild
sex. His erection is like a rock, she's just about to have a sensational orgasm, and suddenly they realize their three-year-old
daughter is awake and has been standing at the foot of the bed
watching the entire proceedings with great interest for the past ten
minutes. That's when the brain slams on the brakes, the man's
penis goes "plop," the woman's vagina goes "clunk" and that's it
for the evening.

There are some other moments when the brain might pull the
plug on erection, excitement, and orgasm.

The man has just inserted his erect penis all the way into the
vagina when the woman speaks:

*"Oh, I forgot to tell you, Dear. Two men came by looking for
you this afternoon. I think they said they were from the FBI
or something . . ."*

or

"Boy, sex is great with you, Mr. Wilson. You sure know how to treat a girl. I can hardly wait until I'm eighteen and it'll be legal . . ."

or

"The doctor said he'd have the results of my AIDS test tomorrow for sure."

It all adds up to one thing. If you want to have the best possible sex, you need to have your number one sexual organ, the brain, in the best possible working order. The hardest penis, the most wildly throbbing clitoris, and the tightest vagina don't mean a thing if the North Pole is boycotting the South Pole. The secret of sexual success is to keep the brain and the sexual organs working together.

How do you do that?

There are two things to be done. First, and most obvious, avoid sexual situations that expose you to fear and danger. There is an old Italian expression that says: "You aren't a real man unless you have had sex in a tree, under water, or with a jealous husband banging on the door."

If you really want to get the best out of sex, it's better to avoid all three of those situations—and any others like them.

The other thing is to practice "Total Sexual Intercourse" (or TSI) to make sure that you give your sexual organs and your brain every possible advantage. That's the way to overcome the self-imposed limitations of the Head. The idea is to supply the sexual organs/receptors and the brain with the greatest possible number of positive sensations to make sex tremendously exciting and to make orgasm sensational.

There's a wonderful fringe benefit too, to TSI. The more you do it that way, the more ingrained the sexual reflexes become. As the months go by, your sexual responses become faster and deeper and much more exciting.

How do you get started with Total Sexual Intercourse?

To get started, you have to keep a few basic concepts in mind.

The first concept to remember is that when it comes to sex,

touching is a two-way street—and sometimes a three-way street. For example, when a woman is stroking a man's penis, he feels the pressure and gentle friction on that organ. Those sensations zoom up to the brain and trigger an increase in sexual excitement. As he gets more excited, impulses from the brain sensitize the penis and the stroking and caressing of his organ feels better and better. Those intensified sensations then are transmitted to the brain, adding to all the previous sensations. That's the two-way street.

But something else is happening. As the woman feels the heat and the swelling and the pulsations of the penis, she begins to get excited. Her brain is bombarded by sexual impulses and begins to fire commands to her clitoris and vagina. The clitoris begins to swell, and lubricating liquid appears in the vagina. Suddenly the two-way street of sexual stimulation and feedback becomes a three-way street. But it doesn't stop there.

If the man then caresses the woman's clitoris with the tip of his index finger, he feels the extremely smooth, extremely soft skin of the clitoris against his finger and the pulsation of the organ as it reacts to his touch. The woman gets another source of sexual excitement, really making it a four-way street!

Then things begin to happen under their own momentum. The stroking of her clitoris feels so good that, by reflex, the woman pushes her entire genital area against his hand. Her stimulation is increased and obviously so is his. So far, only one type of sensation has been involved—touch. Now if she whispers into his ear, "Ohhh, yes! Rub it like that!" a new element has been introduced. As the sense of hearing is brought into action, the man becomes even more aroused, and messages from his brain drive him to excite the woman even more. What started as a two-way street, then a three-way street, then a four-way street, is now a twenty-four-lane super-highway. As the couple rises to each higher level of sensory stimulation, their potential for sexual enjoyment rises with them. The next concept is just as important.

What's that?

It's the basic psychosexual concept known as "recruitment." It simply means that as you gather more and more sources of sensory stimulation, you fire off more nerve cells in the brain. That, in turn, tremendously expands the intensity of the sexual experience. And it even goes further—the closer the sensations are to the brain, the more powerful is their effect. That's where the Cranial Nerves work their magic.

Although most amateur "experts" who write those "do-it-yourself" books on sex have never heard of them, the "Cranial Nerves" can make a sensational contribution to the full enjoyment of sex.

How so?

The "Cranial Nerves" are twelve powerful nerve trunks that run straight from the brain through special little holes in the skull to key points in the body. They are particularly important since they connect the brain directly with certain structures. It's like a private line to Central Control—there are no stop lights, there are no cross streets, there are no obstacles. Impulses go back and forth to the brain instantaneously. Of the total of twelve Cranial Nerves, three of them are vital to sexual enjoyment. They are the Olfactory, Optic, and Trigeminal Nerves and they are only inches away from the brain itself. This is how they work.

The Olfactory nerve runs a few short inches from the brain into the nose and ends in a swelling called the Olfactory Bulb. In most mammals it also connects to a tiny but very powerful sexual organ within the nose known as the "vomeronasal organ." This organ is directly associated with detecting special odors from members of the opposite sex and transforming them into sexual stimulation. In many animals the effects are spectacular!

One striking example is "N-C-E's" or "non-contact erections." If certain male animals are hidden from sexually excited females—they can't see or hear them—the mere presence of the females at a distance and their odor causes instantaneous and powerful erections of the penis in the males. Another example is equally spectacular. If a bunch of female mice are kept together they produce a chemical smell that blocks sexual excitement in the whole group. But it doesn't stop there. Male mice—and other rodents—can produce smells that make adolescent female rodents mature sexually much faster. Imagine what would happen if human beings could do the same things!

Can they?

Maybe. It all depends on that very special vomeronasal sensory organ found inside the nose. Some researchers believe that human beings have that same organ. There is some evidence of that since women who live together—like in college dormitories—gradually begin to have synchronized menstrual periods—something that probably comes from an interchange of very subtle odor-messages.

The important point for us here is that the sense of smell plays a very important role in reinforcing the intensity of sexual excitement. The sexual life of every mammalian creature—except man—is obviously influenced by the sense of smell. Man has concentrated on sanitizing and deodorizing his body until there is nothing left to smell—almost. Fortunately the body does not give up so easily. The odor-detection apparatus of the body is still a direct extension of the brain.

The next Cranial Nerve that helps us to supercharge our sexual experiences is the "Trigeminal Nerve." Part of it, called the "Lingual Branch," goes directly to the tongue and lets us enjoy all those wonderful tastes we love so much. And it's no coincidence that the nose is poised just over the mouth, because taste and smell march hand-in-hand. If you can't smell it, you can't taste it. (Try this experiment—eat an apple while you squeeze your nostrils shut.)

The Cranial Nerves that transmit smell and taste are what make kissing so enjoyable. In kissing, the smell of the lips, their slightly salty taste, the smell of the nearby skin (perhaps mixed with perfume or after-shave lotion), all contribute their share to the rising sexual excitement. As a man kisses a woman's breast, the smell of her skin, and the taste of the nipple, all do their part to facilitate sexual arousal.

The other sexual Cranial Nerve is the Optic Nerve. As its name suggests it goes directly from the brain to the eye. As a matter of fact, the eyes are really a direct extension of the brain itself, bulging out into the face through two openings. The eyes play a powerful and mysterious role in sex. If a man simply sees the naked body of a woman or a woman sees the naked body of a man, the Upper Pole—the brain—sends a flood of messages to the Lower Pole—the sexual organs, telling them to get cranked up for sex. No one understands how a simple image projected on the retina can unleash a torrent of blood and produce a stiff penis or a throbbing clitoris. Even seeing pictures or videotapes of naked members of the opposite sex is sexually stimulating. No one knows why—but that's the way it is—and we should take the very best advantage of it.

How do we take advantage of those three sexual Cranial Nerves?

The ideal way to get the best from all our sexual receptors—and prepare for Total Sexual Intercourse—is obvious. The one form of sex that takes advantage of all the senses is oral sex. If you think about it, it makes all the sense in the world. Other members of the family of mammals don't suffer from impotence in the male and lack of orgasm in the female the way human beings do. In many species, a routine part of their sexual relationship involves some form of oral sex. There is no form of sexuality that jump-starts the sexual reflexes and primes a person for the maximum enjoyment of sex better than oral sex.

But is oral sex all right?

That depends on what you mean by "all right." Until relatively recently oral sex was illegal in many parts of the United States. And one state even had a law strictly prohibiting oral sex with birds. But the United States Supreme Court has wisely decided that what a man and a woman do in their own bedroom is their business and no one else's. But you do have to ask yourself who in society is qualified to set themselves up as "the expert" on what human beings should be allowed to do and what should be forbidden.

Anyway, these days oral sex is legal almost everywhere—except, perhaps, with birds.

But is oral sex really clean?

Why shouldn't it be? The idea that the sexual organs and oral sex itself is "dirty" just doesn't make any sense. The vagina, for example, is one of the only two self-cleaning organs in the human body. (The other self-cleaning structure is the eye.) In a healthy woman the vagina is free of harmful bacteria and contains primarily "lactobacillus" or the same bacteria found in the yogurt that more than two hundred million people eat every day to improve their health. The normal penis is also "clean" and normal semen is sterile—free from any bacteria. (Obviously, enjoyable sex assumes that both participants are well washed and scrubbed.)

When it comes to oral sex, the big question is really not "Should you do it?"

What is the big question?

It's "How should you do it?" To get the very most out of sex, you have to understand the anatomy, physiology, and neurology of human sexual equipment. Fellatio, or mouth-penis sex, is a good example.

When a woman undertakes oral stimulation of the penis, she is supercharging the sexual experience in a way that is unmatched. On her part, she is getting the aroma, the taste, the touch, and the sight of the organ. She can also hear his responses—ranging from simple moans of appreciation to excited and encouraging words. That's about the closest she can get to Total Sexual Stimulation—except for two situations that we'll get to in a moment.

Of course to really make oral sex count, the woman has to know what to do and where to do it. She should recognize that in one important way, the penis is like a lollipop—the real action is at the end. There are two areas of greatest sensitivity—because that's where most of the nerves are. They are the corona, or the ring around the head of the penis, and the frenulum.

The corona is that ridge that encircles the head of the penis—if the head of the penis were a hat, the corona would be the brim. If the woman takes the head of the penis between her lips and runs the corona back and forth between her compressed lips, she'll get amazing results in record time.

The frenulum is the little ridge of tissue just under the head of the organ that ties the head of the penis to the shaft. (That's why it's called a "frenulum"—in Latin it means "little bridle.") If you run the tip of your finger from the urethra—the opening for urine and sperm—down and under the head of the organ, you will find a little fold of skin. That's it. If a woman concentrates her efforts on these two structures, she will provide very interesting and rewarding sensations to her partner.

The female mouth is ideal to excite the penis since it has most of the qualities of the vagina and yet is under conscious control. And of course, it has a very mischievous tongue—which the vagina lacks. The tongue can go round and round the penis, it can poke the opening of the urethra (gently), it can tickle the frenulum, and it can do all sorts of other wonderful things that occur to most women at the appropriate moment.

By the way, there's an interesting historical aspect to the mouth-vagina relationship and it has to do with lipstick. Some people believe that the custom of painting a woman's lips bright red originated in the last century when certain women wanted to give the mouth the appearance of red swollen vaginal lips ready for sex. Interesting . . .

What about the man?

It's obviously his responsibility to do for his partner what she is doing for him. Of course, performing oral sex on a woman is a little more complicated and requires a little more scientific knowledge. On any important trip, if you want to be sure of getting where you're going, you need a map. And performing cunnilingus. ("Vagina-to-tongue" in Latin—you'll notice they got it backward.) is no exception. While the penis is right out there like a lighthouse, female anatomy is a little more complex. Here's a quick review of the most essential points for gentlemen to refresh their memory.

If you think of the female sexual equipment as a stage, the main curtain is the labia majora—or large lips. Once the curtain is opened, that reveals the entire scenario. At the top is the main performer, the clitoris. She dominates the show, wrapped in a lovely cloak of pinkish skin called the prepuce—the equivalent of the male foreskin but far more elegant. Running down from both sides of the clitoris and partially encircling the vaginal opening are the delicate pink labia minora, or smaller lips. Below the clitoris is a broad flat area called the "vestibule." It's composed of very delicate and sensitive pinkish skin with erectile tissue underneath it. Two important structures pass through the vestibule. The first one is the urethra—leading from the bladder to the outside. Below that is the vagina. All of these structures have a tremendous nerve supply, and the clitoris is the most keenly sensitive sexual organ that any human being could have. The penis is a distant runner-up by comparison. That all means that cunnilingus has to be done with sensitivity and understanding.

For example?

Oral sex with a woman is an appreciation of her unique female qualities—it is not a tongue-attack on the clitoris. Think of the labia majora as two lovely gates that open to a world of pleasure. That may be why certain Oriental societies refer to them as "The Gates of Heaven." And you tap gently at the Gates of Heaven and ask for admission—you don't barrel in demanding to see who's in charge.

A gentle nudge of the man's lips against the woman's larger vaginal lips (labia majora) pushing toward the clitoris underneath, a few preliminary swipes of the tongue toward the clitoris, and a lick or two (or more as the situation warrants) directed at the vestibule between the clitoris and the urethra should help those Gates to swing open wide.

Some woman want hard licking on their clitoris—others prefer a more gentle touch. The best way to be sure is—to ask her! It only takes a moment and really doesn't interfere with the proceedings.

The old joke "How can I tell you I love you when I can hardly breathe down here?" is just a joke—nothing more.

There is plenty of time to breathe and to make sure you're on the right track. Cunnilingus isn't a competitive sport—at least not yet. (So far no one has organized the NCL.) Relax and enjoy it—and be creative. There's only one thing you really shouldn't do in oral sex—ever.

What's that?

Blow. Although fellatio is sometimes referred to as a "Blow Job"—which as any man can tell you, it shouldn't be—there is no room for even thinking about blowing in cunnilingus. The uterus has a very rich blood supply, and at certain times—especially during pregnancy—it is very vulnerable to air under pressure. Blowing into the vagina can inflate it dramatically and push air into the uterus. If that air enters the uterine veins, it can end in the sudden death of the woman. It's rare but it has happened. Don't even think about it.

The rest depends on instinct and guidance from the woman. Almost any kind of mouth-tongue-lips stimulation can give her tremendous pleasure, but every woman is different and what is great for one is nothing special for another.

Of course, oral sex is the perfect way to draw back the bowstring.

Draw back the bowstring?

That's right. As anyone who has ever experienced it knows, orgasm is a tremendous release of energy—it is a virtual explosion of heat, pulsation, muscle spasms, sweat, and unbearable pleasure. But that energy has to come from somewhere. It comes from the gradual buildup of tension during everything that happens before penis and vagina come together. It's the equivalent of an archer drawing back the bowstring. The farther back he pulls it, the farther and faster the arrow will hit its target: orgasm. Oral sex draws back the bowstring better than anything else.

The man can see the very impressive female sexual attributes, he can feel the hot hard clitoris pulsate against his tongue and lips, he can smell the very special sexual perfume that comes from the aroused female, he can taste the vagina and clitoris, he can hear the moans and sighs of his partner. Little by little the pathways to his three Sexual Cranial Nerves become supercharged with sensations and he is primed for a mind-blowing orgasm.

There are also a few other creative things you can do.

Like what?

Like the "Venus Butterfly" or the "Three-Headed Turtle." For thousands of years in the Orient every possible refinement of sexual intercourse has been developed. The "Three-Headed Turtle" is an example.

Keeping in mind that the front wall of the vagina and the clitoris are part of the same Center of Sexual Excitement, you can take advantage of this by stimulating them both at the same time. In sex, arousal tends to be cumulative. If you caress the clitoris while sliding a finger or two in and out of the vagina, the excitement is more than if you do the two things separately. It's an interesting variation on sexual stimulation.

If you take it one step further you arrive at what the Asians call the "Three-Headed Turtle." The index finger rubs the front wall of the vagina from inside angling up toward the clitoris, while the thumb gently massages that organ. Meanwhile the third or fourth finger gently tickles the perineum—or depending on the woman's wishes, the anus. The hand is the body of the turtle and the three active fingers are the turtle's three heads. If everything works out well, the result is known as "Setting Foot Into Heaven." Does it sound too poetic to you? Try it first and then decide.

What about the "Venus Butterfly"

The "Venus Butterfly" has become kind of a legend supposed to make a woman wildly and sensationally excited. And it just might do that. It's similar to the "Three-Headed Turtle" but a bit more ambitious. The two hands are placed palms together, and both index fingers go in and out of the vagina, the thumbs work on the clitoris, and the third or fourth fingers are devoted to the perineum or anus.

The clitoris, vagina, and perineum or anus all share the same very sensitive nerve endings, and the simultaneous stimulation of these areas is the perfect preliminary to the main event.

Is there anything else I should know?

Getting the best from sexual intercourse depends on keeping in mind one very important element.

What's that?

Sexual intercourse is hydraulic. Although it may not sound especially romantic, the perfect union of penis and vagina depends on pumping liquid under pressure into inflatable structures until the pressure reaches a maximum. Then suddenly—and explosively—that pressure is released and drops almost to zero. If you raise that pressure to its maximum, the penis gets hard and tense. The clitoris swells to an impressive size, the labia minora and the inflatable tissues under the vestibule and around the vagina become engorged with blood and ready to pop. All that swelling makes them even more exquisitely sensitive. It's as if the penis and vagina develop a sublime itch that has to be scratched—and the more you rub it, the more it itches! The itching and swelling get more and more intense until the Big Bang; then everything returns to normal. All the blood drains out, the penis and clitoris-vagina deflate, and the excitement subsides—until the next time.

That's the physical side of sex—and although it's sensational, there are ways to make it even better.

How?

One way is to change positions. The way that the penis and vagina-clitoris rub together can make a big difference in how fast the explosion happens and how intense it finally is. For maximum sensation, the frenulum of the head of the penis should be in close contact with the upper wall of the vagina and reaching toward the pouch between the cervix and that upper vaginal wall. That stimulates the most sensitive areas in both partners. The "Missionary Position" is probably the worst way to work up to a really great orgasm. (By the way, is that what the Missionaries were supposed to teach the natives? Or was that what the natives were teaching the Missionaries?) Theoretically, one of the best positions is "doggie style," where the man puts his penis into the vagina from behind and the underside of the penis rubs the upper wall of the vagina. But as any lady will tell you, it's a little hard on her knees—among other things. A nice compromise is with the woman on her side, the man behind her and sliding his penis in from behind. Both of them can make all those little adjustments that provide the maximum sensation.

Of course, everyone is different and that's where the homework comes in. Try all the different positions and all the different ways until you find the ones that are just right for you. A penis fits a vagina almost any way you try it—sitting down, standing up, bending over, woman-on-top, and a dozen other possibilities. No one can decide in advance which is best for you. And you will agree that this is a better homework assignment than you ever got when you were back in school.

Is there anything else that a couple can do to increase their enjoyment of intercourse?

Yes, there is and it's been a closely guarded secret in several Asian countries for a long long time. A small group of women have turned it into a profitable career. In some Far Eastern countries male tourists are treated to demonstrations that really should be most interesting to ladies.

These young women come on stage and fascinate their audiences by calmly and expertly smoking a cigarette, a pipe, and a cigar.

What's so unusual about that?

Only the fact that they do it by holding the cigarette, pipe, and cigar at the entrance to the vagina and smoke it by contracting and expanding the muscles around the vagina.

But that's not all. Sometimes they can "sip" a soft drink through a straw inserted into a glass with the other end inserted into the vagina. And a few particularly talented young women can shoot an arrow held in the vagina and hit a bull's-eye several yards away.

Perhaps the most convincing demonstration is the girl who can hold a pencil in her vagina and write lines of poetry with it. This very impressive skill inspired one emotional Englishman in the audience to jump up and exclaim, as only Englishmen can: "By Jove! Her handwriting is better than mine!"

But what these young ladies have accomplished is important to every woman—and to every man who has sex with her.

How come?

Because it demonstrates beyond any doubt that a woman can obtain almost complete control of the muscles surrounding the vagina. With practice and training she can bring these muscles under conscious control and can expertly squeeze, stroke, and pump the penis while it is in the vagina.

It all depends on the anatomy of a woman's sexual muscles. In the female the vagina is supported by a wall of powerful muscular tissue. While their main function is to hold the vagina and the related structures in place, they can also be put to another more exciting use.

Every woman has two groups of sexual muscles and they can be developed with less effort than it takes to do the usual far more strenuous aerobic exercises.

The first group consists of two types of vaginal muscles. The most external pair of muscles is the "bulbocavernosus," or vaginal sphincter muscle. This muscle surrounds the vaginal opening, and as it contracts, the orifice of the vagina is squeezed almost shut. The motion is the same as that made by the lips in pronouncing the sound "wh" in the word "whip." Imagine how that feels on a penis.

The second external pair of muscles are the urethral sphincter muscles. The main purpose of these muscles is to shut off the flow of urine at the end of urination. They also compress the vagina like the vaginal sphincter just inside the vaginal outlet.

Most women can gain control of both these muscles by doing a simple exercise. All she has to do is try to hold her urine back and then let go—a drawing inward and releasing of the pelvic muscles. That exercises the right structures. If she does this about twenty times a day and holds it for a few moments each time, she will soon begin to see interesting results. (Incidentally, it also increases bladder control.)

The second group of muscles which can be trained to increase sexual enjoyment are the levator ani group. These are really three separate muscle groups: the pubococcygeus, iliococcygeus, and puborectalis. They extend from the anal area to the pubic area and surround the deeper part of the vagina. When they are constricted, the walls of the vagina are brought together firmly and squeeze the penis along its entire length. This is a very powerful muscle group and can really make a big difference sexually.

The best exercise for developing the levator ani group is to make the same motion: as if you were trying to stop urinating in the middle of a stream. Proper control and development of these structures also comes with practice; about twenty contractions a day for several weeks should give good control.

How do you use these muscles during intercourse?

Sensationally. It can really make a big difference in sensation both for the man and for the woman. After the penis is all the way up into the vagina, if the woman squeezes it by contracting the external sphincter muscles, it will intensify the erection and increase the man's sexual excitement.

At the same time it stimulates the sensitive nerve endings at the vaginal opening and makes it more intense for the woman. The muscles also expand the clitoris as they contract and contract that organ as they relax. That's the equivalent of constant clitoral massage—which makes everything better. At the same time the woman can alternately squeeze and release the penis using the levator ani muscles.

By using the two muscle groups in combination, some interesting effects can be obtained. With some conscientious practice, the woman can gently and rhythmically massage the man's penis from the base to the tip by contracting first the superficial muscles, then the deeper group. If she really works at her exercises, eventually she should be able to reverse the direction of this caress and stoke the penis from tip to base as well. This can sometimes be enough to bring the man to volcanic orgasm all by itself.

Is there something more you can do to make sexual intercourse more exciting?

Yes. Never forget that sex is a game. In every species, including man, there is a charming "game quality" to sex. It involves teasing, joking, laughing, surprises, and sometimes moments of drama and high emotion. Even in our over-regulated society, there is no law that says you have to do it with The-Man-On-Top-Woman-On-The-

Bottom-At-10:23 P.M.-Every-Tuesday-By-The-Light-Of-The-Pink-Doggie-Lamp-On-The-Maple-Veneer-Dresser. Because sex is so emotional and so symbolic, there are so many experiences and associations that can make sex so much better and so much more exciting.

For example, in the beginning, when sex was new, it was mysterious and very exciting. Sex in the backseat (or the front seat) of a car, sex in a swimming pool, sex on the beach at night—these were all emotionally turbocharged experiences. The way the penis went in and out of the vagina was exactly the same, but the emotional content was what made it so exciting. To make sexual intercourse as good as it possibly can be, you can bring back that same excitement anytime you want to.

How do you do it?

Well, you don't have to drive down to the lake on Saturday night, park in the woods, and have sex with your wife or husband in the backseat of the car—although you can do it if you want to. But you can restore the "game quality" to sex anytime and anywhere.

For example, you can go skinny-dipping at night at the beach or the lake front—or in your own swimming pool if you have one. Moonlight, naked bodies, warm water—that takes human beings back thousands of years to more pastoral times and does wonderful things for sexual reflexes.

Another approach that can infuse sex with excitement is a "scenario." That's when you act out a little story like "The Doctor and the Seductive Female Patient" or "The Nurse and the Handsome Male Patient." The titles should be enough to get you started and you can use your imagination—and the fantasies that everyone has when they visit the doctor or see the nurse. To give you an idea how many millions of people use "scenarios" to enhance their sex life, there are even companies that offer entire scripts for these kind of games—complete with costumes.

Costumes?

That's right. You've seen the stores and catalogues that offer abbreviated Nurse's uniforms and French Maid's uniforms—all with crotchless panties? Well, those outfits aren't for the Fourth of July Parade or because Nurses and Maids need more ventilation on the job than other people. They're to make sexual intercourse more exciting and more titillating by making it full of fantasy and emotion. The possibilities are limitless—"The Amazon Queen and the Lost Scientist," "The King and the Slave Girl," "The Female Sergeant and the New Recruit," "The Belly-Dancer and the Sheik." You can think up better possibilities yourself.

Routine is the enemy of sexual satisfaction. Do you look forward to brushing your teeth every morning? Does your heart beat a little faster when you think of the tingle of toothpaste against your gums? I doubt it. And you have to do everything you possibly can to make sure that the magnificent and earth-shaking encounter that we call "sex" never becomes as routine as—brushing your teeth.

Then the only thing that counts in sex is how much fun everybody has?

Not exactly. The ideal act of sexual intercourse combines reproduction, deep mutual love, and profound physical pleasure. Most people will experience this combination less than a dozen times in their life span. If they are very fortunate, they will frequently be able to combine an expression of love with a real physical enjoyment of sex. But at the very minimum, sexual intercourse should provide the maximum sexual gratification possible for both partners. If they can accomplish that, at least it is the first step toward achieving the rest.

Chapter 5

APHRODISIACS

The following paragraphs were included in the original edition. No one could ever have predicted what has happened since then. Here's the Original—and the fascinating update follows.

> **I've often heard the word "aphrodisiac" used. What does it mean?**
>
> *The word "aphrodisiac," derived from Aphrodite, the Ancient Greek goddess of love, designates something that increases sexual desire or excitement. Usually it refers to drugs such as Spanish Fly and others, but its meaning can also include sexually stimulating books or movies, sexual exhibitions, and even plastic surgery on the sexual organs.*
>
> **Plastic surgery on the sexual organs? Is this kind of plastic surgery common?**
>
> *It depends where you live. In the United States, for example, more than fifty percent of the people have had plastic surgery on their genitals. In some parts of the country the percentage is even higher. There are some areas of the world where everybody has these things done as a matter of course. One is not even considered socially acceptable until the sexual equipment has been remodeled. As a matter of fact, there are more*

than a dozen operations in use today directed at overhauling the sexual apparatus to make sex more fun for everyone.

What are these operations like?

They range all the way from complex procedures done at the Mayo Clinic to primitive surgery performed with a piece of broken glass in the African jungle. One example which falls midway between is the ampallang of Southeast Asia. This is typical of do-it-yourself jobs.

The sportier males of that area make several slits in the loose skin on the underside of the penis near the tip. The openings average about an eighth of an inch in diameter and run at right angles to the shaft. Just before intercourse short rods are inserted into the slits at right angles to the penis. These are usually scraps of copper wire, bits of ivory, or among the jet set, gold and silver. The purpose obviously is to enlarge the business end of the penis and increase its friction against the vagina.

What does the man get out of it?

Clearly there is no increased sensation for him. The only compensation for this sacrifice is likely to be renewed popularity with the ladies. The results must be something special for them if they manage to persuade a proud male to ventilate his precious penis this way.

For those willing to go one step further, there is a somewhat more elegant refinement. Instead of simply poking holes in the organ, a ring of small incisions is made around the head of the penis. Little pebbles are placed into the resulting pouches, and the skin is allowed to heal over them. A month or so later, the result is a penis crowned with a rocky wreath.

Fully healed, the courageous gent emerges to claim his reward: presumably the girls are standing in line to get the benefit of his new equipment. A plain old American penis must look pretty tame by comparison.

Isn't there an operation like this that gives the man more pleasure?

Only if he happens to be a music-lover. The Burmese have added an esthetic note.

They use the same slit procedure, but instead of burying small stones under the skin, they use little bronze bells. Conceivably a talented Burmese lover can do justice to his sweetheart and play a catchy tune at the same time. There are other advantages too. If a Burmese husband comes home unexpectedly and walks in the door to the music of the bells, somebody is in big trouble.

(These lines were part of the original edition and no one could have ever predicted what has happened since then. Here's the fascinating update.)

Is this kind of operation done in any other countries?

Yes, there is another nation where this kind of strange penis-modification is done. It's called: "The United States of America." Nowadays the procedure goes by the name of "piercing" but it is the same ampallang—without the bells. Penis-piercing is now an established part of the sexual scene.

Why do men in the United States do that?

It's not only the United States—it's Great Britain, France, Spain, and a lot of other "modern" countries. One of my patients put it to her boyfriend this way:

"Arthur, you must really hate your penis if you punch holes in it!"

Surprised, he replied,

"Not at all! I love it so much I buy jewelry for it!"

Whether or not it's exactly jewelry is a matter of individual taste. The simplest procedure is called "frenulum piercing." Just under the head of the penis—the part known as the "glans" (Latin for "kernel")—is a little fold of loose tissue called the "frenulum" (Latin for "little bridle"). Some gentlemen poke a hole from left to right through that little bit of loose tissue that lies just below and about ¼ inch behind the glans. They then push a metal rod, threaded at each end, through it.

Finally they screw on a little metal ball at each end. Viola! They are officially pierced!

How did this business get started?

In Western countries most penis-piercing got its start among male homosexuals as well as sadomasochists—both heterosexual and homosexual. Having rods and rings attached to your penis lends itself perfectly to sadomasochistic games. Your friends (?) can tie little ropes to the rings and things and pull and jerk on them to their hearts' content.

You say, "Who likes that?" We'll see about that farther on, in Chapter 10.

Are there other kinds of penis-piercing?

Yes, and some of them are fascinating. For example, there's the famous "Prince Albert." That's the one that makes most men shudder just to think about it. Here's how it's done—but I fervently implore you not to do it.

As they say on television, "Don't try this at home!" Like every physician, I've seen the final results of failed do-it-yourself plastic surgery on the sexual organs. It isn't pretty.

If you were going to do it, you would put the tip of your index finger on the tip of your penis. Then you would move it backward on the underside of the organ about one inch. Then you would poke a hole straight up until it perforated the urethra. (Don't do it!)

The urethra is the tube that goes from the bladder and the prostate gland to the outside. Urine and sperm travel through it and flow or spurt out the tip of the penis. By making this hole, you have now inflicted a fistula on yourself. When you urinate or ejaculate, some of the fluid will dribble out through the hole in the lower part of the penis.

But it's not finished. A metal ring—partly open—is pushed through the hole in the tip of the penis and wiggled (ouch!) until it pops through the new hole you just made. It's like putting a ring in a hog's nose, but instead of sideways, the ring is put on from front to back.

Congratulations! You have just permanently damaged your irreplaceable penis and pushed a ring through the injury to make sure it doesn't heal. You now have a "Prince Albert" on your wee-wee!

The name comes from a hard-to-believe explanation. Supposedly during the time of Prince Albert in England in the last century, gentlemen had these rings installed in their organs so that they could tie them to one side and not have them poke out in their tight pants. If you believe that, you are a customer for the Brooklyn Bridge.

But that's not all. Among dedicated fans, penis-perforating can get pretty fancy. There's the grand finale called the "Apadravya." It's like the ampallang but the metal rod perforates the penis from top to bottom instead of from side to side. It is poked through the same hole as the Prince Albert. (Please don't do it!)

But why do men do this?

Fun and games. Some men believe that anything that makes the penis bigger and rougher can excite a woman more when it's in her vagina. That's the concept behind the more primitive system of inserting pebbles in little cuts made under the skin of the organ. When the cuts heal, the pebbles and scar tissue make the penis fatter and rougher—and supposedly more exciting to women.

Does that sound far out? Sure it does. But the world is getting stranger every day, and the same sort of thing is being done right now—not far from where you sit reading this book.

For men who don't want to go all the way, there are those quaint bumpy-lumpy condoms—the ones that used to be called "French Ticklers." Some women like the way they feel, some don't care, and a lot of them don't express an opinion because their male partners think it's such an exciting toy and they don't want to puncture their balloon, so to speak.

Is there any aphrodisiacal plastic surgery done on women?

Women account for a hefty proportion of sexual reconstruction. Take, for example, the "husband's knot." That's a procedure that most husbands appreciate—even if they didn't know about it until now.

Most women who give birth to their children in hospitals have an incision made in the vagina called an "episiotomy."

At the final moment of delivery, just as the baby is about to come out of the vagina, the mother's skin is stretched tightly over the baby's head. If the head keeps coming that way, it will most probably overstretch and tear the delicate vaginal tissues. In some cases the force of the large head can even tear the muscles around the vagina and the rectum.

After delivery the mother could be left with a large gaping vaginal entrance and torn bleeding tissues. To avoid that, the doctor makes a diagonal cut at an angle of forty-five degrees at the base of the vaginal opening and allows the baby's head to exit without tearing the mother. In a sense, it's a controlled tear that prevents uncontrollable damage.

Then the doctor immediately sets to work repairing the incision by sewing the cut edges of tissue together. The whole procedure takes about five minutes. If the doctor is also sexually knowledgeable, he takes another minute and adds a little plastic surgery. He carefully gauges the size and location of his stitches so that besides closing the wound he takes up almost all the slack in the vagina—caused by years of intercourse as well as the pressure of the baby's head lunging through. In sixty seconds he restores that most vital of all sexual spaces nearly to its pre-copulatory dimensions. He tops it off with a special super-secure-can't-ever-come-loose non-raveling knot that keeps the vagina tight. That's why it's called the "husband's knot."

Doesn't the vagina stretch again with the next baby?

Certainly. But as long as the doctor is there with needle and sutures, neither husband nor wife should ever be inconvenienced. Everything should fit like a glove—or even better.

What if the doctor doesn't do this little operation?

The vagina will continue to stretch more and more with intercourse and childbirth until it no longer firmly grips the penis during intercourse.

The poor penis, dwarfed by the massive vagina, flounders aimlessly within its former home. It also develops the unhappy characteristic of flopping out at the most inopportune moments.

Fortunately years ago a sympathetic surgeon devised a suitable cure. The operation, called "anterior and posterior plastic repair," or "A-P repair" for short, is simple, effective, and solves a lot of problems at one time. It is basically a version of the "husband's knot" technique but more extensive. It stops urinary incontinence—that annoying dribbling when a woman laughs or coughs. And it reinforces, reconstructs, and reorients the vagina at the same time.

That's fine if the vagina is too big—what about something for a vagina that's too small?

A vagina that is really too small is very rare indeed. Usually the difficulty is simply an undersized entrance or "introitus." Most often the hymen is to blame. That small bit of tissue that stands guard at the Gates of Love sometimes does its job too well. Even the most determined midnight battering by a nervous and sweating bridegroom is occasionally insufficient—it will not yield.

The following morning the tearful bride and red-faced groom appear at the doctor's office. In this case the scalpel is mightier than the penis, and in a flash of the gleaming knife the portals swing wide. Nature's Defect undone by Man!

But aren't there some cases where the vagina is really too small?

Very rare. Almost invariably either the vagina is big enough (perhaps with some stretching) or it isn't there at all. Nowadays there is even help for the girl who is born without a vagina. These unfortunate young ladies have a rare deformity that leaves them with a short blind pouch or, in the most severe cases, merely a dimple. Utilizing an ingenious procedure, a man-made but sexually serviceable vagina can be fashioned. There are two drawbacks. Obviously pregnancy is out of the question. And this is a literal case of "Use It or Lose It." The new vagina needs regular, frequent, and energetic sexual activity to keep it open.

Breast operations seem to be getting a lot of attention lately— what sorts of operations are done on breasts?

Breasts were originally designed as organs of nutrition, to feed babies. However, in certain societies they are important sexual organs. The primary female sexual equipment—vagina, clitoris, and associated structures—is well hidden between the legs. But the female breasts are right out there like twin libidinous lighthouses reminding everyone that there is a female attached to them. And in recent years, just like lighthouses, female breasts have been the object of extensive remodeling by ingenious plastic surgeons.

What kind of "remodeling"?

Basically, they have been remodeled to conform to male sexual fantasies. Breasts are mostly fat, sprinkled with glandular tissue that can secrete milk. They are held in place by strong ligaments—sort of a built-in brassiere. When a girl is young, her breasts tend to be like twin globes with a slight upward curvature and nipples pointing straight ahead. But as time, gravity, and pregnancies all leave their mark, the breasts begin to descend. Gradually the nipples begin to point downward and the breasts begin to sag. That's no problem for women and for babies. Slightly droopy mammary glands can still feed babies fine, but they can't feed the fantasies of adolescent and adult males.

What kind of fantasies do men have about those things?

Where shall we start? It's been said that the average man's fantasy of the ideal woman is a nymphomaniac whose father owns a liquor store. And after a night of wild sex, she turns into a pizza at Midnight. That's not far from what most men expect in breasts. They want 36-year-old breasts to suddenly look like a pair of 18-year-olds. And plastic surgeons are only too happy to oblige.

The most popular breast overhaul for many years was simply to insert a plastic bag—not too different from those "sandwich bags" you have in the kitchen—behind the breast tissue. The bag was filled with a liquid—silicone—and pushed the breast upward and outward. The surgery left scars—sometimes under the breast, sometimes in the armpit, depending on the procedure. And some people feared that it left something else. Reports of serious side effects finally caused the U.S. Food and Drug Administration to discontinue the use of silicone implants in 1992 except for testing purposes.

The operation is still done, but the baggies are filled with salt water instead. The idea is that if the bag breaks, what spills out will be relatively harmless salt water rather than silicone.

Do the bags break?

Sure. After all they're just plastic bags. There are also a few other not-so-little problems. For example, the breasts can get hard like a rock if scar tissue forms after the surgery—and it can. The little bags can suddenly pop and the breasts can suddenly drop and then the patient needs emergency surgery to take out the plastic. Or the bags can shift and leave one breast pointing northwest and the other pointing southeast. (In spite of constantly changing styles, so far there are no dresses that take advantage of that look.) There's a far more annoying problem, however.

What's that?

Sometimes the breasts can look great—big, erect, well-separated. But the woman can't feel anything in her nipples or surrounding breast tissue! It's almost like paying eight thousand dollars for a pair of stick-on falsies. Most of these ladies would love to have their old smaller bosoms back—the ones with the sensitive nipples.

There's another problem too—more dangerous than annoying. Implants can confuse the interpretation of a mammogram—that X-ray for breast tumors. That could delay the diagnosis of breast cancer, with the ensuing risks. It's vital for a woman who has these "little bags" to tell her doctor before she has that mammogram.

Then should a woman have her breasts enlarged?

If she wants to, she can. But I would never recommend it to any of my patients. I firmly believe in Dr. Reuben's First Law of Sexual Satisfaction: "If It Works, Don't Fix It—You Can't Get a New One If You Break It!" A woman is a person—she is not just a pair of breasts jiggling down the street. God gave you the breasts you have—enjoy them, feed your babies with them, and don't slice on them if you don't have to.

What about girls with oversize breasts?

In the bosom department it's apparently feast or famine. Very large breasts are not just a cosmetic problem. They are really uncomfortable—tiring during the day, and at night sleeping on your stomach is out of the question. The details of the procedure are a little unsettling, but the results are generally acceptable. First the nipples are cut off and set aside in a container of saline solution. Then a large portion of the fatty tissue of each breast is excised along with a certain amount of skin. The nipples are retrieved from their jar, reattached, and everything is sewn up in its approximate place. Carefully done, the main giveaway is a thin scar underneath the breast—barely visible even in a topless dancer.

Are there any operations like that for men?

Nowadays there are operations for everything. We've already seen the plastic surgery on the penis in a previous chapter. The testicles can be worked on as well. Although they are not directly involved in the sexual act, they play a strong symbolic and psychological role. The truth is that a man with no testicles just doesn't feel right. Even if the hormones that the missing testicles should produce are replaced by injections, with an empty scrotum flapping in the wind, a night of passion just doesn't seem the same.

That scrotum may be vacant for a couple of reasons. Sometimes after birth the testicles fail to descend from their resting place in the abdomen. They may even resist all surgical attempts to bring them down. Occasionally they act like yo-yos, sliding up and down, in and out of the scrotal sac. In other, more tragic cases, they have been permanently lost—accidentally or as the result of a malignant tumor.

There is still an answer. Two egg-shaped artificial testicles of plastic or lightweight metal can be slipped into the scrotum and anchored there so no one will be the wiser. Well, hardly anyone.

What about the "real" aphrodisiacs, for instance Spanish Fly? What is it? What does it do?

Spanish Fly, strangely enough, is a Spanish fly. Almost. Actually it is made from small, shiny, iridescent beetles found in southern France and Spain. The bodies of these insects are dried and pulverized, then treated chemically to extract a drug called "cantharidin." Then, supposedly, the real fun begins. All one has to do, according to the stories, is slip a few drops into your girlfriend's drink. No matter how cold she has been to you in the past, she will be transformed instantly into an insatiable sex maniac begging you to quench her vaginal fires.

Remember the story about the fellow who slipped some Spanish Fly to his date, drove out to lover's lane, and awaited the results? The young lady became worked up, exhausted her boyfriend's resources after four times at bat, and proceeded to have intercourse with the gear-shift lever and most of the knobs on the dashboard? Nice story, but pure fantasy.

Here's a more likely version: Ten minutes after drinking the "love potion" the girl collapses in convulsions—she goes to the hospital and Casanova goes to the clink. If she lives (fifty-fifty chance), he gets off lightly.

If she dies, it's Murder Two.

If it's so dangerous, how did the idea get started in the first place?

Spanish Fly is a truly great aphrodisiac—for farm animals. This is the problem: in humans the dose that works and the dose that kills are about the same. If you are an eighteen-year-old girl, five feet two, and weigh 110 pounds, one drop too much and you've had it. If you're a 1,500-pound cow, it doesn't make that much difference. The stakes are different too.

If your date for the evening won't see it your way, tomorrow night you go out with someone else. If you have a ten-thousand-dollar breeding animal that wants to remain a virgin, some risk-taking is in order.

Well, then, how does it work in animals?

The drug cantharidin is tremendously irritating. After being swallowed it finds its way into the bladder and is excreted in the urine. It burns the lining of the bladder and urethra as it goes by and reflexly stimulates the sexual organs. It causes erection of the clitoris, engorgement of the labia, and tingling of the vagina in females. In the male it causes an immense and painful erection. Animals who get a slug of this stuff copulate mainly to try to get rid of the intense discomfort. No one watching the performance ever wants to try it that way themselves. There is, however, one important use of Spanish Fly for humans. In greatly diluted form, it is a fair substitute for a mustard plaster.

Isn't it true that certain foods are sexual stimulants, like oysters?

That would be too easy. In man's eternal quest for the bigger and better (and more frequent) orgasm, hundreds of foods and food combinations have been tried. Some of them depend on a physical resemblance to the sexual apparatus. For example, oysters, clams, eggs, and onions resemble the testicles. Celery, sausages, and asparagus resemble the penis. The theory, apparently, is "Like breeds like." It could work, but not necessarily the way it's intended. A strict diet of celery might conceivably make the penis resemble a celery stalk—wet and soggy.

One of the problems with aphrodisiacs is that all aphrodisiacs are not equal.

What do you mean?

Some people classify substances that produce an erection in men or swelling and lubrication in women as "aphrodisiacs." But those are really local aphrodisiacs—they target the sexual organs but not the whole person. A true aphrodisiac goes much further—it may trigger a throbbing erection of the penis and clitoris, but it also lights the fires of passion and makes the user eager for sex.

There are dozens of bogus local aphrodisiacs out there waiting for the gullible. Most of them are herbal in origin and go by exotic names like "Panga-Wonga" and "Zulu-Whiz." They come with exciting and romantic legends attached. Take the ad for "Panga-Wonga":

"In the far-off jungles of Burundi, Tribal Chieftains pass on the secret of 'Panga-Wonga' to their first born sons. This magic root has the power to stir the sexual fires in any man. One tablet six times a day will restore your powers to that of a 21-year-old Burundi Warrior!"

Does it work?

Let's ask someone who tried it. Harold is fifty-six years old and owns a cleaning supply company. Here's what happened:

"Well, Doctor, it's no secret that I haven't been having the same kind of erections as I used to. And it's been getting worse as time goes on. I was even thinking of writing a letter to the Army."

"You were going to write to the Army about having weak erections?"

Harold frowned.

"That's right, Doctor. I was in the Service about thirty years ago and we ordinary soldiers always had this suspicion that the Army was putting saltpeter in our food to cut down on our sex drive. I kind of believed it but it sure didn't hold me back in those days. Well, I was going to write to the Army and tell them that it took a while, but the saltpeter they fed me was finally starting to take effect!"

He burst out laughing. "At least I can keep my sense of humor—and with that 'Panga-Wonga' stuff I really needed it. It cost me seventy-five dollars for twenty-five capsules and I took them like it said. After the third bottle I didn't notice any effect—except on my checkbook—so I figured I'd try an experiment. I calculated that if it was supposed to increase the blood supply to the penis like it said on the bottle, then maybe if I rubbed it directly on, it would at least do something."

Harold paused. "Well, it did do something! One night last week just before bedtime, I took the bottle down in the basement where I have my workshop. I opened some of the capsules and mixed the powder with some mineral oil. Then I took out my penis and started rubbing that stuff into the head. I had the light turned off, and while I was rubbing it in, I bumped a can of paint off the workbench. My dog heard it upstairs and started barking. Then Gladys, my wife, got worried. She sneaked down the stairs and suddenly turned this big flashlight on me!

"Wow! There I was with my pants down around my ankles and a big hard erection from all that rubbing. My penis was sort of greenish from the color of the capsules— like it almost glowed. I just stood there kind of stammering. I really couldn't think of anything to say.

"After she got over the shock, Gladys started laughing so hard she had to sit down on the couch. Then she suddenly stopped laughing, reached over and took hold of my penis, and said, 'Well, Harold, we're not going to waste that, are we?'

"So we did it right there on the couch in the basement and since then I haven't had much trouble. So I guess you can say that the 'Panga-Wonga' works—but not the way they advertised it!"

But is there a local aphrodisiac that is more reliable?

Fortunately there is now. And you don't have to go down to the basement to use it. There is a drug—one of the group called "prostaglandins"—that can be applied directly to the penis—either by injection with a small needle or by inserting a tiny suppository directly into the urethra. At the moment, the direct application of this drug to the penis is the most effective local aphrodisiac available.

What about "true" aphrodisiacs?

That's the ideal that men have been pursuing for centuries. If only they could find a drug that would make them irresistible to women.

If there were just some powder or pill that would make women crave sex. From time to time, just that kind of chemical appears—a drug that promises to make any woman who swallows it mad with lust.

In the past couple of years, there have been not one but two candidates for that role. One of them is a drug called Rohypnol® commonly known as "Roofies." It's been in the newspapers and on television as the famous "date rape" drug. Its chemical name is "flunitrazepam" and it's a cousin to a drug called "diazepam," better known as Valium®.

Supposedly it works like this: Just pop a pill into your girlfriend's (or boyfriend's) drink, and in about half an hour, you can do anything you want to them and they'll have a hard time remembering what happened.

Maybe. And maybe you didn't even need to use Roofies! The chemical names should tell the whole story. Once you look beyond the emotional aspect of a headline like:

NEW DATE RAPE DRUG!

you realize that Roofies is just a potent tranquilizer that makes anyone who takes it dopey and lethargic. If they take more, they pass out. But when they are supertranquilized, they may be more relaxed and accessible sexually—just like when they are drunk.

"Date Rape Drug" sounds good in the headlines but there are some other headlines that are even more interesting. Now the same drug is in great demand by young girls who take it on their own!

Why would a girl voluntarily take a Date Rape drug?

Because it makes them dopey and languid—like a lot of other drugs that are called "downers." Girls buy them on their own and take them at parties.

When people start taking mind-bending drugs, no one knows where it's all going to end.

Are there any other "Date Rape" drugs?

There's another drug that has shared the "Date Rape" headlines. It's called "Gamma-Hydroxy Butyrate," known by many nicknames like "Georgia Home Boy," "Grievous Bodily Harm," and for obvious reasons, "Easy Lay."

Here's the real GHB story—and it's an interesting example of some of the confusion that surrounds drugs and sex. Gamma-Hydroxy Butyrate is what doctors call a "hypnotic." That doesn't mean it hypnotizes you—it means it puts you to sleep. It is a legal drug in Europe, where it is used as an anesthetic and for other legitimate medical purposes. Strangely enough, it was sold in the United States for years, without a prescription, to bodybuilders! One of its peculiar effects is stimulating the secretion of human growth hormone, which helps to build muscles. (That isn't a good idea either—for the same reason that taking steroids can cause big problems along with big muscles.)

If you slip GHB into your girlfriend's drink, she will eventually feel relaxed and submissive—the same as if you'd plied her with a few extra martinis or slipped her some tranquilizers. She may even lose some of her sexual inhibitions—just like after she has a few drinks. It has approximately the same effect as the common sedatives. But it is much more dangerous for a reason that has nothing to do with its physical effects.

What's that?

It's too easy to make in your kitchen. Any idiot can buy most of the ingredients at the grocery store—like vinegar and lye. The key ingredient is at least a little bit harder to find. But then that idiot can put them all together and cook up a batch in a couple of days. If the dose is big enough, the final product will knock anyone who drinks it into the next county—or kill them. The illegal stuff you can buy on the street corner or at a dance is usually made that way. You don't know who made it or how—but you can guess. That's the other problem. If the home chemist makes one little mistake in the process, he's selling you a deadly poison, not a ticket to sick sex. But the whole controversy over Roofies and GHB overlooks two little details.

What are those?

First, how much fun can it be to have sex with an unconscious lady? Except for that small group of people who like to have sexual intercourse with corpses, most men like partners who respond just a little to their ardent endeavors. And what kind of man is it that needs to knock a girl out before she gets friendly with him?

The other detail is just as important. It's not exactly brilliant to go out with someone you don't know well and trust—female or male. (It's not just heterosexuals who have heard about GHB and know how to use it.) And if you're not 100 percent sure of your friends, don't let them fix you a drink. And don't eat or drink anything unless you know exactly what's in it. But that's what Mom and Dad have been telling us for years, isn't it? And there's one more thing.

What's that?

GHB and Roofies aren't anything from outer space. "Knock-Out Drops" and "Mickey-Finns" have been around for hundreds of years. In the old days, "ravishers of women" (a more poetic term for "date rapists") and criminals used laudanum (a derivative of opium) and chloral hydrate to doctor their victims' drinks. The effects were about the same. As every doctor knows, there are at least a hundred drugs that can produce effects like GHB and Roofies.

As they say in Spanish:

"El frio no está en las cobijas."
"The cold is not in the blankets."

The problem isn't the drugs—it's the sick people who use them to hurt other people. So whether it's GHB or XYZ, know where you are going and whom you are going with.

Is there anything else like GHB and Roofies?

Sure. There's alcohol, marijuana, cocaine, heroin, amphetamines, and all the dozens of new pills and powders that alter a person's mind and interfere with their good judgment. Sex and drugs? But why? Sex is too much fun to mess it up with drugs. Especially these days. Now it's a whole new ball game.

Back when life was simpler, sex and drugs could mean an unwanted pregnancy—you forgot to use a condom. But now popping a few pills and forgetting the condom can mean AIDS—and AIDS is forever—or as long as you last.

What about all those traditional aphrodisiacs like ginseng and yohimbine?

There's a big problem with substances like that. Sex is as much a "mind event" as a "body event." If you take 100 men and give half of them, say, ginseng pills and the other half sugar pills that look exactly the same, as many as 25 percent of the men who took the sugar pills may report that it helped them sexually. So it's hard to pin down. Some men take yohimbine, prepared from the bark of an African tree, and say it helps them. Some men take it and don't feel a thing. The same is true of ginseng and snake blood and dried deer penis and a hundred other folk aphrodisiacs.

Other foods have a more obvious effect. Feeding your best girl a juicy steak at a classy restaurant may set the mental wheels in motion and land both of you in bed; the secret ingredient is in the atmosphere, not in the steak.

How about powdered rhinoceros horn?

That too was based on the "like makes like" principle. You can almost visualize a poor Asian daydreaming: "If my penis only looked like the horn of the rhinoceros . . ." Obviously if he gazed at the opposite end of the rhino, he would see that the beast had something else going for him too. Strangely enough, among Asian believers, the demand for rhino horn has so outstripped the meager supply that much of the product reaching the market is powdered boar tusk or pig bone.

A true aphrodisiac is the male sex hormone, testosterone. By acting on the entire body it causes a powerful, almost irresistible sexual desire. It works equally in men or women. The onset is slow, but the effect is profound and long-lasting. That's one of the reasons why testosterone and related drugs were so popular among body-builders. As it builds sexual desire, it also builds muscles.

But there's a catch. In men it results in atrophy of the testicles, not a small thing. And as the testicles get smaller, the prostate gland gets bigger—ultimately making it very hard to urinate. In women it can cause masculinization. The clitoris enlarges, hair appears on the face, the voice deepens, and other somewhat unattractive changes transpire. In both sexes it can cause serious liver damage. It also causes mental changes—uncontrolled anger and aggression.

Its use, except by a licensed physician, is illegal and should remain that way. Not as immediately dangerous as Spanish Fly or some of the other drugs, it can make plenty of trouble of the worst kind unless used under careful medical supervision.

What is the ideal aphrodisiac?

It should be safe, inexpensive, non-toxic, available without a prescription, and work in both men and women.

Does that kind of aphrodisiac exist?

Yes, of course, and it's been around for at least five thousand years. People of all nations and cultures have used it and there is no doubt as to its effectiveness. The proof that it works well is that it has been restricted, prohibited, condemned, and destroyed from time to time. Sometimes just possession of this aphrodisiac has sent people to jail—or even the firing squad.

What is it called?

It's called "pornography"—*porne* is the Greek word for "prostitute" and *graphein* is the Greek word for "write." That's the origin of the word, but that's not what it is. Calling sexually explicit pictures or text "pornography" is begging the question. It's like calling a hammer a "murder weapon."

What do you mean?

I mean a better term would be "sexography": "pictures or text about sex."

All sex is not prostitutes, and all sexual material is not pornography.

Let's take a scientific look at what sexography is all about before we finally make up our minds.

Human beings are programmed to react to direct stimulation of the sexual organs. Stroking a woman's clitoris or a man's penis causes sexual excitement. The very sensitive nerves on the surface of those organs transmit the sensation of touch to the brain, which automatically starts the ball rolling. Heart rate increases, breathing gets faster, the pupils dilate, the field of vision narrows, and the sexual organs in both sexes start to produce lubricating liquids.

That's what you might call a very direct aphrodisiac—tickling the penis or clitoris. But there's another program in the human brain—and it wasn't put there by you or me. If a human being sees a member of the opposite sex naked with their sexual equipment exposed, the same set of reactions occurs. Just looking triggers erection in the male, with lubrication, fast heartbeat, and all the rest. Women have the same reaction—although in some societies they are so suppressed that they choke back their responses. But under natural circumstances, women react to naked men and to naked penises and testicles. (We'll see the irrefutable scientific proof of that shortly.)

But if we think about it, it has to be that way. For millions of years there were no hospitals, no obstreticians, no antibiotics, no incubators and a woman had 10 children and 9 of them died before they grew up. It was essential for men and women to have powerful and irresistible drives to copulate just to keep the human race from dying out. Even as recently as 1348, a single epidemic destroyed half the population of Europe!

Men and women also react with sexual arousal to pictures of the opposite sex without clothes on. The image is processed by the brain almost as if they were seeing the real thing. The same is true of text that describes sexual activities. The reader produces a mental image that triggers the sexual pathways in the brain. Of course, these days with television and movies the job is done for you. You can sit in front of the screen and almost feel the sexual action.

Does that mean you are in favor of pornography?

No. Personally, I hate pornography and I'll tell you why later on. But pictures of naked people or people engaged in sexual activities are like a hammer. It can be a tool to construct something or it can be a murder weapon.

Here's an example. A married man might come home from work every night, lock himself in his room, and masturbate to pictures of naked girls. That's hitting himself and his wife on the head with the hammer.

Or a married man can suffer from weak erections—for many reasons—and use sexography as a sexual stimulant—an aphrodisiac—to produce erections that allow him to have sexual relations that satisfy him and his wife.

Forbid him to have that visual stimulation and he can't perform and his wife can't have any sex and their marriage will go down the drain. At the divorce hearing, explain to him and to his wife and to his small children how upright it was for him never to look at pictures of naked people. But that might have kept his marriage together.

The flip side happens too. Many women—more than ever are willing to admit it in public—are excited and motivated by sexography. It makes sex more exciting for them and makes their sexual relationship with their husband more fulfilling for both of them.

But you said you hate pornography?

I do. But "pornography" isn't men and women in all their charm and beauty—either alone or sharing the magic of sex with each other. Pornography is sickness—the hammer used as a murder weapon. It's images of the sexual abuse of children, of sex with animals, of people degrading and abusing other people with sex as the alibi.

We have to respect the people who don't want to look at sexography. That's their privilege in a free society. But that doesn't mean that intelligent men and women can't use sexual images to restore and reinforce their sexual lives. Think of it this way:

Horses and cows can't respond to pictures of other horses and cows having sex. So to stimulate them sexually and keep them from extinction, we have to pump them full of aphrodisiacal drugs. But human beings are different. They can respond to images, so why should they have to resort to drugs when they can get similar results from just looking at pictures?

Then how should sexography be used?

Intelligently. Even simple sexual images can be shocking to children, and sexography is not for them. However, every doctor knows that as they approach puberty almost every child seeks out sexual texts and sexual images as much from curiosity as anything else. Check out the nearest magazine stand and see who's looking at the centerfolds.

Even adult sexography has a powerful aroma of sex education. One of the best-kept secrets of multimedia was this. When Videocassette Recorders first came out, the vast majority of the people who bought them weren't interested in watching videotapes of Uncle Lester's wedding. They wanted to see X-rated videos from the video store. That's what sold millions of VCRs.

Now things have changed. Take a look at that mirror of modern society, the Internet. It's been estimated that people spend vast amounts of time on the Internet watching what they still call "pornography." That's not a surprise because there is a tremendous amount of it available free—pictures, drawings, stories, audio material, and even videos with sound. (Yes, you can hear the moans and murmurs of sex on your own little computer.)

But when you analyze what they are showing in those thousands and thousands of free high-resolution color photos, something amazing emerges. Most of the images of women show them with the outer labia spread apart to show the inner labia, the clitoris, the urethra, and the opening of the vagina. They show them from the front, from the back, on their knees, on their sides, standing, sitting, and squatting. They show them with their brassieres open, their skirts pulled up, and their panties pulled down. And the same poses are repeated over and over and over again—the only thing that changes is the woman who is posing.

Why is that?

The answer can be summed up in two words: SEX EDUCATION.

The millions of men—and women—who spend collectively millions of man-hours (or woman-hours) looking at these pictures are looking for one thing: basic sex education.

If you want an interesting experience, ask the average man to draw a detailed picture of the female sexual organs. You won't believe the result. It probably won't look anything like any woman who ever walked this earth. Most men don't have a clear concept of the female sexual equipment. That's one of the reasons why men are constantly looking for pictures and descriptions of female sexuality.

Of course, at the same time, they are looking for sexual stimulation and something to trigger the neural connections in the brain to set off the sexual reflexes to the penis. But that's what sex is all about—interest, excitement, stimulation, interaction, enjoyment, and good, positive, very human emotions.

Women are also interested—more than many of them admit—in seeing pictures and descriptions of naked men and women. It's a matter of curiosity and comparing themselves to what they see and all the other things that attract men to sex. After all, if only men were interested in sex and women didn't care about it, how long would it take for the human race to die out?

There's another interesting aspect of sexography on the Internet. It's the "voyeur" or "peeping" pictures—and there are thousands of them. This is where women pull up their dresses (without their panties on), spread their legs wide as they sit in beach chairs, and "flash" in public places by suddenly opening their coats to reveal nothing on underneath. The interesting thing about these pages is that almost all the women portrayed are amateurs, housewives, secretaries, female excutives, and professionals—not prostitutes. Obviously they derive some kind of sexual satisfaction by displaying their most personal attributes to the more than 40 million users of the Internet.

> *But specifically, how can a man or woman use sexography constructively?*

If a man feels he needs it, he can read about sex, look at pictures about sex, or view videos or movies about sex. A good time might be an hour or so before he is going to have sex with his wife or his female partner. The visual stimulation lingers in the nervous pathways for at least eight hours or more after exposure.

A woman can do the same thing—although some women prefer reading novels or stories about sexual topics rather than viewing images. That's one of the reasons that "romantic novels" are so popular. While they are not explicit sexography, most women have the ability to fill in the blanks. For example, when the heroine says:

> *"I could feel his powerful hand reaching out for my center of pleasure—and I responded."*

the female reader knows the hero has slipped his hand under her skirt and is just about to reach her clitoris—and she feels her vagina getting wet.

Most men, on the other hand, need to see it all laid out before them so they can respond.

> *But isn't that unfair? I mean, the woman is reacting to a novel and the man is reacting to a video instead of to their real human partners?*

Maybe. But is it better for a man to get an erection by looking at a videotape of two people having sex or is it better for him to stick a sharp needle into his penis, inject himself with a powerful drug and produce a drug-based erection that has nothing to do with any living thing?

Is it better for the woman to have sex without orgasm and without enjoyment to satisfy the puritanical principles of someone she has never heard of and will never meet? And maybe she will wreck her marriage in the process?

If looking at a picture or watching a movie can bring sexual happiness to a marriage, who can be against it? And like the hammer, they can use it to build, not to harm or destroy.

But don't sexual images promote sex crimes like rape?

And the Moon is made of Green Cheese? Are we really supposed to believe that a normal person peeks at a picture of two people having sex and then, crazed with lust, hurls himself into the shopping mall searching for victims?

Here's reality. Sex offenders are deeply troubled people with a serious degree of mental illness. It is their illness that drives them to sexual crimes, not a picture of a naked lady. Besides, most violent crimes—sex crimes included—involve alcohol. Is Prohibition the answer?

For the curious, there is sound scientific evidence that even frank pornography—not to mention sexography—does not increase sex offenses.

A detailed scientific analysis was made of rape statistics in four countries where, because of a change in the law, pornography and sexography suddenly became readily available. They were the United States, Denmark, Sweden, and West Germany. In not a single one of those countries did the incidence of violent sex crimes increase more than the incidence of nonsexual violent crimes. Period.

What about marijuana as an aphrodisiac?

One of the great enemies of sexual performance is anxiety. And there are a lot of things about sex that can make a person anxious.

Here are just a few that affect men:

- "Am I going to have an erection?"
- "Will I lose my erection?"
- "Am I pleasing her?"
- "Did someone do it to her better before me?"
- "Am I going to ejaculate before she can reach an orgasm?"

And here are some that can bother women:

- "Does he care about me or does he just want my body?"
- "Can he keep it up long enough for me to climax?"

- "Will he call me tomorrow?"
- "What will he think if I don't have an orgasm?"
- "If I fake it, will he know?"

Marijuana tranquilizes its users and removes a lot of the anxiety related to sex. That can improve sexual performance in some people. But alcohol and prescription tranquilizers do the same thing. Besides, marijuana is an illegal drug in most places—and it's never a good idea to break the law. And having a clear understanding of human sexuality and a good relationship with your partner makes all drugs unnecessary.

What would you recommend as the best possible aphrodisiac?

The Scottish poet Sir Walter Scott said it about 170 years ago:

> *Love rules the court, the camp, the grove,*
> *And men below, and saints above;*
> *For Love is Heaven, and Heaven is Love.*

The best aphrodisiac of all is: LOVE.

Chapter 6

IMPOTENCE

What is impotence?

Impotence is a penis that won't do what it's told. In spite of an unbelievably complex Copulatory Control System maintained by the body, the penis may fail to respond to its commands at the most inconvenient moments. This upsets the precise progression of events necessary for successful intercourse and the entire undertaking fails. For real Industrial Strength disappointment, nothing matches the frustration caused by a Penis-On-Strike.

Is impotence really a problem?

It can be. Here's one of the reasons why.

Toward the end of World War II, the middle-aged wife of a distinguished French General was visiting the wounded soldiers in an Army hospital. She stopped at the bed of a young officer and asked the doctor who accompanied her:

"And where was this young man wounded?"

The doctor hesitated a moment, then replied: "Uh, well, actually the bullet went through his penis, Madame."

The lady looked dismayed. "Oh! I hope it didn't break the bone!"

The doctor looked astonished for a moment, then quickly recovered his composure. He bowed slightly toward the lady and said:

"Madame, if he has you convinced that he has a bone in his penis I must convey my admiration to your husband the General for his most excellent performance!"

An impressive performance for sure, but in reality the General was lacking something that every raccoon, every coyote, and every American mink has.

What was that?

In Latin, it's called a "baculum" and it is a tiny little bone no more than an inch or two long. What makes it so important is not *what* it is but *where* it is. It is located right within the shaft of the penis. If the General—or any other man—was fortunate enough to have a baculum, he would never have to worry about erections. He could have one anytime he wanted one. (Of course there are some men who possess the equivalent of a baculum—we'll see about them further on in this chapter.)

Most carnivorous animals have this little bone in their penis— and for a very special reason. When they have sexual intercourse, ovulation in the female is triggered by the presence of the penis in the vagina. That means the penis has to make its presence known very emphatically and stay long enough to pop the eggs out of the ovaries. Human females ovulate on their own and don't require a reinforced penis—although many of them would probably appreciate that kind of organ.

As we have seen, erection in the male is basically hydraulic— liquid blood is pumped under great pressure through a complex series of valves. It's a complicated and fragile process and a lot of things can mess it up. So until human males suddenly develop their own baculum or "bone-in-the-penis," impotence will be a major problem that can affect the lives and happiness of both sexes.

Exactly what happens in impotence?

There are several distinct types of impotence, but they all have one thing in common—sexual intercourse becomes difficult if not impossible.

The most frustrating potency defect of all is absolute impotence. In this condition, the penis acts as if it is dead—it just hangs there forlornly. No amount of stimulation can encourage it to become erect. The harder a man tries, the less he accomplishes. Of course there is no possibility of sexual intercourse—it would be like trying to open a lock with a wet noodle. An accurate description can only come from a man afflicted with this form of impotence.

Jerry is such a man. He is forty-one, has been married three times, and is desperate:

"I have been through a lot, Doc. Being married three times and going through two divorces takes a lot out of a guy, but it's never been as bad as this. It doesn't even work! I mean, take last night. Arlene, that's my wife, got herself all dressed up at bedtime—the whole deal. A black transparent negligee, perfume, she even had a couple of drinks to loosen up. And she's really built! Any other guy would give his right arm for a chance to make it with her."

Jerry shook his head in despair.

"Damn it, so would I! If I were still a man. I took it out and let her play with it, I rubbed it against her, I did everything to it but paint it green. All it did was get smaller. I thought it was going to disappear!"

Can a penis actually disappear?

Not really, but some men who are made frantic by relentless impotence begin to think so. In the Orient it may take the form of a disease called "Kuru." A man suffering from impotence may become obsessed with the fear that his penis is receding into his body. He is terrified that it will then be lost to him forever. Impelled by fear he resorts to desperate measures to restrain the wandering organ. He establishes a twenty-four-hour-a-day watch manned by members of the family to keep the penis in sight at all times. Frequently he pierces the phallus with a series of pins, which he attaches to the bedpost with a stout string. Alternatively, the free end of the cord may be entrusted to the most dependable member of the family with instructions to jerk vigorously if the penis begins to wriggle upward into the body.

Is "Kuru" an actual disease?

It is as real as impotence to the man who suffers from it. There is actually no chance that the penis will disappear into the vast emptiness of the abdominal cavity to be seen no more. But trying to convince the victim is no easy task. Fortunately Kuru is a rare and dramatic phenomenon.

Much of the time absolute impotence is simply a cruel practical joke played on a luckless man by his own emotions. But the victim doesn't understand.

Let Jerry finish his story:

"We've been doing the same thing for two weeks in a row. Every night we go to the starting gate, every night I get eliminated before I even get started. If my wife doesn't get some action, this is going to be divorce number three for me."

Jerry's situation is only one example of the toll impotence takes—on the wife, the husband, and the marriage.

How common is impotence?

No one knows for sure because no one takes an advertisement in the *New York Times* to announce they can't get it up. It's estimated that there are between 15 and 30 million men who suffer from this condition in the United States. Strangely enough, 90 percent of impotent men never seek treatment. Probably about 10 percent of all men in any given country around the world have potency problems severe enough to interfere with their enjoyment of sex.

What percentage of men have suffered from absolute impotence?

One hundred percent—but that's perfectly normal. At one time or another, every man suffers from it. Because of the design of the male sexual equipment, after ejaculation the erection usually disappears. (It may linger for three to five minutes on certain occasions, but it eventually recedes.) So, for a variable period of time, no erection is possible and no further intercourse can take place. This is temporary absolute impotence.

But even that transient experience is a little unsettling—no man likes the feeling that his phallus is disconnected from his feelings.

Most of the time, within fifteen to twenty minutes the penis starts reacting again. Actually this form of enforced relaxation protects the sexual mechanisms from being overworked. It functions like a circuit-breaker. When the nerve pathways controlling copulation are overheated by orgasm, the circuit-breaker pops, shutting down the powerline to the penis. After things cool off, power is restored, and another Reproductive Rocket is ready for launching. The average "downtime" is about thirty minutes; the normal range is twenty minutes to one hour—occasionally longer.

Can't some men have subsequent orgasms much closer together than that?

Everyone has heard of cases of super-potency where men have three or four orgasms per hour. This can occur in three types of situations.

After a long period of sexual deprivation, say two to three months, the quiescent period of the sexual reflexes is shortened. After ejaculation, erection can occur again in as little as five minutes. This is a relatively rare situation and is soon replaced (often with some regret) by a more conservative waiting period.

Under circumstances of unusually strong sexual stimulation, it's also possible for re-erection and ejaculation to take place several times in an hour. At the outset of a new sexual encounter or in a relationship with an especially exciting woman, a man can be turbocharged orgasmically. This, too, tends to fade with time as the level of sexual excitement and the novelty of the situation diminish.

An example is the story of the middle-aged couple who were visiting friends on a farm. The wife poked her husband in the ribs and pointed to a rooster in the chicken yard who was mounting hens one after the other.

"Look at him, Henry! He doesn't stop after just one time, like you!"

The husband looked at the rooster and the hens, then turned to his wife.

"That's right, Ethel. But did you notice that he does it to a different hen each time?"

The other explanation for sensational male orgasmic performance is the one that applies more often.

What's that?

A lot of men expect more from their genitals than they were designed to deliver. These fragile structures are controlled by delicately tuned mechanisms oriented to quality, not quantity. There is no category in the Olympics for Copulation—at least not yet.

Still, men who compete intensely in every other area of their lives sometimes find it hard to take sex as it is. Super-potency is dangled before them on television (implicitly), in the movies (explicitly), and on X-rated videotapes (very explicitly). After enough exposure to this sort of thing, they begin to believe that anyone who can't make it every eleven minutes is in big trouble. Their own track record, which actually may be quite adequate, seems pale by comparison. So they do what human beings do when they feel insecure—they tell lies. But the lies make their problem worse instead of better.

How's that?

Say Charlie has sex twice a week with one ejaculation each time. Unfortunately some of the books he's read describe the exploits of supermen with super-penises, and compared to them his performance leaves something to be desired. He doesn't realize that his sex life is about average for his time of life. When the subject comes up in the locker room at the Country Club (every week), he says it this way:

> *"There's never been a night in my life when I didn't go back for a second round!"*

Mike, his golf partner, who is lucky to have one orgasm a week, counters with:

> *"Half the time, I can go all night!"*

Charlie knows he lied and he thinks Mike is lying, but he's not sure. He loses even more confidence in his sexual powers and tells bigger lies the next time. The problem compounds when his lack of confidence really begins to affect his capabilities. Then when the boys start bragging, he just shuts up.

When it comes to sex, it pays to be honest. Like the two eighty-year-old Englishmen who were talking in the Clubhouse after a golf game.

One of them bragged:

"I have sex every month without fail—except in the month of August."

His companion looked up.

"Hmm, August . . . too hot in August?"

The other frowned:

"No, not at all! It's just that August is vacation time for the fellow who puts me on and takes me off!"

When it comes to dealing with impotence, honesty is the first rule and confidence is the second.

Does confidence have that much effect on potency?

More than any other human endeavor, male sexuality is a game of confidence. The rule is:

"If you think you can, you probably can."

An erection is so perishable that a sudden noise, a critical word, even a rejecting look can demolish it. One of the real problems of impotence is the "Vicious Cycle."

How does that work?

Assume that the man fails to get an erection on a particular occasion for some insignificant reason—he's tired, he's worried about a problem, he has a bad cold, or something similar. If his wife or girlfriend ridicules him or compares him unfavorably to other men, the stage is set. The next time he is really in trouble. He failed once—what if he fails again? Just worrying about how his penis will act may keep it from giving any performance at all, confirming his worst fears. He starts to think like this:

> *"When does impotence start?"*
> *It starts the first time you can't do it the second time.*
> *"When is it really bad?"*
> *The second time you can't do it the first time!*

Is that true?

Of course not. As our English cousins would say:

"That's absolute rubbish!"

Potency in a man is not decided by clever sayings. It's based on the normal functioning of the brain and the sexual organs. If you want to rule your sex life by cute sayings, try this one:

Once a King,
Always a King.
But once a K(night)
Is Enough!

And for almost every man—realistically speaking, once a night is enough.

The guiding principle is reality. When it comes to a man's sexual performance no one is keeping score—and no one has to.

Sex has three goals—Reproduction, Affection, and Satisfaction. As you will notice, "Competition" is not on that list. All too often if a man fails just once and takes it seriously, he has two strikes against him. A new conditioned reflex has been established—as soon as he approaches a naked woman he starts to worry and his phallus goes to half-mast. It can be a terrible experience. It happened to Simon:

"I still remember the first time as if it happened yesterday though it was almost a year ago."

As he sat there, Simon slowly shook his head from side to side.

"Damn it, I've been so nervous since I lost my manhood I can hardly sleep.

"It's my own fault. I was out with this woman and I took her over to my place. I met her in a singles bar and I really wish I'd just stayed home and watched TV that night. After we got to bed—we were both a little tipsy—she took my, you know, organ in her hand. It was pretty hard considering how much I'd had to drink, and then she said:

"'Is this all you've got?'

"It was like someone stuck it with a pin—it just collapsed."

Now the sweat had spread to Simon's forehead. He mopped his brow.

"Then she must've realized what she'd said because she did everything to it and put it everywhere she could think of—and she thought of a lot of places. But no matter what she did, all I had to show for it was a wet noodle. She killed my penis!"

He pounded his fist on the table.

"Every time since then I've been afraid! As soon as I bring it out, I'm afraid it's too small. Sometimes the girls don't say anything, but I'm sure that's what they're thinking. The more often I try, the worse it gets."

"Do you ever have erections?"

Simon grinned pathetically.

"Oh, sure. I have them every night—as long as I'm all alone. I can make it every night by myself—but I tried to give that stuff up when I was fourteen!"

What was Simon's problem?

He'd just worked himself into an emotional corner. He hadn't "lost his manhood"—he'd just scared himself. After a few careful and detailed explanations, he began to understand the basic facts of male sexual physiology and functioning. When he finally realized that every sexual experience wasn't his final exam, things started picking up very nicely.

Is there any other kind of impotence?

There is another kind that masquerades as super-potency. It works like this:

Erection is no problem at all. Swift, hard, and urgent, the penis strains toward the vagina. But very soon after penis and vagina make contact, ejaculation occurs! For the man, it's often ten seconds from approach to orgasm. For the woman, nothing. The profuse apologies of her partner are no substitute for a sexual climax.

Does this condition have a name?

The scientific name for this condition is "Premature Ejaculation" although ladies whose partners squirt all over them call it a lot of other things. It comes in many forms, all equally frustrating.

Sometimes the man ejaculates even before his clothes come off—hard on the feelings and on the underwear.

On other occasions, everything goes smoothly until pelvic thrusts begin—with the first forward motion, everything spills out. The variations are almost endless, but they all have one thing in common: ejaculation happens long before there is any possibility of satisfying the female.

Is premature ejaculation really abnormal?

Most women think so. After being stimulated to a high pitch of sexual excitement, their reward is a warm shower of sticky semen deposited on the vulva. Some men try to alibi their problem by insisting that speed of ejaculation is synonymous with potency. "I'm just too sexy!" they say.

If their race is against the clock, they are probably right. But in heterosexual intercourse, the penis is supposed to keep time with the vagina. If the two sexual systems run neck-and-neck and arrive at the finish line more or less at the same time, the race has two winners. If the man always finishes before his girl gets to the first quarter-mile, both of them lose.

One of my patients once observed ironically:

"Doctor, the only advantage I can see to premature ejaculation is that you can double-park in front of your girlfriend's apartment!"

Not much consolation . . .

But don't male animals all ejaculate quickly? If it's normal for them, why shouldn't it be normal for men?

This was the logic applied by some of the sex "experts" of the nineteen-fifties. They noted that many men reported premature ejaculation and compared that to the behavior of animals. They noted that some animal species ejaculated fast and decided that it was fine for men to do the same. That led to the wishful thinking that speed of ejaculation was somehow related to masculinity.

They overlooked a few things. The dog, for example, ejaculates very quickly. He also chases cars, drinks from puddles, and dies at the age of twelve. If it is normal to be like a dog in one way, why not follow his example in all the others?

Another point often overlooked is that during intercourse the dog's penis becomes trapped in the female's vagina. No matter how fast he may ejaculate, the dog stays where he is until his mate is satisfied—unless he wants to leave his penis behind.

One more man-beast distinction: in animals resembling man, the anatomical location of the clitoris in the female brings it into direct and forceful contact with the penis. A minimum of stimulation by the male animal almost guarantees orgasm for his partner.

There is one group of women who adore men with premature ejaculation: prostitutes. On an evening that a girl is lucky to find a dozen gentlemen who are quick on the trigger, she can be home in bed (her own) by nine-thirty.

Is there any treatment for premature ejaculation?

Like remedies for all forms of impotence, they are there in abundance. Because premature ejaculation is such a blight on sexual enjoyment, for women as well as men, virtually every possible cure has been tried—along with some that are obviously impossible.

The most primitive approach is simply to repeat intercourse until the sexual reflexes become sufficiently fatigued to delay ejaculation. This is a tedious business at best and requires sending the lady to the corner to get a pizza while the man is waiting for the next erection to arrive. Some men even masturbate in advance so that what appears to be their first orgasm of the evening is really number two. With this approach, masturbation can become the main event and intercourse an anticlimax. As one sufferer said:

"After I blast off by myself, what do I need a girlfriend for?"

Other men try to delay orgasm by "thinking of other things" during intercourse. This is the technique recommended by some "experts" in the field of marriage counseling who should know better.

A fellow who tried this remedy tells about it:

"I'm only twenty-four, but I felt like seventy-four. No matter what I did, I came too fast. I couldn't find a girl who'd go out with me twice, so I went to this counselor. He told me all I had to do was 'control myself.' I didn't have to pay ninety bucks to hear that. That's what I went to him for. Then he

suggested that as soon as I put it in, I should think about my job instead of sex.

"I sell cars. So I started thinking about my customers, especially the chicks. There's this one who's really built. So as soon as I thought about her and her miniskirts, I went off—even faster than before. Then I went back to him and he told me to do arithmetic problems in my head. So I tried that. I'm not too good at multiplying so I was saying it kind of out loud, like 'Thirteen times eleven is . . .' and the girl I was making it with heard me. She got real mad and pushed me off and went home."

Another variation is to think of something "disgusting" to delay orgasm. If the patient can think of something "disgusting" enough, he may solve his problem by losing his erection completely and throwing up. The whole concept is self-defeating anyhow. How much fun can it be to have sex while you're thinking of dead rats?

Two other wild-eyed methods involve the wife or girlfriend. In one, the woman is asked to masturbate the man almost to the point of ejaculation—then stop. She does this repeatedly until he's had enough. This is supposed to teach him how to last longer. This approach actually has two hidden advantages. It allows her to get even for the times he has disappointed her, and also shows him what it feels like to be left high and dry. As far as curing his problem, it doesn't do much.

The other method calls for the couple to merely lie next to each other in bed naked and think of other things. They are to avoid any sexual stimulation at all. According to the proponents, this "calms down over-excitable men who tend toward prematurity." For the man who ejaculates prematurely and the woman who has to contend with him, lying around thinking of other things instead of having intercourse is not much of a thrill. That's what they've had to do most of the time anyhow.

Are there any methods that work?

There are some techniques that *almost* work. These depend on decreasing the sensitivity of the penis to the friction of the vagina. Unfortunately this is the physical equivalent of thinking of other things in the sense that it takes away much of the physical pleasure of copulation. There are a couple of ways to do it. The easiest (and cheapest) method is for the man to wear two (or more) condoms. The extra layer of rubber may just dull his sensation enough to retard orgasm. They also give him the unmistakable feeling he is making love to a rubber glove.

If that doesn't work, he can put his penis to sleep. In the back pages of some "men's magazines" there are ads for something called a "desensitizer." It's simply an ointment containing benzocaine. That's a local anesthetic that numbs the sensory receptors of the penis and sometimes delays orgasm. It may also prevent orgasm completely and convert premature ejaculation to no ejaculation—at least for the night.

The other disadvantage is that some men are allergic to this chemical. If they are, the entire penis breaks out in red, oozing, itching blisters. That kind of allergy works effectively—it tends to delay ejaculation for a week or more. It can inflict the same kind of allergy on that innocent bystander, the vagina.

The real problem with anesthetic ointments is that in the long run they tend to make premature ejaculation worse. The penis becomes negatively conditioned, and gradually less and less stimulation is required to trigger orgasm. After a few months of using the ointment, just the touch of a woman's hand may be enough to jettison a full load of semen—then and there.

Premature ejaculation is basically an emotional problem—but not a very complicated one. So often men with this condition have an underlying grudge against women—or a particular woman. Some of them merely fear women—or a woman. They utilize sex as a most subtle and yet most satisfying form of revenge—always unconsciously. They bring their victim to the edge of orgasm and then squirt everything they've got all over her. Their penis goes limp, they apologize profusely, and they really feel bad. But they had their orgasm and their partner is left high and dry—or wet. Mission Accomplished.

What's the solution?

Psychotherapy with a good psychiatrist. It doesn't have to be a full-scale psychoanalysis—what we call "goal-oriented" therapy is enough. A few sessions aimed at dealing with the specific problem can work wonders. But sometimes even that isn't necessary. Try this:

The next time you are going to have intercourse and you are worried about ejaculating prematurely, repeat these words silently to yourself over and over, in an emphatic and determined way. It's based on a very effective psychoanalytic formula that has helped many people. If it sounds strange to you, don't worry about it. Consider it a "Magic Formula" and let it work for you. It's effective about 70 percent of the time, and if it works, that's all you care about.

Just say it this way—to yourself:

"I will not spill my milk! I don't want to spill my milk! I am not going to spill any milk!"

Is there any other form of impotence besides premature ejaculation?

Yes. There is another type midway between absolute impotence and premature ejaculation. It is called "copulatory impotence." This is a particularly unpleasant condition because everything seems to be all right—until all of a sudden it isn't. Erection proceeds normally, insertion goes without a hitch. Even pelvic thrusting gets under way nicely. All of a sudden the penis goes limp.

The poor victim has two choices: he can retreat in humiliation by taking his penis out or wait a few seconds and let it come flopping out by itself. Neither choice is appealing. Continuation of intercourse with a soggy organ is impossible. Like all other forms of impotence, the condition is not contagious. The woman remains sexually eager and excited, much to her partner's (and her own) dismay. Once the penis conks out like this it stays down for the count. With luck, another erection can be expected in about an hour.

Fortunately, copulatory impotence is the second rarest potency disturbance. It is difficult to deal with since few men even recognize it for what it is. They blame it on "being tired" or "run down" and hope for better luck next time. Sometimes they're lucky and sometimes they aren't.

What is the rarest form of impotence?

This is another case of impotence sailing under the flag of super-potency. A wife of the victim, a victim herself, can describe it best:

"For the first two years of our marriage, I thought there was something wrong with me. I just couldn't satisfy Chuck. He would get such hard erections and beg me for sex so often I

just couldn't understand it. And he would go on for hours. I'd have a climax and then another one and maybe two more, but he'd still be hard at work. By then it was three in the morning and I was exhausted. When he finally took his penis out, it was just as hard as when it went in.

"In the morning he'd want to try again and it would be the same. I was just happy he had to go to work. Weekends were hell. It was sex, sex, sex, for hours and hours. Finally I got him to go to a psychiatrist and in a few weeks, everything was fine. To tell you the truth, I couldn't have taken it much longer. He was about to wear me out."

This dramatic condition has the equally dramatic name of "Psychogenic Aspermia" (P-A). It is very much as the haggard wife described it. Everything about the man's sexual performance is flawless except that he never ejaculates. Not only does he fail to ejaculate, he never reaches orgasm. It is the male equivalent of female frigidity. The erection stays rigid, sensation is more or less intact (except for soreness after the first hour), but for the man there is no end. Ironically, a man with P-A is almost in the same boat sexually as one with absolute impotence—neither of them can complete the sexual act.

And there's a touch of irony in P-A as well. Some of the world's most famous "lovers" have been men with this condition. In the field of fashion, show business, high society, and similar rarefied atmospheres, there are always half a dozen or so chaps with this problem. Women love to have sex with them—at first. As one woman said:

"They can go, and go, and go, and go—but they never come."

After a while it becomes obvious to most women that there is something wrong and they move on to a more normal man.

The one advantage for the P-A sufferer is that with expert psychiatric help, normal sexual functioning can be restored rapidly. Curing other forms of impotence may take longer.

What about treatment for other kinds of impotence?

The problems of men afflicted with absolute and copulatory impotence are a veritable gold mine for peddlers of nostrums and quack remedies. A hundred years ago it was snake oil, today it is products like "Activated Enzyme Capsules," "Essence of Toad's Toe," and "Pergillium Root." The list of alleged cures is endless. They all have one thing in common: they don't work.

The majority of cases of impotence have some physical basis. The important thing to remember is that the effect of the physical problem can be 1 percent or 100 percent. For example, a man who has a bad case of the flu may have trouble getting a good erection for a week or so. That's a physical basis for impotence, but it's not really significant in the long run. On the other hand, a man who has a spinal cord injury may be totally impotent—no erection and no feeling. That's 100-percent physical and needs to be managed appropriately. That is, no amount of psychiatric treatment is going to restore potency to a man whose spinal cord can't transmit the nervous impulses back and forth from the penis to the brain.

But is there any hope for someone like that?

Fortunately, yes. In recent years medical treatments for serious physical types of impotence have blossomed like flowers after a rain shower. The treatments fall into several categories, but they all have one thing in common. They depend on local reflexes at or near the penis, so they don't rely on messages sent from the brain to the penis and from the penis to the brain. For example, one new and eagerly sought-after oral medication acts on the tiny involuntary muscles that encircle the arteries that supply the penis with blood for an erection. The medicine allows the concentration of nitric oxide to increase. That forces the rings of muscle around the arteries to the penis to relax; the diameter of the arteries then increases, and more blood can flow into the organ.

Since the brain doesn't have to get involved, this kind of medicine works in men who have had accidents that damage the spinal cord—like car crashes or diving headfirst into shallow water. It can also help diabetics whose impotence is due to changes in the spinal cord. But there are some limitations to this kind of drug.

What are they?

It can't restore sensation if the spinal cord is cut or seriously damaged. Rubbing the penis may produce an erection strong enough to have intercourse, but the man won't feel anything. His wife will feel plenty, however—and that in itself can save marriages. Men with partial spinal damage may have partial sensation—each case is different.

Drugs that enhance the effect of nitric oxide are not aphrodisiacs. The man still needs sexual stimulation—the only difference is that he can respond quicker and with a better erection. And the fact that the drug increases the concentration of nitric oxide has made some men who suffer from impotence—both homosexuals and heterosexuals—a little uneasy.

Why is that?

Remember that amyl nitrite and butyl nitrite and similar drugs are popular among homosexual men—and some heterosexuals as well. They use them to help relax the anal muscles to make anal sex easier and also to prolong orgasm. But these drugs—"poppers"—release nitric and nitrous oxide. That's the way they relax the muscles. What happens if someone takes the pills for a better erection and also pops a "popper"? Will they have a super-erection? Will their muscles relax too much? Or won't it make any difference?

As always in the field of medicine, time will tell. There is also a potential problem with men who take other drugs that affect the nitric and nitrous acid metabolism in the body—such as medicines for heart trouble. If you add another drug that dilates blood vessels to nitroglycerine, you have the potential for serious problems. It's always better to consult your physician before you take *any* medication.

There's another interesting aspect too. Certain drugs—including some common antibiotics—can increase the concentration in the blood of the nitrous oxide-enhancing drugs as much as 150 percent. Check with your M.D. for details—or you may have some surprises.

There are other drugs based on the group known as "prostaglandins" that produce an erection more directly. And there are new types of drugs coming to market almost every week that can facilitate an erection very nicely. One problem is getting the medicine where it will do the most good. There are some medicines that have to be injected directly into the penis—although it is not as bad as it sounds. With a tiny needle—smaller than a pin—the man injects a small amount of liquid into the side of the penis, an inch or so away from his body. It doesn't take long for the results to show themselves—his organ grows right before his eyes. The erection ordinarily lasts about an hour and goes on even after ejaculation. But it can also be too much of a good thing.

How is that?

Sometimes the erection just won't go away. It can stay for hours and hours. The worst thing is that repeated intercourse and/or masturbation doesn't make it go away. It's a case of do-it-yourself priapism—the hot hard erection that reaches out, touches you, and won't let go. It's a problem since there is the risk of scar tissue forming and even permanent damage to the penis. If the erection is still there six hours later, it's time to get to the nearest Emergency Room—and prepare to grit your teeth. The doctor may have to appear with a needle—not a little one this time—and suck out the blood that is giving you too much of a good thing. When that rockhard painful penis finally deflates, you can hear the patient's sigh of relief a block away.

There's another way to deliver erection medicine without a needle. This time you simply slide a thin suppository down into the urethra—the canal that carries urine from the bladder to the outside. Pushing it in isn't exactly fun, but most people prefer it to a needle. There is the same small risk of a hard organ that won't settle down, and the treatment for that complication is the same: big needle and let it all out.

However, new treatments are showing up almost weekly, including injections with less risk of uncontrolled erections and even a cream that you can rub into the penis to produce an erection in short order.

Then these treatments have made all the other therapy for impotence obsolete?

Not quite. First of all they aren't "treatments." They are just a way to produce a drug-assisted erection. There are other ways to nudge a reluctant penis without drugs. One of the most popular is the "vacuum method." This has been around at least a hundred years and is amazing in its simplicity. (But remember, anything that you are going to do to an organ as delicate and as important as the penis should be done under the supervision of your personal physician. *Don't try this at home!*)

The man inserts his limp penis into a glass or plastic cylinder with a short piece of tubing at the top and pushes the base of the cylinder against his body to seal it off from the outside. The tube is connected to a rubber ball like the doctor has on his blood pressure machine. By squeezing the ball you can suck the air out of the glass cylinder.

As the air is pumped out of the cylinder, the partial vacuum causes the blood vessels in the penis to expand and fill with blood. Lo and behold! You suddenly have a new item on the menu:

Erect Penis Under Glass!

But then you also have a logistical problem.

How come?

How do you get that hard organ to the vagina without letting it collapse? When you take it out of its glass chamber, the pressure will be equal and the penis will deflate. The answer is a penile ring. If you slip a rubber ring around the base of the penis, you can compress the blood vessels and prevent that blood from oozing out. Once the ring is in place, you can pull out the penis, put it where it can do some good—and that's that. It is a bit inconvenient but not nearly as inconvenient as having a limp organ.

Of course, you should be careful with the ring. If it's too tight it can choke off the ejaculation, which is a bit uncomfortable. It can also cause damage to the penis if it is too tight for too long.

Do men really like the vacuum erection method?

They seem to—and the proof is that almost 85 percent of the men who try it continue to use it. Generally speaking, it allows a previously impotent man to have successful intercourse about 90 percent of the time. It doesn't require inserting needles into the penis or suppositories into the urethra and it is very economical. Once the man buys the vacuum unit and the penile ring, he doesn't have to pay each time he wants to have sex. The other advantage is that the vacuum unit can be used along with pills, creams, and suppositories to enhance their effect.

Some men have tried what amounts to splints for a droopy penis. These take the form of tubular plastic baskets with the head of the penis sticking out. Others are rubber cylinders that hold the limp organ in their latex embrace.

Their basic difficulty is that they don't really solve the problem for either participant. They are halfway measures, and neither the man nor the woman really likes them. Fortunately they are well on their way to being supplanted by the new "erection drugs."

There is, however, one kind of penile splint that lingers on.

What kind is that?

The kind that is worn inside the penis. This is the so-called "penile implant" which is really nothing more than a splint that is surgically inserted into the penis. (This is the equivalent of the baculum found in animals.)

There are several kinds of splints and each one has its problems. For example, there is the "rod splint." These are simply two metal rods, usually made of stainless steel covered with silicone, that are permanently implanted along both sides of the penis. Some models are flexible and can be bent like a coat-hanger while others are hinged. They give a nice erection, but it's an erection that never goes away completely. It can be bent down or hinged down, but it's there forever. When the opportunity for intercourse appears, the gentleman simply reaches down, bends his penis to the desired angle, and forges ahead.

It has certain obvious defects. Since the erection is permanent and you can only alter the angle somewhat, slow dancing with a girl you have just met—or with your wife's sister at a wedding—can give the wrong impression. If your boss stands in front of you in a crowded elevator, he may misunderstand your feelings toward him. And the reality remains that you have a limp penis with a couple of rods sewn inside.

Is there any better kind of splint?

Well there is a *different* kind of splint. There's an inflatable variety that tries to mimic the natural action of the corpora cavernosa—those long twin inflatable cylinders on each side of the penis. The doctor opens the penis and inserts two tubes that resemble the corpora cavernosa. Then he hides a little pump and reservoir containing liquid inside the scrotum next to the testicles and connects the pump to the tubes with a little plastic hose. After the wounds heal, when the patient wants an erection he knows just what to do. As nonchalantly as he can manage, he squeezes his scrotum, pumps the liquid up into his penis, and fills those two balloons. The penis slowly inflates and he has a sort of erection. After intercourse, it's a matter of another squeeze or two and the pumped-up penis deflates. Theoretically it's possible to have sex without telling your partner that you have your own hydraulics installed. But what happens if the lady—in the heat of sex—reaches down and begins to fondle the gentleman's testicles?

If she hits the right spot, there might be a barely perceptible gurgling sound as the erection is drained into that little tank.

There are some other more complex problems with this gadget, however.

About 250,000 of them have been implanted in men in the United States, with about 28,000 more being done every year. The Food and Drug Administration has received about 6,500 complaints of potentially serious problems. They can include infection, migration of the device into other parts of the body, leaks, breaks, and mechanical malfunctions.

Are penile implants a good idea?

It depends on your point of view. Desperate problems drive people to desperate measures and many impotent men consider their problem to be desperate. Aside from all the other disadvantages, penile implants permanently alter the structure of the penis and can make other treatments—like the injection and the pills and the suppository—difficult or impossible. Besides, with the new breakthrough therapies for impotence, there seems to be less and less need for something as extreme as an implant.

There is one other cause of physical impotence—venous leakage. When the penis becomes erect, blood flows inward through the penile arteries. But there are also penile veins that take the blood out of the penis. Unless those veins get shut off, nothing much can happen. Blood will flow in and quickly drain out. When normal erection happens, the amount of blood filling the organ increases about 700 percent and the pressure of that blood squeezes the veins almost shut. That keeps the blood from leaking out. But some men have leaky veins, and too much blood drains out and takes some of the rigidity out of the organ. Doctors have tried surgery to fix those veins, but the results haven't really been sensational. A simpler solution is the rubber penile ring put on after erection, which compresses the veins and holds the blood in the rigid penis.

Can impotence be cured?

That's a good question. None of the techniques that we've described are really a "cure" for impotence. Pumping up the penis in a vacuum chamber, injecting medicines into it, giving it a suppository, or taking a pill that makes it more responsive don't "cure" the condition. They simply relieve a symptom.

The truth lies in the question "What do you call that large structure covered with skin at the end of the penis?" The answer:

"A man."

At the end of every penis there is a man, and just curing the penis doesn't solve the problem. Even the diseases that act directly on the nervous system to zap erections—like spinal cord damage, diabetes, some forms of leukemia, certain diseases of the nervous system, and a few others—have some emotional content. The victim is depressed and anxious about his impaired sexual functioning even if it is because of a physical problem.

The best approach to dealing with impotence is a combination of common sense and sound scientific knowledge.

What does that involve?

First of all, keep in mind that people are not machines. They are complex organisms influenced by physical events, nervous responses, memories, automatic reflexes, and a dozen other variable factors. When it comes to sexual potency, as in every other area relating to human behavior, there is no absolute standard. A man may have a real physical reason for his impotence—high blood pressure, for example—and have trouble getting an erection with his wife. But when he goes to Las Vegas and finds a prostitute in a bar, he may be able to perform perfectly with her.

Other men whose condition is supposed to be caused by some physical disease can perform perfectly well if their wife dresses up like a French maid or wears black net stockings and a garter belt to bed.

Normal satisfying sexual intercourse doesn't have to be that demanding. If a man can accomplish the following three tasks, he doesn't have much to worry about:

1. Deliver the penis into the vagina without losing either the erection or the seminal fluid.
2. Reach an orgasm with a sexually attractive woman and a reasonable amount of sexual stimulation.

3. Make intercourse last long enough for a relatively normal woman to have an orgasm.

Under ordinary circumstances a man should be able to continue intercourse for five to ten minutes. During that time he should have from fifty to one hundred pelvic thrusts. A man who has intercourse more than once a week and less than three times a day is probably in the range of normal.

What's the best way to deal with impotence?

Actively. Modern medicine has a quiver full of arrows that can attack the problem. The first step is to find a sympathetic and understanding medical doctor and explain the problem to him with total frankness and honesty. At the present stage of scientific knowledge it's important to avoid radical treatments that can deprive you of the benefit of future discoveries. For example, as I mentioned, some forms of surgery can make it hard for some of the new drugs to work. Don't panic and rush into a solution—new and exciting treatments are just around the corner.

The next step is to make sure you have the understanding and support of your sexual partner. Potency isn't a battle that you want to fight alone. Just as it takes both a man and a woman to have sex, it takes both to solve the problem of impotence.

The final step is never to despair. Impotence is not a terminal disease. Every day brings new hope and new therapies. Don't give up and your persistence may be well rewarded. Sex is one of the very few renewable pleasures in this life. Don't let anything deprive you of what is justly yours—at least not without putting up a good fight.

Chapter 7
FRIGIDITY

What is frigidity?

Frigidity is a word used to describe impaired sexual feeling in women. It covers the entire range of substandard sexual response from total avoidance of sexual contact to an occasional missed orgasm. The word "frigidity" is a misleading one and was probably coined by a man.

Why is that?

It shows a certain lack of understanding of women's sexual makeup by confusing a symptom with a disease. Inability to respond sexually is not a way of life that any woman chooses for herself. It is imposed on her by conditions beyond her conscious control. Besides, the word already has its mind made up—"frigid" means cold and implies that the lady is deliberately sexually rejecting. That may not be true at all. Perhaps a better term would be "Orgasmic Impairment." This, after all, is what all supposedly frigid women have in common. More important, it doesn't prejudge the situation and assign blame.

What are the different forms of orgasmic impairment?

Like impotence, Orgasmic Impairment ranges all the way from undeniable and obvious sexual failure to the more subtle manifestations that may even masquerade as being presumably over-sexed. The basic problem in Orgasmic Impairment (O-I for short) is that the brain and vagina are not reliably connected to each other. It's like a telephone with loose wires. In some cases the line goes dead in the middle of a conversation. In others the message gets through but is garbled in the process. Sometimes the parties get the wrong number. Sometimes the phone doesn't even ring.

What happens if the phone doesn't ring?

Then the O-I is total and absolute. For all practical purposes the sexual organs don't even exist. A woman afflicted with this condition has renounced all interest in sex and things sexual. She is misunderstood by her family and friends and relegated to the social shadows as a "frustrated old maid"—a title she certainly doesn't deserve. Total orgasmic impairment is a serious emotional problem and deserves to be treated as such.

Why is orgasm so important anyway?

For the answer to that question to that one, ask anyone who has had one. Orgasm is the peak experience in human existence—nothing else even comes close. The things that human beings enjoy most—singing, dancing, eating, drinking—are all pale and feeble compared with the incomparable ecstasy of orgasm. Even Royalty understand that:

> The daughter of a European royal family was about to get married. The young Princess had been briefed by her mother, the Queen, about what to expect on her wedding night, but she was still somewhat apprehensive.
> The next morning she was speaking to her mother.
> "Mother," she said, "it was sensational! It was the greatest experience of my life! But I have just one question."
> "Yes?" said the Queen.
> "Do the poor people enjoy it too?"
> "Of course," said the Queen.
> The young Princess frowned.
> "What a pity! It's much too good for them!"

That, of course, is one of the great satisfactions—and contradictions—of life. The same supreme pleasure of orgasm is available to the richest woman in the world—and the poorest. When it comes to the pleasure of the sexual climax, money, and social standing are of no help.

What does help?

What helps is the sincere wish to enjoy sex to the fullest and the determination that nothing will stand in the way of achieving an orgasm. That, along with a real understanding of what orgasm is and how it happens, almost guarantees that any woman can have an orgasm. By the time you finish reading this chapter, you will have just the tools you need to have the kind of orgasms you have always wanted. If you have never had orgasms, you will learn how to have them. And if you have been having them, you will learn how to have better orgasms than you ever believed possible.

What keeps women from having an orgasm?

A lot of things. One of those things is . . . men. It's obvious that a lot of what happens to a woman sexually depends on how her partner is treating her. Successful sexual intercourse needs more than just a hard penis and tension in the testicles.

For many years it was fashionable in certain circles to say:

> *"A man making love to a woman is like a gorilla trying to play the violin."*

In one sense, it's true. A man's sexual apparatus and functioning are relatively simple. It has to be that way since back in the era of cave men (and women) his primitive role was to ejaculate as quickly and as efficiently as possible. The goal was to keep the human race from dying out as disease and starvation relentlessly reduced the population. To make matters worse, there were always some very large animals in the vicinity ready to make a meal of a man while he was concentrating on sex. Slipping a penis into the vagina, poking it in and out a half a dozen times, ejaculating noisily, and then trotting back to the safety of the cave may have prevented the extinction of the human race, but it didn't do a thing for female orgasm.

If a man is going to help a woman enjoy everything that sex has to offer, at the very least he needs to at least understand the basic principles of female sexual physiology. At the very most, he should be able to get a woman from the dinner table to a wild screaming orgasm time after time after time.

How does he do that?

Well, he can't do it by himself—she has to do a big part of the job on her own—but here's where it all begins.

Both the male and female sexual apparatus are basically hydraulic structures. That means they depend on the pumping of fluid and the operation of valves for their successful functioning.

Sex is hydraulic?

Yes, in more ways than one. Take the penis, for example. It is an empty cylinder only useful as a waterspout until an amazing hydraulic transformation occurs. Under the proper circumstances, one set of valves suddenly pops open, another set of valves snaps shut, and then pumps start inflating the organ with blood. That's when the limp, lethargic organ is transformed into a raging beast with a mind of its own.

The same thing happens to a woman?

Not exactly—but something very similar. Under the right stimulation, some valves open and others snap closed and the tiny clitoris suddenly isn't so tiny anymore. It becomes firm and erect and even begins to peep out from its hiding place under its hood or prepuce. The labia minora (small lips at the entrance to the vagina) also fill with blood and begin to swell. But most important of all, the blood supply to the vagina increases as the hydraulic system is transformed. Since blood carries heat, the temperature of the vagina goes up and the woman becomes very conscious of what's going on just below her pubic bone.

The significance of all this is that a woman's sexual equipment is transformed by sexual excitement. It's almost as if the excited vagina and clitoris are totally different organs from the everyday ones. Most important of all, the way it happens has a lot to do with whether or not she is going to be able to achieve an orgasm.

But how is she going to get there if her partner is like a gorilla playing a violin?

Well, sometimes a clever saying doesn't say it all. First of all, female gorillas seem to enjoy sexual satisfaction. And besides, gorillas are pretty smart animals and they can learn. Men are smarter and they can learn faster.

Then how can a man help a woman reach orgasm?

There's only one way. During sex, he needs to be an instrument whose sole purpose is to allow her to experience the most exquisite pleasure available to human beings: a profound, intense, and powerful sexual climax.

Orgasm in a woman is a very complicated affair that requires a lot of things to happen in an almost perfect sequence. Some women have this sequence programmed into their nervous systems—they can reach a climax with hardly any trouble at all. Others need to learn the steps and gradually make them part of their emotional makeup.

Where does a woman start?

At the beginning—and that means first of all making the decision. A woman who can't achieve an orgasm during sexual intercourse has to decide if she is willing to do what is necessary to get the most out of sex. If she isn't willing to commit herself all the way, her chances of success are limited. If she feels like Vanessa, she is almost sure to get what she wants:

Vanessa shook her long blond tresses, slipped off her sunglasses, and crossed her long tanned legs. She smiled.

"Now we can talk, Doctor. Now that I have assumed the 'glamour pose.'"

"A month ago that wouldn't have been so funny, Vanessa."

She nodded.

"I know. When I think back, it seems so long ago. I can't believe I spent six years of marriage without ever having a climax. I spent hundreds of hours and thousands of dollars making myself into the epitome of glamour and charm—and when it came to sex it was like I had novocaine from the waist down. Well, not exactly from the waist, but you know what I mean. And every time I had sex with my husband, when he was finished, I kept hearing these words over and over again in my head:

'Is that all there is?'

"I couldn't understand what all the fuss about sex was. You got tickled, you got rubbed, and you got wet. Big deal!"
She shrugged.

"Then I started following your program and to tell the truth, it wasn't easy. It made me face the realities of sex for the first time in my life. I mean, I had to really spread my arms wide—and not just my arms—and accept all the wonderful things that sex had to offer. And through it all, I kept remembering the story someone told me many years ago."

"What story is that?"

"A woman who had been single most of her life finally got married at the age of forty. She was a little nervous and asked one of her married girl friends about sex—especially what she could expect to feel.

"The friend said, 'It's like this. When you finally have a climax it's like a gigantic flock of immense birds flying right over you.

"She got married, and night after night went by and she didn't feel anything at all when she had sex with her husband—just like me. Then one night she was really depressed and her husband was going hot and heavy—pumping in and out and panting like crazy. She just lay there staring at the ceiling and mumbling, 'I don't feel anything . . . I don't feel a thing . . . I can't feel any . . . WOOPS! THERE THEY GOOOOOO!'

"And that's what happened to me. I went so many nights without really reaching a climax during sex. Sometimes I started to feel discouraged but I kept at it. Night after night I did what you told me—and just like the story, suddenly it worked and now I have an orgasm almost every single time I have sex. And it more than makes up for what I was missing before."

What does a woman have to do to have orgasms?

She has to devote herself 100 percent to the task. She has to decide that she is determined to get the most that sex has to offer a woman. And she has to do everything that implies.

For a woman, sex happens simultaneously at two locations. A whole series of events is occurring at the vagina, clitoris, and related structures—the Lower Story. But at the same time, a lot of sexual activity is going on in her brain—the Upper Story. If the brain turns off, there's no orgasm. If the vagina turns off, there's no orgasm. (If they both turn off . . .)

There's not much problem in turning on the vagina and clitoris. They are ancient structures, millions of years old, without any moral burden. They have never been to school, they have never been to church, they don't know anything about being "ladylike." No one ever told them that sex was "naughty" or "dirty" or "vulgar." All they want to do is get squeezed, rubbed, licked, and copulated—as intensely and as often as they can.

The Brain has other ideas. In so many women, the Brain has been told that what the vagina wants is indecent, improper, immoral, and depraved. So as soon as the vagina begins to feel like doing what it does best, the Brain clamps down.

How does the Brain "clamp down"?

Just like that. Remember the Brain is the Control Center for everything. For the vagina to get what it wants, it needs blood and plenty of it. When the Brain says "No," it just cuts off the blood supply to the vagina and clitoris. No swelling of the clitoris, no heating or secretion in the vagina, and certainly no orgasm. Even if the woman tries to consciously defy the Brain's veto, anytime along the way the Brain can short-circuit the nervous impulses and derail orgasm. In women with O-I, it happens all the time.

What's the solution?

It's really a double-pronged approach. The first step is to convince the Brain that sex is OK. It's a matter of sitting down and explaining to the Brain that when you're twelve years old and in the sixth grade, sex and orgasm are not a brilliant idea. But when you're twenty-four and married, sex is a most brilliant idea. The Brain also needs to understand that being "ladylike" doesn't mean that you're not supposed to have an orgasm. Having good manners in public doesn't mean that you can't bounce around and scream your head off when you're having sex with your husband.

Remember the old-fashioned advice to girls who were about to get married:

"Be a lady in the parlor and a harlot in the bedroom!"

Some women got that confused and were harlots in the parlor and ladies in the bedroom. Most of those suffered from O-I.

What's the second part of the solution?

The second part is to retrain the Brain. In most women with O-I, the Brain has been programmed to shortstop every bit of sexual stimulation that strikes it. Whenever a sexual fantasy pops up, the Brain squashes it. It screams, "You shouldn't even think of vulgar things like that!"

But sex isn't vulgar.

If a woman feels the urge to "touch herself down there," the Brain screams, "What are you doing? That's dirty!"

That's just not true. Most of the time a woman's sexual equipment is cleaner than her hands.

If a woman wants to sneak a peek at men in tiny swim suits on the beach, the Brain shrieks, "That's immoral!"

What does looking at the human body have to do with moral principles or lack of them?

The first step in bringing the Brain into contact with reality is "Counter-Programming."

What's Counter-Programming?

It involves overwhelming the Brain's roadblocks with healthy input. It means stimulating the normal sexual impulses to the point where the Brain can't slam on the brakes every time a woman approaches orgasm. It starts with the obvious—thinking constructively about sex. Jane tried it:

> "At first it seemed a little unusual, Doctor. I mean, I'm thirty-three, I have a degree in sociology, and I teach at the university. And you suggested that I think about sex all day!"
>
> Jane chuckled, then went on:
>
> "Well, not exactly, but that was what it sounded like at first. I had never had an orgasm—even after seven years of marriage and trying everything. So I figured, what have I got to lose?
>
> "So when I got home from work that first week, I sat down in the den, poured myself a nice cup of tea and began to fantasize. I imagined my husband sneaking up behind me,

slowly pulling up my dress, and then ever so slowly pulling down my panties. That was enough to get me a little excited and I got scared and stopped right there!

"Then the next day I went a little further and imagined that he was sliding his hand up between my legs and tickling me up there. I started to get wet and I really wanted to masturbate. It was amazing how it started making a difference right away."

"Then what?"

"Then I quit the program. I guess I was getting scared because I was doing something 'forbidden.' It took me a week to convince myself that I was thirty-three and married and if I wasn't going to enjoy sex now, when was it going to happen? When I was ninety-nine?

"So I decided to get back to work on my problem. That's when I started watching the X-rated videos."

But isn't it true that women aren't stimulated sexually by watching X-rated videos?

That's what some women say:

"Oh, that's so gross! How could anyone ever watch anything like that! It's a turn-off!"

But as a way of helping to overcome the Brain's destructive prohibitions, X-rated videos and movies have their place. It may be that the Brain is saying "No-No!" but there's "Yes-Yes" down below. And there is solid scientific proof of that.

Scientific proof?

That's right. The irrefutable evidence comes from a wonderfully precise scientific instrument called a "photoplethysmograph." It's a little device about the size of a vaginal tampon that fits into the vagina. By means of a very sensitive photoelectric cell, it very accurately measures the blood flow to the vagina. As we saw before, when a woman becomes sexually stimulated, the blood flow to the vagina increases tremendously. The following experiment has been done many times:

A group of women are fitted with the photoplethysmograph and then an X-rated videotape is shown to them. The tape displays a full range of sexual activity between men and women. That can include fellatio (mouth-penis), cunnilingus (mouth-vagina/clitoris), and the whole gamut of positions for intercourse. During the screening a few of the women expressed distaste at what they were viewing—the Brain said, "Obscene! Vulgar!"

But the photoplethysmograph doesn't lie. In almost every case, in spite of their denials, their vaginas became engorged with blood as the women were sexually excited by what they were seeing. Other instruments detected vaginal muscular pulsations—throbbing of the vagina—and increased groin temperatures. When the vagina and related structures become engorged with blood and the vaginal muscles begin to expand and contract, there's no doubt as to what is going on.

And something else interesting happened. For years it's been said that most X-rated films and videos are male-oriented and turn off female viewers. So a new category of explicitly sexual videos made by women for women has appeared. Those productions are supposed to stimulate women without the "vulgarity" of male-style films. Sounds good but it doesn't work out that way. It seems that women liked the woman-oriented films better but they got just as turned on by the male-style versions.

But is fantasizing about sexual experiences and watching X-rated videos really all right?

Think about it. If a child can't learn to read, we stimulate them in every way to get them interested in reading. If someone loses their appetite, we stimulate them to eat by tempting them with all sorts of goodies. And if a woman can't experience the one thing that feels the best of all in this world, is it wrong to stimulate her to the point where she can feel what other women are feeling?

Listen to what Karen went through. An attractive brunette with bright hazel eyes, she was dressed in a powder-blue suit set off by a pale cream silk blouse. She looked like a very capable Dean of a distinguished women's college—which in fact she was:

"Oh, Doctor! What a dummy I was! I believed everything they told me when they said:

"'When you get married everything will be fine. Just leave it to your husband and you'll gradually learn to enjoy sex.'

"I'm still waiting. It's been eight years and it was the same the first night as it was last night. I just lie there expecting Jeff to bring me to the heights of passion. Of course I've never let him do anything except what I thought was right—nothing oral, no unusual positions, no play-acting. As he says, 'Just a plain vanilla lay!' "

"But what happens exactly?"

Karen looked surprised.

"Exactly? Exactly nothing! I got a nice vaginal rub-down twice a week with a slippery latex-covered penis and I guess the latex got more kicks out of it than I did. But . . ."

She raised a stern index finger.

"But I was a good clean girl who did what I was supposed to do! I was trying the impossible. I might as well have tried to have sex standing on one leg in a hammock in front of the local Shopping Mall. I would have had a better chance!"

"What do you mean?"

"I mean, Doctor, that I stacked all the odds against me. But then I decided to stack them in my favor and the results are totally different."

Karen paused for a sip of coffee and then went on.

"I did everything you told me to. I found a nice quiet place and let all my fantasies go wild. When I got turned on enough, I masturbated to those fantasies and it was really something. Then I rented some of the wildest X-rated videotapes I could find and watched half a dozen of them—one per night. But don't think that I didn't have second thoughts!"

"What do you mean?"

"I guess it was inevitable. After all, I am the Dean of a highly respected Girls' School and I graduated with honors from a leading Ivy League university. My family is one of the most respected in the State. My father is a corporate lawyer and a deacon of the church. And . . ."

Karen raised her eyes toward heaven in a gesture of bewilderment.

". . . And here I am wanking off to some filthy video tapes! I'm sitting there in my impeccably decorated Early Colonial style apartment watching some bimbo with immense breasts spread-eagled on a fur rug getting a workout from a hunk with a rock-hard penis! And it's getting me so turned on that I

*have to play with myself to keep from going out of my mind!
At the same time my Brain is insulting me by screaming,
'Slut!' 'Cheap!'*

"Then what did you do?"

*"I pulled the plug on the damn video recorder, poured
myself a nice hot cup of tea, and had a little talk with myself."*

Karen smiled and then went on.

"It was basically a monologue and here's how it went:

*"'OK, Karen, you say you want to enjoy sex. How do
you think it's going to happen? When your husband is duti-
fully pumping away trying to make you come, is your
father's law firm or your college diploma going to get you
off? When Jeff can't hold back any longer and finally ejaculates, can you climax with him by reciting your very distinguished family tree in chronological order? No? Well then,
what are you going to do about it?"*

Karen looked me straight in the eye.

*"There was only one answer to that, Doctor. I was going
to do anything I had to do to enjoy sex the way I have a right
to enjoy it. Why should anyone or anything interfere with my
access to the greatest pleasure in life? I also remembered
what you once told me."*

"What was that?"

*"You said the French nobility used to refer to sex as
Opera for the poor people.*

*"Well, if the poor people can enjoy sex, why not me?
And if I have to watch videotapes and masturbate and think
about big hard hot penises and throbbing vaginas and anything else to let me enjoy what I have a right to enjoy, then
I'm going to do whatever I have to do. That's what I decided
and that's what I did.*

*"I went back to those videotapes. You know, they aren't
exactly Academy Award stuff, but once you get into them,
they can be a turn-on. After awhile I could play with myself
while I watched them and even climax that way. I know it
doesn't sound like much, but for me it was a tremendous
sexual awakening and a relief at the same time."*

"Then what happened?"

*"Well, it all would have been silly if I hadn't applied it
where it would do the most good. When Jeff and I had sex, I
turned my mind back to the videos and it really helped. I got*

a lot more excited and I started to feel things that I had never felt before. It was great!"

Why do X-rated videos and pictures help?

Human beings are programmed to respond to certain sexual cues. When a man sees a naked woman the image hits his brain and starts a chain of mysterious responses that end up at the end of his penis. Why just looking at breasts and vulva should open all the valves and flood the penis with blood is still a mystery—but that's the way it happens.

And the same thing can happen with women. For decades women were told they weren't supposed to react to the naked male body—and often they didn't. But if they open themselves up to their inner responses, their normal healthy sexual reactions will point them in the right direction. For most of their lives so many women have choked back their sexual instincts—and with them, their orgasms. Now they can reverse the process and enjoy what every woman so richly deserves.

What's the next step after fantasy and X-rated stimulation?

Getting down to the nitty-gritty of sex—with orgasm. The basic purpose of sexual fantasies and X-rated videos and masturbation is to promote and reinforce the messages between the brain and the sexual organs. It's like learning to play tennis. The first time you're standing behind the net and the ball comes at you, you don't know what to do. But after hitting the ball back fifty times or so, you don't even have to hesitate—you respond instantly.

That's the way it should be with sex. Those nervous impulses have to race from the brain to the clitoris and the vagina without a second's pause along the way. When your clitoris is being gently massaged by your husband, you don't want to have to think:

"Am I feeling anything? Should I be feeling anything? Is it right to feel anything?"

You just want to let that clitoris get harder and hotter until you can't stand it any longer—and the faster it happens, the better!

Once the Brain and the vagina are working in harmony—more or less—it's time to start working on penis-vagina orgasm. And that brings up the question of the famous "G-Spot."

The "G-Spot"? What's that?

A lot of people who have tried to find it have asked exactly that question. Back in 1950 a German gynecologist by the name of Ernst Grafenberg announced that he had discovered a particular spot on the wall of the vagina that was extremely sensitive and could produce a very powerful orgasm when it was correctly stimulated. Apparently "Grafenberg" was a hard name for a lot of people to remember, and the area became known as the "G-Spot." But that was only the beginning.

Almost immediately the world was divided into two opposing camps—those who welcomed the "discovery" of the "G-Spot" as the "Gateway to New Sexual Satisfaction" and those who insisted that there was no such thing and it was all someone's wild fantasy. Some women—about 30 percent of adult females—thought they had a G-spot and could have better orgasms than the other 70 percent.

Other women insisted that all women are created equal and there is no such thing as a special spot of privilege in the vagina. Even today—after nearly half a century has gone by—the debate rages on in the pages of distinguished medical journals. And the burning question is:

"Is there a G-Spot or isn't there?"

Is there?

The answer is simple and very precise: "Yes" and "No." There is an area of heightened sexual sensitivity in the vagina of virtually every woman. When it is stimulated, all the reflexes that lead to orgasm are accelerated. That's the "Yes" part.

The "No" part is this. The "Spot" doesn't necessarily have to be precisely where Dr. G. located it. He put it on the upper wall of the vagina about an inch or two from the entrance. It can be somewhere else—and that "somewhere" is what can make orgasm possible for nearly every woman who wants one.

How is that?

Very careful scientific studies of female sexual sensitivity and response—not the ones that show up in popular books written by nonscientists and self-styled experts—have recently revealed some fascinating and extremely useful information. These studies prove that Dr. G. was right—but he stopped too soon. There very definitely is an area of increased sensitivity in the vagina that can make all the difference between "Go" and "No-Go"—or as one of my female patients referred to it, "Come" or "No-Come." But that strategic area extends all the way from the entrance to the vagina to a point just above the cervix—all along the anterior or upper wall of the vagina.

Where is it exactly?

Right here:

If you insert a finger into the vagina and move it upward behind the pubic bone until you reach the cervix (the neck of the uterus that extends into the vagina) you will move along a strip of tissue that is woman's most sensitive sexual area.

Stimulation of this area targets the vagina, the urethra, the clitoris, and the little corner of the upper vagina where it meets the cervix. This area is sexual dynamite. If the "G-Spot" is considered the "Orgasmic Spot," then this is the true "Orgasmic Highway." The right kind of stimulation of this four-lane non-stop "Orgasmic Interstate" virtually guarantees a bone-rattling orgasm.

Then why doesn't every woman have all the orgasms she wants?

Because they never get on the right road. Instead of the Freeway, they're plugging along on some bumpy old back road full of pot-holes. Think about it. Most women have sex in the so-called "Missionary Position." That's with the woman on her back, knees raised, legs apart, and the man lying on top of her. From an orgasmic point of view, it probably should be called, "The Missionary Impossible Position."

The penis vigorously stimulates the back wall of the vagina that has hardly any sexual sensitivity and is as far from the clitoris and the front cervical-vaginal pocket as possible. If the woman has any trouble at all reaching a climax, this is the one position that makes it even harder for her. It's about as accurate as trying to feed someone a banana while you're blindfolded.

If the man's erection is hard, if the vagina is tight, if the woman is really excited sexually—and about half a dozen other "ifs"—the woman can reach an orgasm. But that's stacking all the odds against her. It's much better to shave the odds in her favor.

How do you do that?

By taking advantage of the realities of human female anatomy and physiology along with the latest scientific and medical findings. If a woman really wants to have an orgasm or if she wants to increase the frequency and intensity of her orgasms, this is what she can do about it.

First, in a quiet place and a quiet moment, she can learn the route. Get the kids out of the house if necessary, lock the bedroom door, and get ready for some interesting discoveries. Lie on your back and slowly insert a finger (lubricated if necessary) into the vagina. Keep it along the upper or anterior wall and move it slowly upward until you reach the cervix. You'll feel it as a tubular structure with the consistency of the tip of your nose. There is a space between the cervix and the upper wall of the vagina that is sensitive in many women. Run your finger around there to get used to it. Then move your finger up and down from the entrance of the vagina to the pocket by the cervix. You should feel sensations along the clitoris, the urethra, and the vagina. If you feel like it, you can keep moving your finger around until you have an orgasm. Rubbing the clitoris with your other hand might help too.

But is it all right for a woman to play with herself like this?

She isn't "playing with herself." She's learning the location of the most sensitive parts of her sexual structures so that she can enjoy what she has a right to enjoy—sexual orgasm. If she's going to give a speech to the Parent-Teachers Association, she will be very careful to rehearse it. That's a very minor event in her life. If she wants to have an orgasm—easily one of the most important events in her life—shouldn't she rehearse that at least a little bit too?

What's the next step?

Ideally, more practice. It's worthwhile repeating that stimulation of the "Orgasmic Highway" until the woman is sure of her response. When she has the reflexes well rehearsed, she's ready for the next step.

That's when she can try it out with her husband. The basic idea is to bring his hard penis into the closest possible contact with the upper wall of her vagina, getting that organ to press as hard as possible against that vaginal wall. It's important to press hard because there are nerve endings deeper in the vaginal tissues that need to be stimulated at the same time. And for all of it to work ideally, she has to make the penis as hard as possible. That's another part of the woman's job at that stage.

Why does she have to do it?

Because at that point, the penis is the key to her orgasms and the job is too important to leave to a man. She has to make sure that she gives him a good hard erection—that means whatever it takes. If it's oral sex, do it. If it means stimulating him in a particular way that you know always turns him on, do it. If you're going to reach your goal, you need that penis, and you need it hard.

The next step is to make sure that you are turned on to the maximum as well. Encourage your husband to do whatever you know excites you the most. Let him rub your clitoris the way you like it best—and tell him exactly how you want it done. If you don't tell him, he'll probably rub it the way he rubs his penis—and you probably won't like that very much!

Then encourage him to perform oral sex on you—if that's what you like. Remember to explain to him that it's all for a good cause—orgasm. And you can show him the route to the Orgasmic Highway while you're at it. Just make sure his finger has enough lubrication by then. When you get to the point where you can't hold back much longer, take hold of that penis and put it where it should go.

Is that all there is to it?

Not quite. Sliding the penis into the vagina isn't enough—it has to travel that orgasmic route if it's going to do the most good. That's where picking the right position comes in. One of the best positions is with the woman on her side and the man lying behind her. That way the underside of the penis rubs right along the front wall of the vagina. At the same time, the man can push downward against the vaginal wall to increase the pressure and thus the stimulation. But that's not the only way.

Try several different positions until the penis rubs the vagina just the right way. It's a good idea—and not exactly the most difficult assignment in the world. Depending on the relative size of the man and the woman, sometimes if the woman lies on her stomach with a pillow under her to raise her hips, the penis can fit just the right way. For other couples, if the man lies on his back and the woman rides him facing him, penis-vagina alignment is just right. (Among aficionados, this is called the "cowgirl" position, for obvious reasons.) Sometimes it's better if the woman rides her man facing his feet—this is the "reverse cowgirl."

Is all that really necessary?

No, none of it is necessary—unless a woman wants to have an orgasm. Think of all the time and effort a woman puts into selecting just the right makeup. Eye liner, powder, base, eye shadow, lipstick—all have to be chosen carefully and applied meticulously. The final result is enjoyable and satisfying. But it can't compare with the enjoyment and satisfaction of a wild and frantic orgasm. Doesn't it make sense to devote as much time and effort to achieve orgasm as you devote to make up your face?

With dedicated experimentation, eventually almost every woman will find the combination of foreplay and position that gives her the right kind of Super Highway stimulation to bring her to a climax almost every time. But that's not the end of it. Once she discovers it she has to repeat it as often as she can to nail down the reflexes. It's like playing basketball. Once you can get the ball in the hoop, it's not time to stop. It's time to do it as many times as you can so that you can do it without even thinking about it.

Is there anything else a woman can do to make sure she has an orgasm?

Yes. Recent scientific and medical studies have given us some very interesting clues. It seems that a woman's ability to reach a climax in sex is increased if her "sympathetic nervous system" is stimulated before intercourse. The whole concept of the "sympathetic nervous system" is fairly complex. However, as a practical matter, it turns out that twenty minutes of intense physical exercise—like aerobics— stimulates the sympathetic nervous system and can produce a big increase in sexual responsiveness. But don't do what Natalie did.

What did she do?

Let her tell it:

> *"You know, Doctor, you really saved my sanity. I did exactly what you suggested and I started having climaxes for the*

*first time after four years of marriage and it was terrific! I
never imagined that sex could be that great! But I was never
satisfied and I was looking for something even better. You
know, as a computer programmer I'm a perfectionist, and I
thought I could go for the max.*

"What do you mean?"

*"Well, you said that twenty minutes of exercise could make
my orgasms even wilder so I did it. Well, maybe I overdid it."*

"What happened?"

Natalie paused, shook her head, and smiled.

*"I go to this great aerobics class and so I figured if
twenty minutes is good, forty minutes is twice as good. So I
gave it my all, rushed home to Dan, my husband, pulled off
his clothes, dragged him into bed as I undressed on the way,
threw myself on top of him, and . . ."*

"And what?"

Natalie lowered her eyes.

"And—I promptly fell asleep!

*"But I learned my lesson. You said twenty minutes, and
twenty minutes it is!"*

Is there anything else that can make orgasms better for a woman?

Yes. Remember the story about the young man carrying a violin
case who stopped an old lady on the street in New York. He was lost
and anxious to get to his appointment. He said:

*"Excuse me, ma'am. Can you tell me how to get to
Carnegie Hall?"*

She looked at him, glanced at his violin case, put her face close
and said:

"Practice, my boy! Practice!"

Practice may not get you to Carnegie Hall, but constant, conscientious practice will take you straight to the kind of orgasms that
you never dreamed possible—orgasms that will transform your sex
life and your life as a whole. Try it—you have nothing to lose and
everything to gain.

Chapter 8

HOMOSEXUALITY

Important Note: *Homosexuality isn't what it used to be. Years ago it was simply a set of Sexual Practices. Now it is tied in with human rights, civil rights, political correctness, job rights, freedom of expression, military service, sexual harassment, and a lot of other things. What follows is a medical-scientific description of homosexual practices. It is taken from ample material supplied by practicing homosexuals as well as current medical-scientific studies of homosexuality. You may believe that homosexuality is good or you may believe that it is bad. But as a physician and a scientist, I cannot pass that kind of personal judgment. Therefore nothing in this chapter should be—or can be—interpreted as being against or in favor of homosexuality.*

What is homosexuality?

Homosexuality is a condition in which a person of one sex has a driving emotional and sexual interest in those of the same sex. Because of the anatomical and physiological limitations involved, there are some formidable obstacles to overcome. Most homosexuals look upon this as a challenge and approach it with ingenuity and boundless energy.

Is homosexuality good or bad?

The answer to that is a philosophical judgment and far beyond the scope of this book. In recent years homosexuality has become an emotionally charged political issue. Let's take a medical-scientific look at what homosexuality involves and leave the value judgments to the philosophers.

What causes homosexuality?

Like every complex area of human behavior, there's no simple explanation. Some people say it's "genetic"—you're born with it and there's nothing you can do about it. Other people call it a form of mental illness curable by psychotherapy. Still others believe it's a personal decision—a person simply decides to be a homosexual. Some people say it's a sexual perversion. Other people, most of them homosexuals, say it's normal—just like being heterosexual. To complicate matters further there are about ten other points of view.

Who's right?

Everyone. Because we're talking about opinions and everyone is entitled to their own personal opinion. From a scientific standpoint, thousands of research projects are constantly under way, so let's just concentrate on what homosexuality *is* rather than *why* it is.

Has homosexuality changed in recent years?

Yes and no. The things that homosexuals do with each other sexually haven't changed since sex began because, from an anatomical point of view, there aren't too many choices. But something else very important has changed.

What's that?

Homosexuality has come out of the closet. A gigantic homosexual subculture has suddenly blossomed in America. Homosexuality used to be in the shadows—now it is front and center. There are homosexual churches, homosexual movies, homosexual beach resorts, homosexual restaurants . . . even sitcoms on TV with homosexual themes.

Is that good or bad?

That's the strange thing about homosexuality. It has become so politicized that everyone wants to know if you are for or against it. But to physicians and scientists that's not the point. Homosexuals are human beings and this chapter is about what they do—not whether it's right or wrong. Based on the facts and their beliefs, everyone has to make up their own mind.

What percentage of the population is homosexual?

No one knows for sure because it isn't the kind of thing you take a full-page ad in the paper to announce. Some people say that 2 percent of men in the United States are homosexual. Others insist on 10 percent. The real number is probably somewhere in between. The number of female homosexuals is probably about the same—more or less.

I've read a lot of articles about homosexuals, but they all seem to leave out what I really want to know. How do homosexuals actually have sex?

That's the key question. The majority of people think of "having sex" as penis-vagina intercourse. But by definition, male homosexuals have eliminated the vagina as an option. If they are going to have any sex at all, they need someplace to put their penis. That's the problem. If they're just going to have sex with other men, from an anatomical point of view, their choices are somewhat limited. That's why homosexuals need a lot more imagination in sex than the average heterosexual couple.

An obvious activity is masturbation. There are a lot of ways to masturbate and a common homosexual experience is mutual masturbation. Some chaps like to masturbate while their partners watch. It gives both of them a certain kind of sexual satisfaction. Others prefer to stroke each other's phallus until they both ejaculate. But there are many more forms of imaginative mutual masturbation.

For example?

Well, then it gets interesting. There is the "Princeton Rub"—an elegant name to say the least. The procedure is vaguely reminiscent of the "dry hump" so common among high school heterosexuals. That's when two teenagers out on a date, after kissing and squeezing a little, become so aroused that they rub their sexual organs together through their clothes. It often ends in ejaculation by the young gentleman and a lot of (wasted) lubrication by the young lady. The degree of satisfaction has to be weighed against the amount of damage to the underwear.

(Perhaps that's what they mean when they say, "Rubbing someone the right way.")

Grown-up homosexuals do the same kind of thing, but they usually get undressed and find a relatively comfortable position. One homosexual lies on his back with his legs pressed together while the other lies on top of him and inserts his penis into the gap between his thighs just below his testicles. Technically it's called "interfemoral intercourse."

Of course, the fellow on the bottom can lie face down while the other puts his organ into the same space. Some kind of lubrication is a good idea and sometimes one of the fellows covers his body with grease or oil. Some guys also use the armpit and the space behind the bent knee as a place to rub their lubricated penis to the point of ejaculation.

Another possibility—and probably not the last one—is for one man to lie on his back with his knees up while his friend rubs his penis against his perineum (that's the area between the testicles and the anus).

But aren't those strange ways to have sex?

That depends on your point of view. As the French say:

"Chacun à son goût."
"Each one to his own taste."

Of course the one on the bottom isn't really getting the same kicks as the one on top who is rubbing his penis against some part of his body. To make up for that, the bottom half often masturbates or is masturbated by his buddy.

Don't homosexuals do other things too?

Certainly. The next common variety of homosexual behavior is oral intercourse. This is also known as fellatio, which means the same thing except in another language. In this variation, one man sucks the penis of the other. Sometimes they then reverse roles, sometimes not. Both fellatio and masturbation play a big role in one area of homosexual activity.

What's that?

Casual sex. It's part of the bond—almost like a fellowship—that many male homosexuals have. That makes casual and spur-of-the-moment sex easy and possible. In traditional places for homosexual encounters like public parks at night, gay bars, public restrooms, adult bookstores, and homosexual clubs, the usual male-female sexual flirtation doesn't take place. When two "cruising" homosexuals meet and choose each other, sex follows promptly.

It can be a quick masturbation or fellatio in a park or a public restroom or a longer encounter in one fellow's apartment. It's quite different from what most heterosexuals are accustomed to. As a matter of fact, if heterosexuals could do the same thing, for young male bachelors it might sound like a dream come true.

Imagine if after work on Friday one of the fellows from the office could stroll down to a secluded spot in the park and find half a dozen or so attractive young ladies loitering there. After a word or two, one of the girls, without exchanging names or even introductions, would proceed to unbutton the gentleman's trousers and fellate him to orgasm. It can't happen, right?

But if they want to, homosexuals can do that almost every day of the week. Of course there are some problems involved.

Like what?

Well, it's not exactly a lasting relationship. There are no introductions, no names are exchanged, and if it's nighttime, sometimes the fellows don't even see each other clearly. And there is always the problem of the uncooperative police who tend to be on hand in those kinds of places. One never knows if that charming and cooperative young lad is a police officer ready to clamp on the handcuffs.

And that's a big problem. Being arrested can be a nuisance. It's especially inconvenient since some men who seek this kind of anonymous instantaneous sex want to (or have to) conceal their homosexuality. If they get arrested, it compounds their problem. Sometimes they resort to "glory holes" to minimize the risk.

"Glory holes"? What's a "glory hole"?

Homosexuals have a rich vocabulary of their own—and a lot of it is touched with a wry humor. It's part of the ever-expanding homosexual sub-culture. A "glory hole" is an opening in a partition between two spaces that can be used for sex. For example, there are "glory holes" in tea rooms.

In tea rooms? Do homosexuals spend a lot of time drinking tea?

Actually you don't drink tea in a "tea room." A "tea room" is a men's public toilet where homosexuals go to find other men for impromptu sex. It can be in a shopping mall, a bowling alley, a military base, a hospital, an office building—almost anywhere.

Where else do you find "glory holes"?

In certain gyms and health clubs, in some truck stops, at certain movie theaters and in some "adult bookstores." Those holes in the partitions between the toilet stalls are there for a very special purpose and it's somewhat complicated. Actually there is a fairly rigid etiquette that "glory hole" neophytes have to learn.

How does it go?

Well, it can vary from city to city but basically it's something like this. Let's take a cubicle in a "health club" as an example. Monty, who knows about those kinds of things, explains it:

> *"You see, Doc, you go into one of the cubicles, but first you make sure there's another guy in the one next door. Make yourself comfortable. Then find the 'glory hole' and decide what you want to do.*
>
> *"If you want to suck someone's penis or just masturbate it, you put your finger in the hole and wiggle it. Then if they're interested, pretty soon you'll see their penis—it should at least be half erect or they're not really serious—coming through that hole.*
>
> *"Then you can go ahead and do what you want. You can suck it or play with it until he comes. Oh yeah, if you want them to use a condom, you should push one of them*

through the hole after you put your finger through. Some guys stick the condom on the end of their finger and that's OK too. But the way things are these days, it's dumb not to use a condom."

What if someone wants to be masturbated or sucked?

Let's ask Monty.

"Well, if you want it done to you, wait for the finger to come through that hole. You don't know what's on the other side. It could be a cop just waiting to bust you! Or it could be a Straight Arrow who just came for a workout. Be patient and avoid embarrassment. And it's not too bright to put your wee-wee through that hole if you don't know what to expect in that other cubicle!

"But if you see that friendly finger wiggling at you, it's probably going to be OK. Then you can push your own organ through the hole and get sucked or masturbated. If you want to play it safe, put the condom on first."

Monty said, "If you want to play it safe," but is having sex that way really safe?

It doesn't seem that way, does it? There are a lot of risks to casual sex. Especially the "glory hole" kind.

What are they?

For one thing, it takes a lot of courage to push your erect penis through a hole in the wall and wait for someone to do something to it—someone you have never met and can't even see. You're betting that they are a kind and gentle person like you just looking for an anonymous orgasm—and not a sadistic killer or someone who has just escaped from a mental hospital.

There is also the ever-present risk of infection, either AIDS or hepatitis—or anything else. It's hard to check someone out if you can't even see them. And although most homosexuals will want to use a condom in the "glory hole" there's one situation where you can't be sure if your partner is "condomized" or not.

What's that?

Anal sex. Some "glory hole" users want to have their neighbor's penis in their anus so at "Show Time" they put their buttocks up against the hole. But they don't have any way of knowing if their new friend is going to use a condom or not. And by the time they find out, it's too late. And even if he uses a condom, they can still get infected with AIDS or hepatitis.

How can they get infected if he uses a condom?

A lot of ways, as we'll see in the the chapter on Sexually Transmitted Diseases (Chapter 14), but there's one little-known way that a homosexual can get infected even with a condom. Suppose his invisible new friend across the way is nervous or a little tipsy or high on drugs or just clumsy. He pulls on a condom—one of those reservoir tip types—and discovers he has it on backwards! (It can happen . . .) He then quickly pulls it off, turns it inside out, and slips it back on his penis. Then he slides his condom-covered penis through the hole into his neighbor's anus—and gives him AIDS!

How come?

There was just enough secretion at the tip of his penis to contaminate the inside of the condom. When he turns it around, the wetness is now on the outside. And when he pushes his penis into the anus of his acquaintance, the virus of AIDS finds a new place to grow.

For fast, frequent, anonymous sex, there are safer places than "glory holes." There are the bathhouses.

Bathhouses? Is that where they take a bath?

No. Just as you don't drink tea in a "tea room," you don't take a bath in a "bathhouse." A typical "bathhouse" looks a lot like a health club. There may be lockers, whirlpools, a sauna, hot tubs, sometimes even a small swimming pool. But there are a few other conveniences as well. For example, there are the usual booths, a TV room, and an "orgy room."

Once again, "the baths" is the kind of place that heterosexuals looking for women can only dream of. (There have been occasional attempts at heterosexual "bathhouses" but most closed for one reason or another.) The procedure varies according to local customs and individual preferences, but typically it works like this:

A customer enters, goes through the usual routine: paying, getting a locker, etc. Then he emerges clad only in a towel. He walks around the club—"cruising"—or lies down on a cot in his cubicle. Eventually another man makes eye contact, comes up to him, and they go off together into a cubicle. They decide between them what they are going to do and they do it. A few minutes later they separate and find other partners.

What about the "orgy room"?

That's a special kind of place. Anywhere from three to five or more homosexuals may congregate there and have sex together. Some of them simply lie around the room masturbating or fellating or being fellated or having anal sex. But sometimes they get together in "daisy chains," where groups of homosexuals link together, each one simultaneously sucking a penis and having his penis sucked. They can do the same sort of thing with masturbation or anal sex.

Is anal sex really safe?

In these circumstances, "safe" is a relative word. If you go to a place where half-naked strangers are strolling around and you have sex with them anonymously, "safe" wouldn't seem to be uppermost in your mind. But of course, anal sex is the least safe of all sex.

Why is that?

The anus is the tail end of the digestive system—it isn't part of the reproductive system—and it's not ideally-designed for sex. For one thing, it's full of super-bad bacteria like the deadly *E. coli*. It can also harbor the virus of hepatitis—the same hepatitis that kills more people every year than AIDS. And there's another little detail that's hard to overlook. The anus and rectum are home to the residue of the digestive system—feces. Bacteria, viruses, and feces—not exactly the ideal place to insert your penis. Or put your mouth.

Put your mouth?

That's right. Some homosexuals enjoy anilingus, or licking and tonguing the anus. It's obviously an acquired taste and not everyone's choice. The downside of course is that you're almost guaranteed to get hepatitis sooner or later—probably sooner.

But then why do homosexuals engage in anal intercourse?

Because they don't have a lot of choices. (Incidentally, some heterosexuals engage in anal sex—and they do have a choice. But that's another story.)

As any man will testify, the erect penis screams for total stimulation if the sexual experience is going to be really satisfying. Rubbing it in your hand or having it sucked or pushing it between someone's legs is not enough. For real sexual release, the penis has to be engulfed by a warm grasping structure that can massage it intensively—and at orgasm squeeze out the last drop of ejaculation. The vagina is tailor-made for the penis, but that's the area that homosexuals don't want to get involved with. The closest structure available to them is the anus. In addition to the viruses, bacteria, and feces, the anus has another problem.

What's that?

Well, it's designed to keep what's inside from getting out, not to let what's outside get in. It has two powerful sphincters (muscular valves) that work to keep feces in the rectum until it's necessary to dispose of them. That's exactly the opposite of what homosexuals want to do. They want to push a long, hard (more or less) cylindrical penis into the anus. To do that, they have to fight two muscular rings—the external and the internal sphincters. The external sphincter is voluntary—a person can control it. But the internal sphincter is involuntary—beyond conscious control. That's one of the reasons that "poppers" are so popular.

"Poppers"? What are poppers?

As we saw in the chapter on Impotence, "Poppers" is the slang name for amyl nitrite, a common drug once used by doctors to dilate blood vessels. People who had heart disease cracked a little glass ampoule about the size of a peanut that held a few milliliters of transparent liquid. The liquid flowed onto cotton netting enclosing the ampoule and the patient inhaled the vapors. The blood vessels dilated and the pain cleared up. But devotees of anal sex discovered something else.

What did they discover?

Amyl nitrite also relaxes all the muscles in the body—including the anal sphincters. At the same time it seems to prolong orgasm—making it attractive to heterosexuals too.

But amyl nitrite isn't harmless, especially when you use it a lot, so it was gradually restricted in many countries. It frequently brings on a pounding headache and it can have more serious side effects as well. But the demand was still there, and substitutes like butyl nitrite quickly appeared. The chemical has since surfaced as "video-tape recorder head cleaner" and "carburetor cleaner" although most people use it for sex. As a result, the immense sales of amyl nitrite make it seem that Americans are fanatics about keeping their video-tape recorder heads and carburetors spotlessly clean.

So if you give your "bottom" partner (the one whom you are penetrating) a "popper" to pop, that will relax the muscles guarding his anus and anal sex gets a lot easier. Other things get easier too.

Other things? Like what?

Like postillioning, inserting objects, and "hand-balling." Those are three variations on anal sex that call for intrepid participants. Postillioning is a relatively mild activity where one homosexual inserts one or more fingers up into the anus of his partner. He can do it during masturbation, fellatio, anal sex, or just for fun. It's also possible for two chaps to do it to each other. The risks are the usual ones—inflicting cuts, tears, and infections on the anus and the delicate lining of the lower rectum. That's a relatively minor risk compared with those of the next step.

What's that?

Inserting objects into the rectum. As any surgeon will tell you, the rectum wasn't designed as a playground. It's really the far end of the large intestine. It starts at the anus and extends about 5 inches upward where it becomes the descending colon. It is tender and delicate and the walls are relatively thin—it's easy to poke a hole in them. When that happens, the feces spill out into the peritoneal cavity causing a very serious infection—and sometimes a permanent flat line on the electrocardiogram.

Homosexuals aren't the only ones who insert things into the rectum. Heterosexual couples do it too, but homosexuals seem to do

it much more frequently and with much more ingenuity and origi-
nality. Most doctors have had this kind of experience:

It is 2 A.M. Sunday morning. A young man stands forlornly at
the Emergency Room door. He is about twenty-six years old, short,
thin, with long bleached blond hair. He is drunk but sobering up
fast. Sweat clings to his pale pink silk shirt. He wants to see a doctor urgently. The intern motions him over to the examining table.
The patient walks with a strange, bent-over, crablike gait. As he
walks he talks—fast.

"Ya see, Doc, it was an accident. I couldn't help it, I . . ."

*"It's OK. You don't have to explain. Just get up on the
table."*

Obviously the intern has seen this problem before.

*The patient does as he is told. Pants off, on his hands and
knees, chest on the table, anus in the air. He is still talking.*

". . . slipped in the shower . . ."

*The intern is hardly listening—he knows it didn't hap-
pen that way and he is more worried about what he's going
to find. He inserts the anuscope, flicks on the light, and there
it is: a whiskey glass. He breathes a sigh of relief. Whiskey
glasses are easy, relatively speaking.*

*He snaps on a special rubber-cushioned clamp, squirts
in some lubricant, the patient gives a little gasp, and it's out.*

*Then things slow down a little and the doctor doesn't
mind talking:*

*"I always worry when I see these fellows come in. You
can spot them across the street—they all have this same
sideways walk. And they almost always say the same thing:*

" 'I slipped in the shower . . .'

*"It would have to be the world's most amazing shower!
You know it didn't happen that way. I just pray it's a shot
glass—they're a cinch. It usually happens like this: Two
chaps are having a big time on Saturday night—you know,
drinking or taking drugs and whooping it up. Finally one of
them rolls over and waits for his friend to mount him; only
his buddy slides in the first thing to come to hand instead,
often a whiskey glass. They're both so wiped out by then
they don't know what they're doing.*

*"I don't mind those things—they go in small end first,
and when you turn them they come out small end first. It's*

*the offbeat stuff that gets me. Like the time this old gentle-
man hobbled in. I flipped him over, popped in the scope,
started to snap on the light, and almost flipped—his whole
rectum was as bright as day! Someone had slipped the poor
fellow a flashlight—he was literally the most turned-on gent
in town. I had a devil of a time getting it out!"*

Flashlights aren't the worst—light bulbs are. Occasionally a
homosexual manages to pass one of these into the rectum. No
clamp can get a grip on them. Major surgery is urgently indicated
and there is real danger. If the bulb bursts, the result may be intestinal perforation, peritonitis, and death.

From time to time, articles appear in the medical journals listing
the objects removed from the rectums of patients, mostly males.
Some of the more routine items that enter the gastrointestinal systems of homosexuals via the exit are:

Pens, pencils, lipsticks, combs, pop bottles, tennis balls, electric
shavers, and enough apples, bananas, carrots, cucumbers, onions,
parsnips, potatoes, salamis, turnips, and zucchinis to stock a small
grocery store.

The most common items, as you can imagine, are bottles,
broomsticks, vibrators, and dildos.

Do all homosexuals do these things?

No. Sometimes they work the other way. Something that seems like a
good idea one moment may turn out to have unexpected complications.

The penis-in-a-bottle trick is an example. Occasionally a gentleman decides to masturbate by lubricating the mouth of a suitable
bottle. It seems like a handy substitute for an anus. He forces his
penis in (everyone likes a tight fit), thrusts in and out, finally ejaculates, and then tries to take his penis out.

Not so easy. As the penis is stimulated by friction against the
bottle, the erection gets harder. This squeezes the base of the organ
tightly, cutting off the circulation. After ejaculation the blood
can't drain out, the penis stays hard, and the bottle stays on.
You've seen the famous ship-in-a-bottle? Well, here's how it is
when a very anxious chap shows up at the hospital with a penis-
in-a-bottle.

The first time you see it, it's really quite impressive. A big red-
dish swollen phallus trapped in a glistening bottle. The doctor does

what the victim was afraid to do—he breaks the bottle. He usually explains the dangers and sends the repentant masturbator on his way. But there are more dangerous games than that.

For example?

"Hand-balling" for example. This is a strange kind of practice that has become more and more common and it works like this:

It usually requires a man who has had his anal sphincters fairly well stretched. (After enough anal sex, the "bottom" gets the external anal sphincter "broken in.") His partner, using a lot of lubrication, goes through the postillioning routine. The one who is being fingered—the "bottom"—often has his amyl nitrite "popper" ready. He inhales the chemical, the muscles of the anus relax, and the "top" squeezes his fingers together and slowly pushes his entire hand upward into the rectum. Once his hand is up there he can open his fingers, move around, and do anything that comes to mind. It's really quite impressive to watch, and of course, there are people who do it several times a day every day.

Who's that?

Doctors in hospitals. But they work under sterile conditions, use sterile gloves, give the patient anesthesia, and have other things in mind. For example, they might be retrieving some of the objects we mentioned before that found their way into the rectum.

Hand-balling is a risky business. It's possible to mutilate the inside of the intestine, poke a hole in it, introduce a bad infection, and inflict other kinds of trauma. You can damage these delicate structures on the way in as well as on the way out.

The best advice about hand-balling is what they say on some of those TV commercials:

"For professionals only. Do not attempt this at home!"

How do homosexuals meet each other?

Many different ways. In that vast homosexual subculture we mentioned, there are homosexual support groups, homosexual social clubs, and homosexual affinity groups. There are also specialized homosexual organizations dedicated to gardening, sports, music, political issues, employee groups, legal problems, and dozens of other areas.

Homosexuals also meet at other places.

What kinds of places?

Sometimes they meet informally and casually like heterosexuals do—at parties, sports events, at work. But they have a problem. A man can recognize a woman across the street. But if two men meet at a heterosexual party, how do they identify each other as homosexual? It isn't easy—but it's not impossible either. Frank tells his ideas:

> *"We call it 'gay-dar'—it works like radar but it's for identifying other gay people. It's mostly eye contact, Doctor. If you look at a fellow just a little bit longer than usual and he keeps up the glance, that's a clue. Sometimes the handshake is just a little too warm, or these days everyone is into the 'abrazo'—you know, men hugging each other. If he puts his cheek against your cheek and presses, that's another clue. It's really a subtle sort of thing, but you hardly ever make a mistake.*
>
> *"And then you can always wait around and see what happens. I mean, when you're sitting together eating like at a barbecue, you can sort of put your hand on his leg and see what happens. If he pulls back you can say, 'Sorry!' and pretend it was just a mistake. But if he doesn't pull away, then you just might have a new friend!"*

Are there any other places for homosexuals to meet?

There's always the gay bar. There are as many different gay bars as there are varieties of homosexuals. Some are sedate establishments, some are not so sedate, and some cater to very special tastes—like "leather" and "S&M" (Sadism and Masochism). There is one problem that has to be solved in these places. That's the question of identifying personal tastes. Since there are so many individual preferences in homosexual activities, when a fellow goes into a gay bar, he has to have some way to know what the other fellows want and are looking for. Homosexuals have evolved a very ingenious solution.

What's that?

The "hanky code." Although some people say that it's more of a put-on than a reality, it has solved some problems. It works like this:

Just pop a colored hanky in the back pocket of your jeans. If it's on the right-hand side it means you're interested in the passive form of whatever homosexual activity it indicates. If you wear it in the left pocket, it means you want to be active, or "on top." Here are some examples:

Color	Left Pocket	Right Pocket
Light blue	Wants to suck	Wants to be sucked
Red	Hand-baller	Hand-ballee
Light pink	Puts object in anus	Wants objects in
Gold	Two men looking for one	One man looking for two
Black-and-white check	Safe sex top	Safe sex bottom
Medium blue	Cop	Wants cop
Mustard	Big penis	Wants big penis
White	Wants white bottom	Wants white top
Black-and-white stripe	Wants black bottom	Wants black top
Black velvet	Takes pictures	Poses

The list goes on and on, but you get the idea.

Homosexuals can also meet new friends via personal ads. There's some risk involved—you're going to be alone, naked, and defenseless with someone you don't really know anything about. A typical ad might run something like this:

Seeking Friendly Sex . . .

GWM, 25 y/o, 5'11", 196#, abundant curly chest hair, 7 inches cut. Bottom. Moderately passive. Bears OK. Looking for kix. Men or Tourists welcome. Making out, sucking, anal with condom. Kinky OK. I want broad shoulders to sleep on afterward. No lasting ties. HIV Neg. Call Chet.

What does that mean?

It means that Chet is a Gay White Male. His measurements follow. His penis is 7 inches long (At least he says it is . . .) and he is circumcised. He will accept a large hairy partner—a bear. The rest is self-explanatory except for the last item: "HIV Negative." That was presumably on the day he wrote the ad. Do we know what has happened since then?

Sometimes these ads work out fine—and sometimes they trigger another item in the newspaper:

> Police found the nude body of Zinz Zoblinzt, a graduate student, in his apartment early this morning. According to the Medical Examiner he had been beaten to death with a heavy candlestick. Neighbors reported seeing him admit an unknown man shortly before midnight. No motive was immediately apparent.

Do homosexuals have their own language?

Not precisely a language, but a private argot that has its own fey humor. Here are a few examples:

- **Auntie**: an aging homosexual.
- **Bear**: a large, hairy male homosexual.
- **Breeder**: an impolite way of referring to heterosexuals.
- **Buns**: buttocks.
- **Butch**: a masculine, usually supermasculine, homosexual.
- **Camp**: be obviously and obnoxiously homosexual.
- **Chicken**: a young homosexual.
- **Chicken Dinner**: sex with a teenager.
- **Chicken Hawk**: a homosexual who looks for underage boys.
- **Closet Queen**: a homosexual who denies or suppresses his homosexual feelings; usually intended as an insult; can also refer to a homosexual who is not currently active.
- **Do**: suck a penis.
- **Do for Trade**: give him some homosexual action.
- **Drag**: female attire worn by homosexuals and transvestites.

- **Drag King**: derived from Drag Queen; a woman who likes to dress like a man.
- **Drag Queen**: a homosexual who comes on in drag.
- **Drag Show**: a performance by female impersonators.
- **Fag Hag**: a woman who is attracted to male homosexuals.
- **FI**: a female impersonator.
- **Fish**: a woman (contemptuously).
- **Fishwife**: a male homosexual's real wife.
- **Fruit Fly**: same as Fag Hag.
- **Gay Dirt**: a play on the expression "pay dirt"; an attractive young man paid by the police to trap homosexuals.
- **Girl**: an effeminate homosexual.
- **Golden Retriever**: a urinal.
- **Grimm's Fairy**: an older male homosexual.
- **Hustler**: a male prostitute.
- **Meat**: a penis.
- **Nelly**: an effeminate homosexual.
- **Queen**: same as Nelly.
- **RG**: a real girl (in contrast to an effeminate homosexual).
- **Rough Trade**: a vicious or dangerous homosexual.
- **S&M**: sadomasochism or slave-master.
- **Sappho Daddy-O**: a heterosexual man who likes to associate with lesbian women; the male equivalent of a Fag Hag.
- **Seafood**: a homosexual sailor.
- **Straight**: a heterosexual.
- **Trade**: a homosexual looking for action.
- **Trick**: a partner for a transient homosexual encounter.
- **Troll**: a homosexual who is cruising and forces himself on other gays.
- **Trouble**: a Butch who is likely to cause trouble.
- **Twinkie**: a young, fresh-looking homosexual.
- **Wrinkle-Room**: a gay bar frequented by aging homosexuals.

This is just a small sample—the list goes on and on.

Are there many female homosexuals?

As we mentioned, no one knows the exact number, but there are probably about the same percentage of homosexual females as there are homosexual males—between 2 and 10 percent and probably closer to the first figure.

Female homosexuals are called "lesbians"—a charming and poetic name taken from the Greek island of Lesbos. Sappho, a talented female poet, lived there and was thought to be homosexual. Lesbians are not quite as high profile in society as male homosexuals.

How come?

Social customs. If a male accountant shows up at work wearing a red evening gown and a pearl necklace plus high heels, there won't be much doubt about where he's coming from. But if a female accountant appears at the office wearing a blue pinstripe double-breasted suit with a masculine cut, a white dress shirt, and a blue necktie, no one will give her a second glance.

Women can cross-dress and no one blinks. And a "Butch" lesbian can wear masculine clothes with ease.

"Butch"? Does that mean the same as in male homosexual slang?

Not quite. "Butch" is a term used to describe a masculine type lesbian and "Femme" is a term used to describe a feminine type lesbian. But things have changed and the distinctions can be very subtle. These days, some lesbians don't want to be stereotyped.

Notwithstanding, there are many subtle variations of these terms. There are "soft butches" and "hard butches," "top butches" and "bottom femmes." There is also a rare category known as a "top femme"—an effeminate lesbian who nevertheless takes the initiative in sexual matters.

What do lesbians do to each other sexually?

They do the best they can. Technically, it's complicated. Male homosexuals have a penis and they can put it wherever they can find an opening. But although lesbians don't have a penetrating organ, they do have a tremendously sensitive structure—the vagina—that is designed to be penetrated, filled, and frictioned. They use ingenuity and inventiveness and come up with some solutions.

Lesbian sex often starts off with breast caressing and nipple play. Then it usually moves on to stroking the clitoris and the area at the entrance to the vagina. Then it may progress to inserting a finger or two into the vagina and sliding them rhythmically in and out.

One of the most popular moves in lesbian sex is cunnilingus—applying a hot wet tongue to the clitoris and vagina. Most lesbians pride themselves on their clitoris-licking technique. They claim that they can satisfy women better than men can because they know exactly how it feels when someone does it to them and they know where to aim their tongue and lips. It may be true—but only up to a point.

Up to what point?

The next step. A lesbian can do anything a man can—until it comes to the last little detail—pushing a hard penis into an eager vagina. That's where most—but not all—lesbians have to stop.

Not all lesbians? Some women can go beyond that?

Yes, a very few. There are a very small number of women with hypertrophy of the clitoris. Their organs can be 2 or even 3 inches long when they are erect. With some acrobatic contortions, they can get their clitoris to the entrance to the vagina and come closer than any other woman to heterosexual intercourse. But some lesbians have another solution.

What's that?

The magic of electronics. These days the electric vibrator has reached new heights. It's no longer just a battery and a buzzer. Now high tech is knocking at the Gates of Love with hummers, ticklers, tappers, zappers, and every possible programmed sensation known to the electronic geniuses of Hong Kong, Taiwan, and points east.

And that news is not lost on lesbians. They apply various styles and sizes of vibrating plastic penises to the clitoris, urethra, vagina, and anus of their friends.

Do lesbians go for anal sex too?

Yes, since the anus has an excellent nerve supply. But they're not as involved with anal sex as male homosexuals. It's really a matter of individual preference with them and it's not "center stage" like with their male counterparts. Of course, there are many different tastes among lesbians, but for most, the main action is at the vagina. And that brings up a problem.

What kind of problem?

The problem is what to put into the vagina. Most women, when they get to a certain level of sexual excitement, have a desire to feel something filling their vagina and massaging it more and more vigorously until they reach orgasm. That's a challenge to lesbians.

The vibrator helps solve the problem, and its intense electric vibrations spread over the clitoris, the vaginal walls, the urethra, and radiate downward into the anal area. That is usually enough for orgasm. And there's another ingenious way too.

What's that?

The strap-on-penis. It's usually about 6 inches long and about 2 inches in diameter, made of foam-filled latex or plastic. The apparatus is rigged to a leather or nylon harness that you sort of step into and fasten with straps. It isn't cheap—the combo can run about a hundred dollars or more. One lesbian slips into it, and then slips it into her partner. As the catalog says:

> *"Guaranteed not to shift—even if you're on your back, on your side, or on your knees."*

That should take care of every foreseeable situation. And there's even a rubber penis with a snap-on cap that is a miniature vibrator for more stimulation.

Do some people actually use these things?

Certainly. And it solves a problem for them. (Remember, this is a medical-scientific book and we're seeing what happens—not whether it's "right" or "wrong." That's another book to be written by someone in another profession.) Dildos and vibrators and all the rest of the sexual gadgets serve a purpose.

And a lot of thought goes into them. For example, there is another type of rubber penis that you can strap on—but not to your pubic area. You fasten this one onto your chin. It has straps that go around your neck and the back of your head and the penis pokes forward from the chin. It sticks straight out and as you slide it into the vagina, your mouth and tongue are right in front so you can lick the clitoris. Some lesbians like it for the new outlook it gives them. But not all lesbians like imitation penises or dildos.

Why not?

They just don't like to have anything in their vaginas during sex. They don't like the idea of being "penetrated." So they go for trib-adism—where one woman lies on top of another and they rub pubic areas and clitorises together. Lesbians can achieve orgasm this way without anything resembling a penis getting in the way.

Do lesbians cruise like male homosexuals?

Not usually. Women homosexuals tend to be more reserved— besides, women have more latitude in relating to each other. They can kiss on meeting, hold hands, share clothes, and all the rest with-out seeming out of place. If you see your local gas station attendant giving a male customer a peck on the cheek as he's filling the tank, you'll wonder. But if you see the lady who has the flower shop greet a female customer with a kiss, you won't even blink an eye.

Of course, there are all kinds of lesbians. Some are calm and laid back, others are militant and aggressive. Lesbians have their own subculture as well. Their slang illustrates it well.

For example?

These days, some lesbians call themselves "Dykes." It used to be an insult, but they have wisely taken the sting out of it. They also have special—and very descriptive—names for lesbian topics.

For instance, a "Granola Dyke" is a natural-organic-ecology oriented lesbian, often well-respected by other lesbians. Some les-bians speak of "Serial Monogamy." That's a polite way of referring to someone who changes partners frequently—plenty of "friends" but one at a time.

If bad news strikes a lesbian relationship it can come in the form of the dreaded "LBD"—"Lesbian Bed Death." That's when two lesbians who are getting bored in a long-term relationship one night undress and get in bed together. And much to their disappointment, instead of sex—they just fall asleep.

Is homosexuality increasing?

It's hard to tell because the statistics aren't reliable. The visibility of homosexuality is increasing because more and more homosexuals are openly displaying their homosexuality instead of denying it. The awareness of homosexuality is increasing as more homosexual social issues appear in the media.

The most important thing is not whether there are more homosexuals or fewer homosexuals in this world. It seems clear that homosexuality is here to stay. For that reason it's important for everyone—parents, children, teachers, and government officials—to learn about it and understand it.

Chapter 9
MASTURBATION

What is masturbation?

Masturbation is sexual stimulation designed to produce an orgasm through any means except sexual intercourse. The term comes from the Latin word *masturbari,* which means "to pollute oneself." It is also known by such imposing terms as self-pollution, manustrupation, and onanism.

A lot of people have always felt guilty about masturbation, and these ominous words haven't made them feel any better. Especially onanism.

Where does that word come from?

The Bible. In Genesis 38:8–10, Judah tells his son Onan to marry and have sex with his brother's wife. Onan is reluctant.

> *And Judah said unto Onan, Go in unto thy brother's wife, and marry her, and raise up seed to thy brother.*
> *And Onan knew that the seed should not be his; and it came to pass, when he went in unto his brother's wife, that he spilled it on the ground, lest that he should give seed to his brother.*

*And the thing which he did displeased the Lord: where-
fore he slew him also.*

For hundreds of years this passage was used by clergymen and
parents to scare the daylights out of little children who masturbated. Their translation was "If you masturbate, God will come and
kill you."

Careful reading of the passage makes it appear more likely that
Onan was engaging in a primitive form of birth control—pulling his
penis out at the moment of ejaculation and spilling the semen on the
ground. His execution seems to have resulted from his refusal to
fertilize his sister-in-law rather than from "spilling his seed."

Should children be kept from masturbation? Is masturbation harmful?

The only thing harmful about masturbation is the guilt that is
drummed into children who admit to masturbating, by parents who
may themselves masturbate but don't admit it. Virtually every
human being, at one time or another, in one way or another, has
masturbated. Most of them have felt overwhelmingly guilty
because of it. But most of them have kept on masturbating.

Some of the "terrible" things masturbation is supposed to cause
are pimples on the face, "loss of manhood," "pollution," and weakness. Of these afflictions only pimples are a recognized disease.
Virtually all children develop pimples at puberty. Virtually all children are actively masturbating at that time. Therefore it's much
more reasonable to conclude that "Pimples cause Masturbation."
No minister, moralist, teacher, or scientific researcher has ever
shown any evidence that masturbation is harmful in any way.

Why do people masturbate?

The primary reason is—masturbation is fun! Certainly not as much
fun as full-fledged sexual intercourse, but pretty close. And of
course, that's precisely what masturbation is supposed to be—a substitute form of gratification when sexual intercourse is impossible.

Masturbation is most common in early puberty when sexual
objects are unattainable and social prohibitions against intercourse
are enforceable and enforced. As social and sexual maturity proceeds,
masturbation gradually recedes and is replaced by copulation. At

times when sexual opportunities dwindle, it may reappear, and later in life it sometimes predominates again. Childhood and old age have been called the "Golden Years of Masturbation," since sexual feelings are present but the means to satisfy them are sometimes lacking.

When does masturbation usually begin?

Deliberate masturbation may occur in children as early as six months of age. Usually by two or three the pattern of masturbation is well established. From that point on, things don't change much until puberty.

Young boys usually masturbate by grasping the erect penis gently with the hand and stroking it repeatedly from tip to base. Others simply pull at the glans or head of the organ. Less often, childhood masturbation takes the form of lying prone on a bed and rubbing the erect penis against the mattress.

Masturbation in little girls centers around the clitoris; many very young girls are unaware of the existence of the vagina. Rubbing is the most popular form of activity, and any object can be pressed into use. Pillows, dolls, and balled-up sheets or blankets all serve the purpose for the time being. One of the favorite targets for masturbation is a nice soft cuddly Teddy-Bear. Strangely enough that cute little Teddy-Bear can show up again in the sexual activities of adult life! And in a most fascinating way. (See "Sexual Perversions.")

Why do children begin to masturbate so early?

Because their mothers teach them to. Frequently it develops like this:

Marie is in the pediatrician's office. She is worried. Her four-year-old boy, Jimmie, in her words, "plays with himself." This is how she tells it:

"But doctor, it's the most embarrassing thing in the world. I just can't stand it any longer!"

"What seems to be the trouble with Jimmie?"

"The trouble? Why he does this horrid thing to himself all the time! He takes his . . . his . . . his male, you know, and plays with it, right in front of me!"

"How long has he been doing this?"

"For about a year now but it's getting worse! Last week he did it in front of my mother!"

"Perhaps he has some irritation of his penis—that's common in young children."

"Why, I can't imagine how that could happen. I wash his . . . his . . . organ very carefully at least twice a day. I spend at least fifteen minutes each time cleaning it."

"Twice a day? That's interesting. How long have you been doing that?"

"Oh, about a year."

Just in case Jimmie didn't figure it out for himself, his mother showed him that gentle rubbing of his penis feels good. He got the message and started to produce these good feelings himself. But he finds it hard to understand the rest. If he plays with his own penis, his mother gets furious. If she does it, it's OK. Besides, there must be something really great about the whole business if mother won't let him do it. The other things she forbids, like candy and staying up late, are a lot of fun too.

This is the characteristic pattern of masturbation: discovery (or revelation by mother) of pleasant sexual feelings and the start of masturbation—prohibition (usually by mother)—guilt—continued masturbation with added guilt. The same thing happens, of course, with little girls.

Do children really have sexual feelings?

Certainly, although not in the adult sense. The combination of pleasant sensations that come with genital stimulation and curiosity about sexual mysteries is plenty to keep them occupied for most of the childhood years. For small children, sex is really a mystery.

Remember the story about the three-year-old who gets up one night for a drink of water? He walks by his parents' bedroom and hears some noises. He peeks through the door and sees that they are having sex. He shakes his head in amazement and says to himself:

"Look at that! And they punish me for sucking my thumb!"

At puberty, things begin to change.

What happens then?

The sudden surge of hormones causes dramatic alterations in the sexual organs as well as the sexual feelings. This is the period of preoccupation with sex. For the first time, in an important way, orgasm enters the picture. Up until now, masturbation was primarily self-fondling with pleasant sensations. Now something new has been added—the big payoff.

In boys the first orgasms are dry—no seminal fluid, no sperm. Later on fluid appears, followed by sperm in increasing numbers. Girls begin to feel real genital tension for the first time. Erection of the clitoris and engorgement of the labia minora force their attention to their sexual organs. Menstruation also makes them gradually more conscious of sexual matters.

Do girls have orgasms at this time too?

They can but not nearly as frequently as boys. Their masturbation is usually not as direct either. They tend to continue to rub against things like playground equipment, especially swings and slides. Haven't you noticed that girls spend a lot more time on the swings in the playground than the boys? Climbing trees and sliding down poles are also very effective mechanical means of rubbing their clitoris and labia.

Boys are much more active sexually at this stage and are beginning to branch out into other forms of masturbation.

Other forms of masturbation?

Yes. Group masturbation and mutual masturbation. A certain percentage of boys around the age of twelve to fourteen, besides masturbating alone, also masturbate in groups. That's the famous "circle jerk." It works like this:

Three to six boys get together at a clubhouse, in a field, or any other private place. They usually bring cigarettes and girlie magazines. This adds to the "forbidden" atmosphere.

Gradually they bring out their penises and begin to masturbate. There's generally a competition; the one who reaches orgasm first is the winner. (An interesting contrast to later life, where the man who climaxes soonest is usually the loser.) Sometimes two boys will go off by themselves and masturbate together. Occasionally they work up to masturbating each other.

Isn't group and mutual masturbation similar to homosexual behavior?

Not really. The sexual pressure that builds up in adolescent boys is tremendous. It has to find some outlet, and, at least in our society, approved sexual outlets for thirteen-year-old boys are few and far between. Somehow basketball and volleyball just don't do the trick. The testosterone is pouring into the bloodstream, their penis pops to attention at a moment's notice, and something has to give. These types of masturbation are a reflection of this period. Usually they are replaced by heterosexual activity as the boys mature.

Do girls do the same thing?

In a slightly different way. Adolescent "crushes" and close physical contact with other girls, such as hand-holding, arms-around-the-waist, and occasionally kissing, are common at this stage. Group and mutual masturbation are rare but do occur. Although parents don't usually think about it that way, "pajama parties" lend themselves to masturbatory experiments. These activities actually pave the way for bigger things to come. In the middle teens, adult-type masturbation usually begins.

What is that like?

In boys, it is masturbation with sexual fantasies. During the process of stroking the penis, the boy thinks of sexual scenes. It may be an imaginary episode or a reliving of a particularly exciting sexual experience. One boy, Ted, describes it this way:

> "I started 'doing it' about a year ago when I was twelve. Some other guys told me about it but I didn't believe them so I tried it myself. I don't think it's right, but I just can't help it—I get the urge and then before I know it I'm doing it again. I feel lousy afterward.
>
> "Most of the time I just think about different girls I like— you know, their bodies and everything. Then I think about the party when this girl let me put my hand inside her panties. Every time I think about that I want to do it some more."

In many cases masturbation acts as a bridge helping to make the transition to adult sexuality.

What about girls?

Adult-type masturbation in girls serves a similar function. This is one way the sexual equipment is, so to speak, broken in. The nervous pathways are established and the idea of sexual stimulation proceeding to orgasm is reinforced. At that stage most girls masturbate this way:

Gentle stroking of the pubic area just above the vulva initiates erection of the clitoris and swelling of the labia minora. As sexual excitement increases the girl begins firmer pressure downward toward the clitoris, without actually touching it. With approaching orgasm, the shaft of the clitoris is sometimes gently kneaded with the index or third finger. Rarely do girls manipulate the head of the clitoris because of its extreme sensitivity. At this point, and especially in virgins, masturbation by insertion of objects into the vagina is rare.

Some girls masturbate by merely rubbing the vulva. Enough pressure is transmitted to the clitoris to begin the cycle and carry it through to orgasm.

Isn't it bad for a girl to masturbate like that? Doesn't all that attention to the clitoris interfere with her sexual responses later on?

Girls who masturbate are often threatened that they will have trouble getting "adjusted" after marriage because their sexual interest is fixed on the clitoris instead of the vagina. Like many sexual threats, this one is in far left field too. Since the focal point of sexual gratification in the female, before, during, and after marriage is the clitoris, masturbation of the clitoris can only help her to *get* "adjusted." There just isn't anything bad about masturbation—with one exception that we'll see in a moment.

Is it true that some girls can achieve an orgasm just by stimulating their breasts?

It is true that a number of women masturbate by fondling their breasts, especially the nipples. And it's possible for some women to reach an orgasm just that way. But often there's something else going on. Because of their anatomy, women can masturbate anywhere at any time. All they have to do is cross their legs and rub their thighs together. This moves the labia and clitoris against each other and soon triggers an orgasm. Very often, some women who say they have orgasms while playing with their breasts are also doing a little thigh-rubbing—sometimes without even being aware of it. A lady on the verge of orgasm doesn't think about all those little details. After the heterosexual preliminaries have begun, the pattern of masturbation changes to imitate more closely the mechanics of petting.

What are "the mechanics of petting"?

"Petting" is the nice word for mutual masturbation. Just as you "pet" a pussycat you can "pet" a clitoris and vagina. And just like you can "pet" a dog, you can "pet" a penis. Masturbation, in the broadest sense, is sexual stimulation leading to orgasm except by penis-vagina or oral contact. Whether a girl strokes her own clitoris or her boyfriend caresses it for her, if that's how she is going to reach orgasm, it is masturbation. That doesn't make it bad, it just describes it.

At a drive-in movie or at a summer beach party, teenage girls are introduced to all kinds of new experiences. They become aware of the sensitivity of the inner part of the thighs, the mons veneris (the pubic area), the prepuce of the clitoris, and if their dates are bold enough, the vagina itself. These are the necessary preliminaries leading to normal mature sexual activity.

Later, when she masturbates, the girl tries to reproduce these feelings. She may begin to explore the vagina herself and determine the most sensitive areas.

Isn't it better if she finds this out after she's married?

That's fine, if she can get married at the age of fourteen. Otherwise it's asking a lot to expect a healthy, sexy young female to wait seven long years to find out what it's all about. In certain other cultures, she would be initiated into the intricacies of her own sexuality by the older women of her tribe. They would teach her to masturbate and ceremonially help her to destroy the hymen at the onset of menstruation. In some tribes, gigantically elongated labia from masturbation are considered desirable and extremely attractive sexually.

In our culture the older women of the tribe simply tell a young girl:

"Don't touch yourself down there!"

and

"Save it until after you're married!"

It doesn't seem to be the kind of help she needs. . . .

What kinds of things do girls insert into the vagina?

The most common object is the most available one—a finger. Many women learn by experience that stroking the roof of the vagina also stimulates the clitoris and intensifies orgasm. Some women like to insert objects into their vagina to masturbate and some don't. There is no problem of lubrication, unlike the male, since adequate supplies of natural lubricant are available. Candles, cucumbers, carrots, darning eggs, and many other household items used to be among the favorites. But things have changed. These days, women who are serious about masturbating have a whole new world at their fingertips.

Like what?

Like twenty-page catalogs of high-tech artificial penises for ladies. An imitation penis, for some unknown reason, is called a dildo. No one seems to know where the name originated—it might just be the sound that one of these makes as it goes in and out of the vagina.

The earliest known dildos have been found in ancient Egyptian tombs; they were made of clay. Since the Egyptian nobility had buried with them only things of great value that they planned to used in the next world the dildo must have been very important to Egyptian ladies.

Apparently these devices were popular in biblical times too. They are mentioned in Ezekiel 16:17:

> *"Thou hast also taken thy fair jewels of my gold and of my silver, which I had given thee, and madest to thyself images of men, and didst commit whoredom with them. . . ."*

Obviously the reference to "images of men" does not refer to the entire man but merely to a very special part of the male anatomy. While few dildos have been made of gold or silver, for economic reasons, nearly every other material has been pressed into service at some time. In the Middle Ages sealing wax was cheap and plentiful. It quickly took on the warmth of the body and softened just enough to provide a "natural" feel. Some primitive tribes used clay, unglazed for the common people, glazed for the wives of chiefs. Unglazed clay is a little rough and has the disadvantage of shattering under vigorous usage; cleaning up can be painful.

With the discovery of vulcanization of rubber, the French, who have always displayed ingenuity and verve in sexual matters, developed what they cheerfully called the *consolateur,* or consoler. Made of natural gum rubber in the shape of a long, firm but pliable penis, the device was fitted with a reservoir made in the form of a scrotum. This was filled with hot water (some ladies preferred milk), which circulated through the entire apparatus to give the effect of body heat. With the deluxe model, at the moment of orgasm, all the lady had to do was to give a good hard squeeze to the testicles, which pumped a jet of warm fluid into the vagina at the perfect moment. It had its disadvantages: some ladies got so excited during real sex with their husbands that, by the force of habit, as orgasm approached, they reached out and gave a good hard squeeze. . . . You can imagine the rest.

Asian technical know-how now dominates the field. Gone are the days of cream-colored plastic cylinders discreetly hidden in the drawer of the bedside table. Now there are dildos for every taste— including some very special ones.

For example?

How about a soft pink plastic penis 7 1/2 inches long and 1 1/2 inches in diameter? It's made of special "jelly" plastic so that once it warms up it feels more like a real penis. That's an important point. Like the gynecologist's speculum, all dildos need to be warmed before using. Otherwise it's like having sex on the slopes of Mount Everest with Big Foot.

Some women just want to masturbate to relieve sexual tension if their husband or male friend is away or unavailable. They usually simply rub, roll, stroke, fondle, and massage the clitoris to the point of orgasm. But other women like the feeling of being penetrated while they massage the erect clitoris. For them, the plastic penis gives satisfaction. But there's more to it than that.

More than that?

Yes. There are women who find that adding fantasies to their masturbation increases the excitement. That's one of the reasons dildos come in so many amazing forms—to satisfy so many different sexual fantasies. For example, most artificial phalluses for masturbation are the color of Caucasian skin. But you can also buy dildoes in several other shades. A woman who puts fantasy foremost can buy a penis that is—supposedly—an exact duplicate of any famous porn star's. Here's the advertising copy that accompanies it:

> *"Finally! Stan the Man can be yours! All of him! A full 9 inches of Stan's Manhood cast from his actual endowments in yummy soft plastic! Complete with suction cup at the base. In a plain wrapper."*

When you undo the plain wrapper, you find a plastic replica of a penis complete with engorged veins and oversized plastic testicles. Actually it looks like Stan had a bad case of priapism (see Chapter 2). And it looks like the folks in Hong Kong who made the casting put Stan's wee-wee under a big magnifying glass when they molded the plastic. But that's what fantasies are about, isn't it?

What about the suction cup?

Oh yes, the suction cup. Since the phallus isn't attached to Stan anymore it can be hard to manage, especially at the moment of orgasm. So just wet the big suction cup where the penis used to be hooked to Stan, and slap it down on any smooth surface at any angle.

Some women like to sit on the phallus since it gives them more freedom of movement. Since it is flexible, others bend it upward, stick it against the wall and walk into it backward. It also has a vibrator inside, so the idea presumably is that you turn it on and then it turns you on. The possibilities ignite the imagination.

What about vibrators?

Almost all the upmarket penises include battery-powered vibrators—there are even some variable speed models for those who want to start slow and work up to a climax. Almost every problem has been solved by modern dildo designers.

For example, what do you do if you like to masturbate in a nice tub of warm water? The motor in an ordinary vibrator will give one quick sizzle and stop forever. But don't worry, you can find a "totally waterproof" dildo with vibrator that purrs along like a nuclear submarine. But it's not only for tub-time. The ads for this item say:

"Drop it in your purse for fun-filled hours in the pool!"

You may have fun-filled hours in the pool but you can also get a no-fun vaginal infection. Even the most sparkling pool water isn't something you want to pump into your vagina. If a woman is going to masturbate with these "toys" she has to be meticulous in the way she manages them.

What should she do?

Simple hygiene is usually good enough. Just wash everything with soap and water before and after using them. And keep them to yourself. A shared dildo is like a shared penis—it can bring you surprises you never imagined.

If you want to keep water-fun less intrusive, there's a sponge with a vibrator inside. Slip into the shower, put the sponge against your clitoris and vagina, and feel all your worries fade away—and you get clean in the process.

Incidentally, the vibrating sponge is one of the several masturbating "toys" that a woman can share with a man. (More about that as we go along.)

But isn't it abnormal to masturbate with dildos and vibrators?

And immoral? And indecent? That's the problem with sex. Doesn't it seem that someone always wants to know if you're having too much fun—so they can put a stop to it? When sexual tension builds up in a man or a woman and they have no satisfactory way to express it, what should they do? Take a cold shower?

Who has the right to say that standing under a torrent of frigid water and freezing your already tense and overheated body is better for you than just to masturbate and relieve the normal sexual tension? Masturbation serves an important purpose in human sexuality. It's not a substitute for sexual intercourse, but sometimes it has to do until real sex comes along. And some of these ingenious and innovative devices can make getting relief simpler and more satisfactory. Of course, some of them shouldn't be taken too seriously—as the signs in the Penny Arcades used to say, they are "For Amusement Only!" Take the "Passion Panties" for example.

What are they like?

They look like any other pair of ladies' undies—black lace and skimpy cut. The big difference is the little vibrator the size and shape of an egg sewn into the crotch where it nuzzles against the clitoris. A wire goes up the lady's sleeve and controls the speed and intensity of the vibes. So, at work while she's typing up the boss's speech, she can just press a button and vibrate herself to another world. Or at the bus stop—when the bus is late and it's boring to wait—just tap a button and who cares about the bus?

There's an even more fascinating variation on the "Passion Panties."

What's that?

"Pager Passion." These are the same kind of panties but instead of a vibrator they have a little pouch for a pager located where the vibrator used to be—right up against the clitoris. When your "significant other" calls your pager service, the pager vibrates and you know that he is thinking about you. And in this case, you know *exactly* what he is thinking about you.

The ladies have some obvious advantages when it comes to vibration. Their orgasms can be inconspicuous and dry. They can do things that no man would ever attempt. The Wild Butterfly is an example of the female advantage.

What's the "Wild Butterfly"?

It's a nice soft plastic gadget that looks like a butterfly with its little wings spread apart. It's about 3 inches by 3 inches and fits right over a lady's sexual equipment. The head part of the butterfly sits on the clitoris while the body reaches about to the vaginal opening. The vibrator is built in. But the interesting thing about the "butterfly" is that it comes with a harness so you can wear it under your clothes. That means—like the "Passion Panties"—you can press a button and blast off anywhere and anytime. In some universities female students sit through lectures on things like "Post-Modern Concepts in North African Existentialistic Philosophy" with an ecstatic expression on their faces. The professor still hasn't figured out their little secret. But there's something even more advanced.

What's that?

The "Secret Scorpion." It's like the "Butterfly" except as we all know, the scorpion has a tail. In this case the tail hangs down between the lady's legs. As the clitoris and labia are vibrated by the body of the "Secret Scorpion," the tail can find its way into the wearer's vagina—or into her anus if she feels like it.

Do women combine anal play with their masturbation?

Some do, although it's usually the exception. But there are dildos for every taste, and those ladies aren't left out. One of the most impressive units has two penises. One is the usual 7 inch phallus with another penis below it about half the size—and the usual central vibrator. The idea is to lubricate both of them well and slide one into the vagina and the other into the anus. Obviously a device like that is an acquired taste. And speaking of acquired tastes, some of the dildos seem more in fun than serious masturbation tools.

For example, after all the jokes about sex and rabbits, there's a vibrating dildo in the form of a soft plastic penis with little bunny ears coming out of the base and pointing upward. The bunny has an elongated body and long pink ears. You are supposed to insert the penis in your vagina, turn on the motor, and that cute little bunny tickles your clitoris with his ears! Of course, if you're sentimental about Peter Rabbit maybe you don't want such an intimate relationship with his ears.

There are other dildos with talented animals mounted alongside. There's one with an elephant. While the dildo goes in and out, the elephant's trunk tickles your clitoris—and guess where that nice long elephant's tail is going?

There's also a plastic phallus with a miniature beaver clinging to the side. When you insert the main shaft and turn on the motor, the little beaver licks at your clitoris. All these animal dildos can be reversed so that the critters enter the vagina and massage the so-called "G-Spot." (More about that in Chapter 7.)

Do women really use those dildos?

Yes, they do but not necessarily the way they are advertised—or portrayed in those porno videos. Alice describes her experience. She is a commercial artist, twenty-eight, married five years, and the mother of two children:

*"Doctor, I have to be honest with you. I do masturbate
sometimes, especially when my husband, Bill, is out of town.
I miss him and I miss sex. So I have one of those, I guess you
call them 'dildos,' and I use it.*

*"But really it's more of a vibrator than anything else. The
first thing I do is get comfortable in bed. Then I turn it on and
rub it against me just above my clitoris. It's too much to stand
if I put it right on the clitoris itself. Then my clitoris starts getting bigger and I gradually slide the thing up inside myself."*

Alice paused for a moment to think.

*"Before I had the children I never needed anything
inside when I masturbated but now it feels good to have
something in there. I never push it in and out. Just having
something inside me is enough. I rub my clitoris with my
other hand faster and faster until I climax and that's it!"*

Is that the way most women do it?

No, some are very inventive. Quite a few women masturbate in the
bath. You know those "pulsating shower heads" with the choice of
sprays that you can unhook and hold in your hand? Many women
spread their legs just a little bit and direct the spray between their
legs. The warm water jet pulsing against their clitoris can bring on
an immense orgasm. And by choosing different types of sprays,
they can have a whole range of exciting feelings.

But it doesn't stop there. You know those hand-held jets they
sell to clean between your teeth? Just imagine how that tiny pulsating stream of warm water feels against a throbbing clitoris.

Masturbation serves an important purpose—it relieves sexual
tension, it's enjoyable, and sometimes it can be therapeutic.

Therapeutic? How can masturbation be therapeutic?

Here's an example. Take a man who is seventy-one years old. His
wife, age sixty-nine, has had open-heart surgery and needs about
six weeks to recover before she can have sex again. What does the
gentleman do while he's waiting? Take a cold shower every night
and every morning?

That won't solve his problem—and it'll give him two more
problems. One of them is dry skin. The other is more serious: possible
impotence. The truth is that a man in his seventies who doesn't have

an ejaculation for a month is unlikely to be able to have one ever again. There are exceptions, of course, but in the seventies, more than ever before, it's a matter of "Use It or Lose It!"

If he masturbates at least once a week—and preferably twice a week—he will have every chance of keeping his sexual equipment working.

What if he can't get an erection?

There's a way around that too. The important thing at that stage is to exercise the whole set of ejaculatory reflexes—it's a kind of sexual calisthenics. You might call it "orgasmic aerobics." Even if he doesn't have an erection, all he has to do is carefully lubricate the head of his penis—cold cream, petroleum jelly, almost anything will do. Then he applies a vibrator to the head of his organ. The ideal vibrator for this is one that has a soft rubber suction cup on the end. If he places the suction cup on the head of his penis, he should get the results he is looking for. He can experiment with the setting—slow, fast, whatever feels the best.

In a few moments—even without an erection—he will feel an orgasm beginning to build, and shortly afterward he should have an orgasm and/or an ejaculation. If he practices his "orgasmic aerobics" regularly, he may find that he will have stronger and more frequent erections. There are other benefits too.

What are they?

Fewer prostate problems. Infrequent—or nonexistent—orgasms produce congestion of the prostate. A swollen congested prostate is no fun—ask any man who has had one. Masturbation can also be therapeutic for women.

How is that?

There are some women who just can't reach an orgasm (see Chapter 7). Some of them can't have an orgasm during regular intercourse and some just have never been able to have an orgasm at all. Masturbation with a vibrator and/or a dildo can almost always trigger an orgasm. For the women who have never had one, it opens the door to a whole new world. For women who have trouble reaching a climax during intercourse, there's another trick that sometimes helps.

She and her partner start off in the usual way. It's important to make sure that she reaches a reasonable level of sexual excitement. The best indicator is the clitoris—it should be tense and swollen, the equivalent of an erect penis. If that doesn't happen with the usual stroking and gentle rubbing, she can gently put the tip of the lubricated vibrator either above or below the clitoris—not on it. That should make the clitoris come to attention promptly. At this stage it's better if she controls the vibrator rather than her partner because she knows what she's feeling better than anyone else.

Then it's time to insert the penis and start the action. As intercourse proceeds, she should feel a mounting level of excitement. If she doesn't, she can use the vibrator around the clitoris as she goes along. If things work out as expected, she should have a resounding orgasm along with her partner.

As time goes by she should be able to reduce the amount of vibrator stimulation and react more and more to penis-vagina-clitoris sensations.

What are the masturbation tools for men like?

Well, most of them are the opposite of dildos in that they are spaces instead of objects. Generally they are artificial "jelly-like" vaginas with a motor and a soft lining. The man lubricates them, inserts his penis, turns on the motor and off he goes! Mirroring the plastic penises of your favorite porn star, men can buy a plastic replica of the vagina, clitoris, and labia of their favorite lady porn actress, complete with built-in vibrator.

Do men use these as much as women use dildos?

Not really. Many men feel strangely guilty about using artificial vaginas. That's reflected in some of the jokes they tell.

A good example is the story about the traveling salesman who had been away from home for a month and one night found himself in a hotel in a small town. Next door was an exhibit of vending machines. Late that night he ventured in and came upon a bright pink machine labeled:

"Your Wife Away From Home."

It had a small hole at waist height and a sign that said,

"Deposit One Dollar And Carefully Insert In Opening."

Since he was alone in the showroom, he took out his swollen penis, slid it into the hole, deposited a dollar, and waited eagerly.

There was a loud humming of motors and a whirring sound and when he pulled out his penis, he found a button sewn on the end of it!

The message is clear: the man who is tempted to resort to an artificial vagina instead of a real one has some very unusual experiences in store. In reality, most men masturbate the old-fashioned way.

What's that?

They just take hold of their penis and slide their hand up and down until they finally ejaculate. One reason they don't resort to complicated techniques is that the male sexual impulse is primitive and direct. The penis wants what it wants when it wants it. Like the old joke: Why do men sometimes act so silly when it comes to sex? Because all the blood drains out of their brain and goes into their penis. (Male readers will understand that in a flash.)

But some fellows, especially in their teens, go to great lengths to put together scenarios that simulate sex with a woman. Arthur is an example. He is nineteen and studying computer programming:

"You know, when I was fifteen I'd never had sex with a woman and I was really excited to see how it felt. I was masturbating once or twice a day at that time and I figured I'd try something new. So one Saturday afternoon when my parents were out, I tried this:

"I took a cantaloupe and made a hole in it big enough to take my penis. Then I went into my parents' bedroom and pulled the mattress off the box spring. I lay down on my back on the box spring, put the melon on my penis, and then pulled the mattress down over me.

"It was terrific! It felt like some woman was lying right on top of me and I really went crazy! Just as I was about to come, the door swung open and my parents walked in!"

Arthur sat there slowly shaking his head.

"That was four years ago and I still haven't been able to explain to them what was going on!"

Are there any other types of masturbation besides genital and anal?

Yes. No one talks very much about urethral masturbation, but it is more common than most people realize. In this form of sexual stimulation, the passage from the bladder to the outside is stimulated by inserting objects and moving them back and forth gently. So far no one has come up with a mechanized way to do this, but with transistors and miniaturization, it can happen any day.

This type of sexual play is most common in women, probably because their urethra is more sensitive sexually. Located between the clitoris and vagina, it is well-supplied with nerve connections to these structures. The most common object used for urethral stimulation is the handiest one—a hairpin. Inserted gently and slid back and forth, it rarely brings on orgasm itself but facilitates and intensifies clitoral and vaginal masturbation. Safety pins (closed), pencils, rubber bands, and even lipstick cases will do the trick. As the urethra is used more and more this way, it stretches until it will admit the tip of the finger. Women who enjoy this technique then masturbate with one finger on the clitoris, one in the urethra, and one in the vagina. They say that each area multiplies the sensations from the others.

Men also use urethral masturbation but to a much lesser extent. The greater length of the male passage requires longer objects, but they're easy to find. Small pieces of wire, lengths of plastic tubing, large-caliber pencil leads, all find their way into the urethra.

Don't these things ever get lost?

Occasionally they do, and then it requires a trip to the hospital. The doctor who extracts a bobby pin from a woman's bladder usually doesn't have to ask how it got there. If he does ask, he should be prepared for an original answer:

> "Why, Doctor, I must have sat on it! I'll have to be more careful in the future, won't I?"

This excuse isn't available to men, of course. When that pencil lead slips into their bladder, all they can do is mutter something about an "accident" and let the doctor get on with the retrieval. Because the urethra is such a delicate structure, urethral masturbation is never a good idea. It can cause serious and permanent damage. Don't do it!

Is there anything a man and woman can use together?

Yes. Probably the ultimate in masturbation toys is the "Double Whammy." This is a soft tube of plastic with a tiny vibrator at each end. The gentleman slips it onto his erect penis with one of the mini-vibrators toward his partner and slides his penis into her vagina.

Then the "fun" begins. He can turn her vibrator on with his remote control and vibrate her clitoris while he moves his penis in and out. And she—with her own individual remote control—can vibrate the shaft of his penis. Or he can put the "Whammy" on upside down and she can tickle his testicles with the vibrator—urging him on to greater efforts. Or they can both vibrate each other at the same time.

Is that a good idea?

To be honest, sometimes you can go overboard with sexual electronics. From time to time these gadgets can help, often they can entertain, occasionally they can solve a problem.

But if we carry the idea to its ultimate extreme, all we have to do is take the perfect replica of a male porn star's penis, lubricate it well, insert it into the perfect replica of a female porn star's vagina, turn on both their motors, and jump quickly to one side.

Do you know what would happen? Nothing. Nothing. And more nothing. Absolutely nothing. And that's the key.

Masturbation is fine—up to a point. But it gets lonesome very quickly unless there's someone else there at the end of the penis or the beginning of the vagina. Sex isn't sex unless there's a human being with real human feelings and emotions at the other end. That's really what sex is about—the closest, most intimate, most fulfilling relationship that two members of the human race can ever have. And besides, it's more fun.

Chapter 10
SEXUAL PERVERSION

What are sex perverts?

Those are people whose sexual attention isn't really focused on penis-vagina sex. The word "pervert" is precisely descriptive: it's made up of the Latin word, *pervertere* which means "to turn away." So a sex "pervert" is someone who turns away from normal sexual instincts.

These days no one likes to call things by their real names—short people are "vertically challenged" and criminals are "ethically challenged." "Sexual pervert" is an accurate descriptive term for a particular pattern of sexual behavior. But the new politically correct way to refer to these folks is "paraphiliacs"—which may sound worse. Take your choice.

There is a tremendous amount of variation among perverts/paraphiliacs. Their "turned away" sexual impulses can steer them to things as light and fluffy as ladies' underwear or to something as terrible as raping little girls. They may like to be tickled or dressed up in diapers or to tie up other people and whip them.

The category of sexual pervert includes a little bit of everything—relatively harmless masochists, fetishists, voyeurs, and exhibitionists as well as dangerous child abusers, rapists, and sex murderers. The world of sexual perversion is bizarre and grotesque.

From a medical point of view, we can understand sexual perverts. But sometimes their effect on our personal lives—and the lives of our children—is unsettling and even dangerous.

How do people become sexual perverts?

Sexual perverts start out the same as everyone else—but they just never quite grow up sexually. Think about it for a moment. Growing up is tough. You are under the total control/domination of your parents for the most important years of your life. They control your clothes, your eating, your sleeping, and your relations with other people. They even control such intimate aspects of your life such as toilet-training, spanking, and punishment. If those experiences are not assimilated and put behind you as you get older when your sexual hormones begin to percolate, those emotionally charged experiences can become overloaded with sexual content. The average person advances from one stage of sexual development to another. The pervert gets stuck at one point and never moves from there.

The Peeping Tom is a good example. (Now they're called "voyeurs" which is French for "lookers.") Everyone in the world starts out sexually as a Peeping Tom/voyeur.

How is that?

The only sexual activity ordinarily available to small children, except for masturbation, is peeping, or looking at other people sexually. At about the age of three or four years, little boys and girls become interested in each others' bodies. The boys want to know "How come girls don't have one?" And girls want to know "How come boys have one?"

Even at this first tentative moment, sex is mysterious and alluring. From that point on children seize every opportunity to observe the sexual makeup of their companions. Mutual inspection of genitalia is the reason for those childish games, "Playing House" and "Playing Doctor." That's the basis of the joke:

A little boy and the little girl next door go out to play. The little boy says, "What shall we play today?"

The little girl thinks a moment and says, "Let's play Mommy and Daddy. You shave and I'll have PMS."

But playing Mommy and Daddy doesn't stop there. While mother is busy in the kitchen studying a new recipe, the children are busy in the playroom studying each other.

This is a normal and essential part of the process of sexual maturity. There is really nothing naughty about it. The childish pastime of "You show me yours and I'll show you mine" is a phase most children pass through rapidly and safely.

It soon gives way to more advanced peeping. At school the boys watch the girls and the girls watch the boys. As puberty begins, sexual interest becomes more refined and centers around breasts and buttocks. In high school, girlie magazines are passed around among the boys and mutual sexual exploration begins on dates. Ultimately, observing the body of the opposite sex becomes part of the enjoyment of sexual intercourse. Looking at the body of the sexual partner becomes one of the pleasant events leading up to copulation.

Then isn't everybody a voyeur?

When it comes to sex, maybe everyone is a "looker," but not everyone is a sexual pervert/voyeur. We all like to look at sexual things, but we don't all creep through the bushes on a Saturday night peeping in the neighbors' windows hoping to catch a glimpse of someone undressing or taking a shower. In voyeurs, the normal evolution of the sexual instinct gets short-circuited along the way. The natural sequence "Sexual Interest—Sexual Stimulation—Sexual Intercourse" doesn't happen. When a man watches a woman take off her brassiere and step out of her panties, his heart beats faster, he gets an erection, and he can't wait to have sex with her. When the voyeur is standing on an orange crate watching the lady next door step out of her panties, that's it right there! He may masturbate while he's watching, but his sex really stops at the childish peeping stage and the childish masturbation stage. And peeping isn't all child's play.

Why not?

Some peepers devote tremendous energies to their hobby. They keep track of the best places to go and the best times to be there to get an "eyeful." Listen to an expert:

Ralphie is a fry cook. He is thirty-two and never married. He doesn't go out with girls anymore. He went on a few

*dates when he was younger, but they made him nervous. He
is thin, well dressed, and very tense. As he talks, his eyes
dart about the room.*

*"Well, I don't know. I don't think there's any harm in it.
I don't touch nobody, I just look. It ain't against the law. I
mean everybody's got a right to look, don't they? I just sit
there and look. Like on the subway, for example. I know the
right stops. I get on where all the girls from the offices get
on and I just sit there. The train stops, they come in, they sit
down and cross their legs. That's when you see it! When
they cross their legs! Last summer I even saw one without
any panties on!"*

*Ralphie gets a little excited at this point as he remembers
what he has seen. If Ralphie were in the second grade and
going through that two-week period when he wanted to look
at little girls' panties, it wouldn't be a big deal. Well, that's
exactly where he is, only he's twenty-five years too late.*

*"Then after I ride around for about an hour I get pretty
excited. So I go home and play with myself."*

That is the extent of Ralphie's sex life—looking at women's
underwear and then masturbating.

But things are changing fast for voyeurs.

How come?

Two reasons—technology and the Internet. Now you can buy a
"spy camera"—a tiny video camera the size of your thumb (or
smaller) that you can hide anywhere. Dedicated peepers put them in
the changing rooms at ladies' dress shops, girls' locker rooms,
ladies' public toilets, hotel rooms, and anywhere else they can think
of. They also use video cameras with infrared and zoom lenses to
peek into bedrooms—maybe your bedroom!

Then they publish their photos on the Internet where they also
exchange tips and techniques. Some of them even send in pictures
of their own wives naked or having sex with them—or other men.

But that's weird, isn't it?

Not weird, just perverted. Their sexual instincts are turned in
another direction. Most voyeurs have stopped evolving sexually

about the age of twelve. Of course some of them are frozen at earlier ages.

Those are the ones who don't even want to see breasts and vaginas. They are the "upskirt" boys. They shoot pictures up a woman's skirt—either when she is standing on a balcony or walking upstairs. They are turned on by photos of legs and ladies' panties. That's what they used to see when they were four years old and playing on the floor while Mommy had some lady friends over.

Many perverts are very specialized. Some of them are only interested in pictures of pantyhose and nylon stockings. And some are turned on to bathrooms.

Turned on to bathrooms?

That's right. They hide their video cameras in public washrooms and hotel bathrooms waiting for the chance to see women undressing and urinating. They buy wireless video cameras that transmit the signal without wires to a video recorder a hundred feet away.

That's an important element in perversion—often overlooked in attempts to understand it. Most perversions have a big element of curiosity. The voyeur is curious—he's trying to find out what women look like and what they do "down there." That's the part he missed somewhere along the way. He can't get into ladies' washrooms and locker rooms to learn what nobody ever taught him—but his camera can.

And the women don't even suspect they are being filmed?

Most of them don't know—but some of them *might* know. That's the flip side of the coin. For every peeper, there's an exhibitionist lurking somewhere around the corner. If you check the Internet again, you will find thousands of pictures of "amateurs"—women who take pictures of themselves before they put their clothes on and send them in to be shown to the more than 40 million folks who can dial in to the Internet.

What are those pictures like?

They are like anything you can imagine. One woman sends in photos of herself in a bathing suit sitting in a deck chair by her backyard swimming pool. She's pulled aside the crotch of the swimsuit and is showing you her vagina. She's holding a drink in one hand and smiling into the camera.

Another woman sends in a picture of herself taken from behind. She's looking over her shoulder and winking at the camera. You notice that her skirt is pulled up to her waist in back and she's not wearing any panties.

A third woman is sitting on top of her clothes dryer with her legs spread wide apart. She isn't wearing any clothes.

The interesting part of these photos is that most of these women are middle-class housewives, most of them married. The photos often include their names and addresses.

That seems so strange. Why do these women do that?

Part of the explanation is a simple one, summed up in one word: Power. A lot of sexual perversion is related to power. Remember, little kids are powerless, and if they're still little kids inside when they grow up, they find that sex gives them the power to manipulate other people.

There are few things more powerful—as far as men are concerned—than a head-on view of the female sexual attributes. In history, on more than one occasion, a determined group of women have stopped an advancing enemy army simply by lining up in front of them and raising high their skirts. (No panties.)

So a slightly overweight housewife in Iowa who doesn't even get a second look at the supermarket can get hundreds of letters when she appears naked on the Internet holding her vibrator in one hand.

And it's power that drives the most popular sexual perversion of all.

Which one is that?

BDSM, the King of the Perversions. Those innocent initials stand for an immense shadow world that exists in every city and suburb in America and probably reaches right into your own neighborhood. The letters translate to "Bondage-Domination-Sado-Masochism." They include all the people who like to tie other people up, whip them, paddle them, tease them, and humiliate them. That's the "Sado" part—short for "Sadist."

But each "Sadist" has his or her "Masochist" counterpart who loves to be tied up, whipped, paddled, teased, and humiliated.

BDSM used to be clandestine and furtive, but now it has come out of the closet—in a big way. There are BDSM clubs all over the United States and all over the world. There are BDSM stores that sell the tremendous variety of equipment that the BDSM fans need. There are mail-order catalogues for BDSM folks and even weekend courses and seminars for "newbies" to learn the "ropes."

The BDSM "scene" has evolved into a sub-culture with its own language and customs.

For example?

Well, here's a list of a few of the most common BDSM expressions:

- **Asphyxia**: A "game" in which the "Bottom" is deprived of air by ropes, gags, masks, plastic bags, etc. *See* Edgeplay.
- **B&D**: Bondage and Discipline. Hurting people and being hurt.
- **Blood Sports**: A group of techniques in which the Submissive's skin is broken and blood is allowed to escape. Since the advent of AIDS and the spread of hepatitis, interest in blood sports has declined and those who practice it have developed techniques to try to protect themselves. The most common blood sport is Cutting. *See* Cutting.
- **Bondage**: The way you tie people up—ropes, handcuffs, straps, and wrapping them in tape, plastic wrap, etc. A group of techniques for rendering a Submissive physically helpless. These include rope ties, handcuffs and manacles, wrapping, and mummification.
- **Bottom**: The one who is whipped, tied, or tortured.
- **Branding**: Marking a "Bottom's" skin with a hot iron similar to the ones used to brand cattle.
- **CB/T**: Penis and testicle torture. (The actual words are more graphic.)
- **Consensual**: Agreeable to all involved.
- **Cutting**: A technique in which cuts are carefully made in the Submissive's skin to produce an aesthetically pleasing pattern and stimulation to the Submissive. The cuts are sometimes made into permanent markings by placing foreign substances in them before they heal.
- **D&S**: Domination and Submission.

- **Decorative Binding**: Using rope or cord to compress or tie a portion of the body where struggle will not cause it to tighten or cut into the submissive. *See* Immobilization.

- **Discipline**: Whipping, spanking, and strapping.

- **Dominant**: The one who intimidates and humiliates the "Submissive" or "Sub." Also known as "Dom" or if female, "Dominatrix."

- **Edgeplay**: These are dangerous D&S "games" that are looked upon with some trepidation. They can bring the victim to the "edge" of death. Because there is no formal "ruling body" in D&S, what is called Edgeplay is up to the individual. Therefore, something that to one person might be considered Edgeplay might not be Edgeplay to another. But Blood Sports and Asphyxia can be considered Edgeplay.

- **Fistee**: Someone who welcomes an entire fist in their rectum or vagina.

- **Fister**: Someone who inserts their entire fist into the rectum or the vagina.

- **Go Word**: A signal by the Submissive that everything is all right and you can continue with or increase the present level of stimulation.

- **Golden Showers**: A humiliation technique where the Dominant urinates on the Submissive. Consumption of the urine may be part of this scene.

- **Immobilization**: Using rope or other bondage tools to render a Submissive relatively helpless despite his or her struggles. *See* Decorative Binding.

- **Limits**: The point at which something fun becomes not-so-much-fun.

- **Masochism**: The ability to derive pleasure from pain. Derives from the writings of Leopold von Sacher-Masoch.

- **Masochist**: One who enjoys pain and humiliation. Usually the "Bottom."

- **Negotiation**: Agreeing on terms and conditions before a scene.

- **Panic Snap**: A linking device used with cable and chain that allows two lengths to be disconnected even when there is tension in the system. A safety device.

- **Play Party**: S&M sex party.

- **S&M**: Sadism and Masochism; a term often used to describe the D&S scene; however, it is falling into disrepute because it is both inaccurate (Dominants are not Sadists) and overly limited (all Submissives are not Masochists).

- **Sadist**: An individual who enjoys causing pain in a nonconsensual manner or regardless of the presence or absence of consent. Derives from the writings of the Marquis de Sade, a disturbed French nobleman.

- **Safe Word**: A word or phrase which permits the Submissive to withdraw consent and terminate the scene at any point without endangering the illusion that the Dominant is in complete control. *See* Slow Word.

- **SAM**: "Smart Ass Masochist." A pseudo Submissive who attempts to control everything the Dominant does. A term of contempt. Example: "She's cute and willing, but she's a real SAM; you will spend most of your time trying to keep her from telling you which whip to use and how to swing it."

- **Scene**: An individual session of whatever duration where the participants are in their D&S roles. Example: "It was a tremendously hot scene last night when Master Jim waxed Lisa at The Vault."

- **Slave**: Often used interchangeably with Submissive. However, generally reflecting a more intense level of submission or sexual plus non-sexual submission. For example, a slave might be someone who remains in a 24-hour-per-day submission and cooks, cleans and, otherwise, takes care of a Dominant's house.

- **Slow Word**: A signal by the Submissive that things are getting too intense and you should change or decrease the stimulation.

- **Squicks**: Pushes a Bottom beyond his or her limits.

- **Strapple**: An elongated paddle with a bit more flex that is something intermediate between a strap and a paddle.

- **Submissive**: An individual who gives up power in a D&S relationship for the mutual pleasure of those involved.

- **Suspension**: A set of techniques for suspending a Submissive using ropes, webbing, or chain so that no part of the body touches the floor. This is a highly specialized technique and great care must be used to prevent damage.

- **Switch**: Alternates between being the "Top" and being the "Bottom."

- **The Scene**: The gamut of D&S activities and people considered as a whole. Example: "The Scene contains some of the nicest people I have ever met."

- **Top**: The one who inflicts pain and suffering.

- **Topping from the Bottom**: For a Submissive to dictate the precise action in a scene. A term of contempt. Example: "She's cute and willing, but she's always topping from the bottom; you will spend most of your time trying to keep her from telling you which whip to use and how to swing it." *See* "SAM."

- **TT**: Breast torture. The term applies to both males and females. (The actual words are more graphic.)

- **Vanilla**: Not in "The Scene." A term used to describe ordinary, conventional life both sexual and otherwise. While it can be used in a pejorative sense, it is more often used to distinguish between scene and non-scene activities and people. Example: "I have to be careful in my vanilla life that people don't find out that I'm a Dominant."

BDSM folks also use their version of the "Hanky Codes"—a colored handkerchief sticking out of their back pocket. The idea is that someone looking for "fun" can pick their partner quickly and accurately. Here are some of the common ones:

Color	*Left Pocket*	*Right Pocket*
Black	Heavy S&M top	Heavy S&M bottom
Gray	Bondage top	Bondage bottom
Red	Fister	Fistee
Yellow	Golden shower top	Golden shower bottom
Black-and-White Check	Safe sex top	Safe sex bottom
Purple	Piercer	Piercee
Dark Blue	Anal sex top	Anal sex bottom
Light Blue	Wants oral sex	Expert at oral sex
Light Pink	Dildo user	Dildo receiver

Ladies who are wearing dresses can just hang their hanky from their belt or in a pocket. If they want to be less subtle, they can wear miniature handcuffs as a pin or earrings. That should get the message across.

But how does BDSM actually work?

The basic arrangement goes something like this:

The "Top," who is "Dominant," hurts and punishes the "Bottom," who is "Submissive." The "Bottom" has a "Safe Word" if things get out of control—which they often do. When the "Top" hears the "Safe Word" he or she is supposed to stop—which they usually do. With those terms in mind, we're ready to visit a "Play Party."

What goes on at these "Play Parties"?

A lot of things you'd never imagine. Let's peek into one of these get-togethers and see what's happening. There's also a very formal etiquette that governs "Play Parties" when BDSM fans get together—and we'll see that in action as well. There's one other thing to keep in mind as we enter the Party Scene—in spite of their costumes and poses, all the participants are ordinary people—the kind of men and women you have contact with every day. Let's check it out.

We pull up to a modest house on a quiet suburban street. It's 9 P.M. and there's a quiet party going on. A dozen cars are parked on the street and in the driveway.

Let's go inside. As we ring the doorbell and peek through the window into the living room we see a typical middle-class suburban home. Beige drapes. Maple furniture. Pale green nylon carpeting. But when the door opens . . .

Standing there is a short plump woman dressed in black leather. She is wearing a leather mask that covers the upper half of her face. She has a leather mini-skirt and above the knee leather boots with 6-inch heels. Her face is stark white with blood red lips. In her right hand she holds a whip—braided black leather and 3 feet long.

Her voice is warm and inviting:

"Gee, I'm sorry I kept you waiting. But I was giving a lesson to one of my pupils. I'm Mistress Pain. Come on in!"

There are nine people in the combination Living-Dining Room. As we enter they all turn to look at us.

One by one they speak:

"Hi!"

"Glad you could come! "

"Join the party!"

"Make yourself at home!"

Then they turn back to what they were doing.

Closest to us is a man—naked and on his knees. His hands are bound behind his back with handcuffs. He has a leather collar around his neck attached to a leash. A woman is standing above him jerking on his leash. He is straining to push his face into her crotch—she isn't wearing panties. Every time he gets close, she jerks the leash. Little rivulets of blood are running down his neck and we notice that there are steel spikes inside the collar.

Across the room there is a wooden cross made of two-by-fours. A naked woman is tied to the cross in the crucifixion position. Another woman in a floor-length black gown is putting clothespins on her breasts and erect nipples. As she clamps on each new clothespin, the woman shrieks in pain.

Lying on the rug nearby is a man done up in plastic wrap—the kind you use to wrap leftovers in the refrigerator. But he's no leftover. He's squirming like a fish out of water and grunting loudly but no one pays any attention to him. Only his head is out of the plastic and he has a black leather gag in his mouth; fastened to the front of the gag is a dildo. A tall thin woman in a topless maid's outfit consisting of a microscopic miniskirt and apron is squatting over him and just about to sit on the dildo. He is squirming and grunting.

Mistress Pain is at our side again.

"The refreshments are in the kitchen. Our Slave made some great cookies and there's punch—it's okay, it's all organic—nothing artificial."

She pauses a moment and points down the hall with her whip.

"Oh, by the way, there's Watersports in the bathroom—if you're into that."

There are two things that impress us so far.

What are they?

First, everyone is friendly. They seem like ordinary people—not wild-eyed perverts. Secondly, in spite of the screams and moaning, they seem to be getting some kind of enjoyment out of their bizarre suffering.

We open the door to the bathroom and there is a fat naked man lying in the bathtub. There is no water in the tub—rather there is no *tap* water in the tub. Two naked women are perched on the edge of the tub holding onto the shower rod. They are both urinating on him.

One of the women—about 30, blonde and Nordic—turns to us:

"Hi! You must be new here! Is Golden Showers your scene? If you want it we'll save some for you!"

We smile and shake our head.

She smiles back.

"Okay! When you get to the kitchen, turn left. The Dungeon is through the white door."

Then she turns and nonchalantly sprays her urine all over the fat man's chest.

We pass through the kitchen where there is a buffet of snacks laid out on the counter. We see the white door to the Dungeon and go through it. The "Dungeon" is really a two car garage entirely closed in. It has imitation brick paneling and it very busy this evening.

In one corner is a small cage with a naked woman in it—she is lying on her back. An elderly man in a black cape—and nothing else—is pouring melted wax from a candle through the bars onto her breasts. Every time the wax hits her she screams:

"Stop! Stop! Stop! I love it! Hotter!"

"Stop" is obviously not her "Safe Word."

As we walk away we notice that the gentleman is masturbating with his free hand.

In another corner a naked woman is chained to the wall—her arms held high above her head. Two other women are bent over her buttocks. One holds a small branding iron— a miniature of the kind used on cattle. As the other grabs the victim's buttock, she presses the iron against it. We can smell the burning flesh and we see the brand: "S-L-A-V-E."

It's about time to leave and we make for the front door. Mistress Pain meets us there.

"Gee, thanks for coming. Maybe next time you'll get into it with us."

She smiles cheerfully.

But that seems like such strong stuff. Does it ever get worse?

Actually what we saw was very mild—mostly play-acting. BDSM can really get rough. For example, some fans get into torture— politely called "genital torture" or "genitorture" for short. They whip the penis and clitoris with small cat-o'-nine-tail whips, tie heavy weights to the testicles and labia, and sometimes edge toward the borders of insanity.

Other BDSMers use electric shocks and slicing and slashing with very sharp knives. Then there are the "hand-ballers."

What are "hand-ballers"?

As you can imagine, they are not devotees of the game called Handball. These are the folks who like to insert—not a finger or two—but an entire hand into the vagina. With careful lubrication, they insert one finger at a time, then the folded hand, then the entire hand. For the "Bottom," it can be quite a sensation. There are both male and female "hand-ballers."

But that's tame compared to the homosexual variety. That's when they insert the whole hand through the anus into the rectum. It's the equivalent of the medical procedure of a proctoscopy except that the proctoscopy instrument is just a narrow metal tube. The person who has someone's hand well up into their large intestine is really engaging in "Edgeplay."

Is there much Edgeplay in BDSM?

It's a matter of degree. How do you know where to stop? Some BDSMers push beyond the Play Party to "Slavery" where they have a "Slave" living in their house 24 hours a day. They keep the "Slave" in a cage at night. It can cause problems if the "Slave" is underage. Or if the "Slave" gets loose.

Have you ever seen a headline like this one:

YOUNG GIRLS ESCAPE FROM HOMEMADE JAIL—TORTURED

Could that have been BDSM out of control?

How about this headline:

14-YEAR-OLD HONOR STUDENT SUICIDE BY HANGING—POLICE PUZZLED

What does that mean?

It means the police *weren't* puzzled. And it wasn't suicide. It was just another case of Asphyxiophilia. That is a strange type of sexual perversion where an individual hangs himself while masturbating. The idea is to partially strangle himself to try to accelerate his orgasm and make it more intense. Some fellows use plastic bags over their heads while others use rope around the neck—padded for comfort. But sometimes things get a little wild and their Edgeplay plays them right over the edge. When the cops get there, they find a dead naked teenager who has ejaculated. Out of consideration for the family they call it an "unexplained" suicide. It was BDSM gone awry.

Rarely women engage in Asphyxiophilia and for a unique reason. They hope it will accelerate their orgasm and maybe produce a "female ejaculation," where women actually ejaculate a type of liquid at orgasm.

Sometimes a "Top" will choke a "Bottom" during sex or masturbation to try to increase the sensation. But choking someone is a delicate business, and squeezing can quickly turn into "Squicking" and send your "Bottom" to the Next World. Then you go to jail—which may not be a totally disagreeable place for a devoted Masochist. That paradox actually caused a problem for law enforcement in the nineteenth century.

How come?

The stern and religious law enforcers back then punished those guilty of sexual offense by whipping them in public. The problem was that many of the sex offenders were masochists and savored every single lash.

But there's still a real problem because the outer limits of BDSM are rape, torture, and ultimately murder. When you read about people who kidnap and torture little children, who rape infants, who cut their victims into little pieces and/or eat them, you are seeing cases of BDSM far beyond the Play Party stage. Paddling someone on their backside with a Ping-Pong paddle in your book-keeper's garage is one thing. But the Spanish Inquisition and the Nazi concentration camps are the other end of the spectrum.

This BDSM stuff makes me nervous. Why do I have to know about it?

Because it is much closer to you than you ever imagined. If you have children, if you have coworkers, if you have employees, if you have relatives that you care about, you need to know what BDSM is all about—because it is all around you.

In recent years BDSM has become big business and part of the "cultural scene." Children as young as three and four years old are being exposed to it, and older children are being bombarded with it.

Three- and four-year-olds exposed to BDSM? How can that be?

Check the Saturday morning cartoons on TV. The BDSM content is amazing when you focus on it, especially the bondage component. The most frightening part is that most of the time it's little girls who are tied up. Bad examples for your daughters and for your sons. Here are just a few examples—there are dozens and dozens:

- Watch the cat being flattened by the steamroller!
- Look at the dog being blown to bits by a stick of dynamite!
- See the cute bunny thrown off the roof of a high building!

Then watch the terrified expressions of the tots in the audience as they are being prepared to enjoy Sado-Masochist good times.

Isn't the message:

"Getting tied up is fun! All the kids do it!"

And getting slashed to bits with a big sharp hook! Doesn't that make you quiver all over?

What about older kids?

They watch movies loaded with BDSM. Bring them up the very best you can and then send them to sit in a dark movie theater where they can absorb lessons in Sado-Masochism. But you say you never allow them to watch those horror films where people are tortured and bound? You only send them to adventure films and comedies? See if you can identify any of these "adventure films" and "comedies." How many of them did your children see?

- A male actor is raped.
- A male actor is tied up and something is stuffed in his mouth.
- A young girl is put in chains by an evil magician.
- An actress teases a tied-up cop, then an actor ties her to a table and teases her.
- One of the actresses is tied up with her hands high above her head.
- An actress is tied up by the cops who half drown her by submerging her head in a bucket of water.
- An actress is pushed toward hot lava.
- The two male stars are tied up together.
- Kidnapping and captivity with bondage.
- Female actress acts like a slave.
- Actors and actresses are tortured and tied in various jail films.
- A male actor is tied up and his female costar is raped.
- An actor slaps a half-naked woman who is tied to a steel bar.
- A doctor is tied up by one of his patients.

These are only fourteen examples—there are hundreds more. The next time you and your children watch TV or go to the movies, play a little game. See how many indicators of BDSM you can pick out. Look for these unmistakable signs in the context of Bondage-Domination Sado-Masochism:

- Leather or rubber clothing or accessories.
- Skin-tight black clothing or black masks.
- Very prominent and heavy shoes or boots, sometimes with spikes or chains.
- Actors being dirtied with slime, gooey liquids, mud, or food (these are often "nicer" substitutes for the urine and feces common in some BDSM "games").
- Knives, razors, axes, or saws used to menace human beings.

- Actors being handcuffed, tied with rope, hung upside down, or confined in very small spaces.
- Children being threatened or terrified.
- Actors who are helpless and menaced with rising water, fire, or smoke.

The BDSM message is in clothes as well as actions. Black leather, iron and steel jewelry, piercing jewelry, big boots, chains and more chains—all transmit the message:

"BDSM is OK! We want you—and your child!"

Is that what you want for *your* child?

Are clothes important in paraphilias/perversions?

Yes, they are. There's an entire category of paraphilias/perversions that centers around clothes. They're called "fetishes"—a strange word that comes from Portuguese. The word in that language is *feitico* which in turn comes from the Latin word *factitiius*, meaning "artificial." That pretty much sums up a fetish.

Basically a fetish is a sexual perversion that substitutes the part for the whole. For example, there are men who are sexually excited by women's shoes. The usual explanation is that these chaps have "substituted the shoe for the woman." Not quite. More precisely they have substituted the shoe for the organ that it most closely resembles: the vagina. (Incidentally that's the real basis of the Cinderella tale. In the original version the Prince isn't going around trying a shoe on all the girls—he gets his thrill by getting them to put their foot into a fur slipper.)

The closer the object is to the female sexual organs, the more exciting it is to men with this perversion. That's why ladies' panties are so spine-tingling to guys with this fetish. Fetishes even get into advertising sometimes. Remember the ad for women's panties that went like this:

"Our panties may not be the very best thing in the world. But they're next to the best thing in the world!"

It sold a lot of panties.

But what causes a fetish?

Like the other sexual perversions, a fetish is a case of arrested development. Little boys gradually develop an interest in sexuality. They see their mother's and sister's and aunt's stockings and underwear and clothes and shoes all around them. They pass through a phase—often about the age of 7 to 9—where these items are vaguely interesting sexually. Most men go beyond this very quickly but some are stranded at that point. These are the ones who become fetishists. It's not the woman but the item of clothing that turns them on.

A classic example is the story about the two dumb brothers on the beach. Suddenly a beautiful and totally naked woman comes out of the water and walks by. One brother nudges the other and says:

"Wow! Wouldn't she look great in a bathing suit?"

To these fetishists, the bathing suit is as important—or more important—than the woman.

What items of clothing turn these men on?

Brassieres, panties, stockings, pantyhose, and shoes are the most common. Some men use them for masturbation—rubbing the items against their penis until they ejaculate. That's why they like soft silky undies.

But perversions are detours from ordinary sexuality, and some men take bigger detours than others. For example, some men get their kicks from stealing women's underwear. In the days before clothes dryers, more than one woman saw her panties and bras disappear from the backyard clothesline.

Other men have different tastes. They like to smell the items—and that has given birth to a fascinating and little-known industry.

What's that?

Reselling used ladies' undies at fabulous prices. Men who consider it important to their happiness will pay up to $20.00 each for used ladies' underwear. They will pay more if the panties are stained with various bodily secretions. These same gentlemen also buy old feminine shoes and socks—the older the better—and stockings and pantyhose. At the farthest reaches of paraphilia/perversion, there are customers for used tampons—at $25.00 each.

What about men who like to actually wear women's clothes?

That's an interesting group—or to be more accurate, an interesting collection of groups. There are several categories of transvestites, or men who wear ladies' garments. The first group is the "female impersonators" whom we've all seen in the movies and on TV. These are men—known in show business as "FIs"—who do their very best to imitate women. By means of makeup, padding, and sometimes surgery, they can fool all but the most perceptive observers. In transvestite slang, they are harder to "read" or "clock."

The next group is the fetish group of transvestites or "TVs" who dress as women primarily for the sexual excitement that the bras and panties they wear give them. They may also be after other things—we'll see about that in a moment.

Then there are the "Drag Queens," usually homosexuals, who are role-playing as females for homosexual reasons. Normal men sometimes have trouble "clocking" Drag Queens, especially if they're at a club, it's late at night, and they've had too much to drink. Maybe that's how the term "rude awakening" originated.

The last group is very interesting. These are men who want to live as women. They are transvestites because they wear female attire but they go far beyond that. They claim to suffer from "gender dysphoria"—deep dissatisfaction with being male and not female. They don't want to be men anymore. They want to be changed into women.

Is that possible?

In one word: "No." Gender—male or female—doesn't reside in the sexual organs. It is present in every cell of a person's body—males have a male chromosomal arrangement and females have a female chromosomal arrangement. That's it.

But transsexuals, or the transgendered as they prefer to be called, don't want to accept that. They go to amazing lengths to try to prove the opposite. In a real sense it is tragic because of the tremendous suffering they go through in the process.

What do they do?

It's a long, complicated affair and it's much the same for most of them. Strangely enough it follows a fairly uniform pattern.

It usually starts with a powerful surge of mixed emotions as they first begin to collect and wear women's clothes. Then they frequently go through the "Purge" stage. In a fit of guilt, they throw all their female clothes away. That's followed, sooner or later, when in a fit of regret, they buy a whole new wardrobe of ladies' outfits. That's called "Bingeing."

Sometimes they marry, in an attempt to solve the problem somehow. Then, almost inevitably, comes what transsexuals call "The Talk." That's when they confess to their partner that they are really transvestites or transsexuals. That's rarely successful and frequently leads to what transsexuals refer to as "The Fit"—the emotional explosion when a woman discovers that her husband likes her clothes better than his.

Being a transsexual isn't fun. They suffer from a lot of internal conflicts and it's tough for them to fit into society. Normal men and women find it very perplexing to have someone that they thought was a man suddenly present himself as a woman.

What happens next?

Some transsexuals opt for "Sexual Reassignment Surgery" to make them into women. That's a big step, and they usually take it by stages.

First they do the "RLT" or "Real Life Test" where they try to live like a woman. That can involve taking female sex hormones, having their beard removed, using makeup, and wearing a wig. They usually take a "femme" name at that stage. "Mark" can become "Marlene," "Glen" can become "Glenda." They may also go to "Finishing School."

What is "Finishing School"?

It's a very unusual training course, usually taking an entire weekend, that teaches men how to act as women. They learn how to walk like a woman, how to talk like a woman, how to react like a woman. Remember in *Huckleberry Finn* when Huck is dressed like a woman and he closes his legs to catch an object when a lady throws something to him instead of opening them wide to catch the object in his skirt? That and many other little details is what men learn in that kind of course.

For example, they learn that they can do a pretty fair imitation of female breasts by filling their empty brassieres with birdseed. (Presumably they are also told that gentlemen wearing bras filled with birdseed shouldn't hang around in the park, especially when the birds are roosting.)

They learn to hide their penis by taping it down inside their panties and wear loose dresses to hide the occasional erection before the female hormones start to work and make an erection unlikely.

They learn about makeup—little things that most men wouldn't know. Like:

"Don't pick cherry-red lipstick!"

and

"Stay away from strawberry-colored rouge!"

They are also coached on how to use makeup to cover their beards and to emphasize whatever cleavage the female sex hormones have given them. In applying makeup to their faces and chests they are constantly reminded to "be subtle." It isn't easy.

They also get good advice like this:

"If you are dressed as a female when you have to use a public washroom, don't forget the new 'you.' Don't stand up when you urinate."

It can be hard to explain to the girls in the office why the new secretary stands up and faces the toilet with "her" toes toward the wall while everyone else is sitting down.

Then, when they are all through, to celebrate the successful conclusion of the course and their new role as women, all the graduates go shopping together.

Do some people make fun of transsexuals?

They shouldn't. Transsexuals have a lot of obstacles to overcome and the little details above are just a few of the easiest. The tough one is the surgery. The hard fact is this: you can't make a man into a woman. And transsexual surgery is not for the faint-hearted. The SRS (Sexual Reassignment Surgery) goes something like this:

First, the testicles are cut off. Then the penis is cut off. Then an artificial clitoris is put together—it has more or less sensation. An opening to simulate a vagina is made and sometimes lined with what is left of the scrotum. The man now has a simulation of female sexual equipment. But he still doesn't really look like a woman.

If he wants to pursue the process he has to have part of his cricoid cartilage cut away in his neck—that's the "Adam's Apple." And of course he'll need breast implants, and probably liposuction. He will be a steady customer of his surgeon for a couple of years.

But will he be able to have sex?

Well, he can receive a penis in his artificial vagina. As far as orgasms are concerned—maybe. It's hard to know exactly because few transsexuals like to discuss that detail in public. But it's fair to say that having their penis and testicles cut off doesn't improve their chances of reaching an orgasm.

Are there female transsexuals too?

There are some—but not nearly as many as the male variety. Women don't really have to struggle to be cross-dressers. A woman in trousers wearing a sport coat and a necktie and wing-tip shoes on her feet hardly rates a glance as she walks into her office. Short haircuts, no makeup, work boots, and worn jeans all have their place in women's fashion—"butch," but fashionable.

There are some women who want to "go all the way" and they face the same hard road as men. They go through the male hormone routine and bodybuilding to give them male-type muscles. They don't have to worry about makeup like male transsexuals but the beard is a problem. Some women put a light coating of petroleum jelly on their face and then pat on finely powdered tea leaves. It may work from across the room, but tea leaves in petroleum jelly on the cheeks don't do much for intimate moments.

The big step is, of course, "the operation." SRS for women is pretty drastic and goes something like this:

The first step is cutting off the breasts. However, the nipples are saved and stuck back on. Then the uterus and ovaries and fallopian tubes are removed. Then there is the matter of the penis. That's tough. It's such a complex organ that it's hard to make one that really works. Most plastic surgery penises are tubes of skin or tissue and are more decorative than anything else. Female transsexuals often use a dildo attached to a harness to interact sexually with their new partners.

All in all, transvestites and transsexuals have a difficult situation and for most of them, there is not really a happy outcome. But there is one paraphilia/perversion that has a superficially brighter tone to it.

What's that?

Plushiephilia. That's the fascinating yet poignant sexual attachment to stuffed animals. There is a small group of people—men and women—who are sexually aroused by stuffed bears and bunnies and monkeys. You may love those cute little critters, but they liter-ally *love* them.

What do you mean, "literally **love** *them*"?

They actually have sex with these stuffed animals. Of course, it's not that unusual when we consider that many little girls have their first experience at masturbation by putting their teddy bear between their legs and rubbing their clitoris against it. During the early years of childhood, almost everyone develops an emotional attachment to the plushie that they take to bed every night. If they get "stuck" at that stage of emotional development—and that's what "perver-sions" are all about—they keep their love affair with their favorite "plushie" as warm as ever—or warmer.

Listen to what Arnold says. He is an insurance executive and vice-president of a big agency. He is 46 and unmarried.

> *"My big bunny, Ginnie, is really my best friend. She's so warm and huggable. I just love to feel her fur against my bare skin. She never rejects me, and when I've had a hard day at the office, she's there to console me and make me for-get all my problems. It's just pure happiness—perfect love."*

But do these folks really have sex with their stuffed animals?

It's not the usual kind of sex, but they do something. They cuddle with them, they kiss them, they rub their penis or clitoris against them, and they hold them tight. Sometimes they do more.

Arnold continues:

"Sure, I have sex with Ginnie. Her insides are foam and I've made a nice little opening where it should be. She gets down on all fours and we do it 'bunny-style.'"

He paused a moment.

"I know what you're going to ask, and the answer is, of course I worry about her. I always use a condom!"

But not all "plushie-love" is just masturbation. Some people go much farther.

Martha is thirty-nine and teaches gourmet cooking. She does it this way:

"Doctor, it's really wonderful. It's just like being a little girl again and yet it's sexy and exciting. Milton, my husband, is into it too, thank goodness. On weekends he gets dressed up in his fur suit—you know, it's a costume that makes him look like a big teddy bear. Then his name becomes 'Bigfoot.' I get undressed and we take out a big white gorilla plushie—he's nearly six feet tall and his fur is really long. His name is Jo-Jo."

Martha paused with a faraway look in her eyes.

"Well, I take all my clothes off and we put Jo-Jo on his back. Then I lie down on top of Jo-Jo and he kind of puts his arms around me. Then Milton, I mean, 'Bigfoot,' gives it to me from behind. You know, we have sex. It's so beautiful with all that nice cuddly fur in front and behind me!

"Then, just when I start to have my orgasm, Milton pulls a cord and a spring makes Jo-Jo's big arms grab me tight, tight, tight! It's wonderful!"

Then plushie-love is really harmless?

Well, nobody gets whipped by a plushie. But there are two problems. It's the substitution—in most cases—of a stuffed animal for a human being. That's not the ideal relationship. And there's one more problem.

In shopping centers and stores and amusement parks all over the country there are people dressed in fur suits representing animals and products. They are very attractive to children, who are constantly touching them and being touched by them. Most of these are probably normal men and women earning an honest living. But one out of a million might not be. It's a good idea to keep a very close eye on your children when you take them to a place where fur suits abound.

What's the best way to deal with sexual perversions?

It depends. The ones that are dangerous—child molestation, rape, murder, and violent and destructive perversions—have to be stopped. The infantile perversions like voyeurism, collecting ladies' undies, shoe fetishism, and others like them respond to education. When the paraphiliacs understand that grown-up sex can be a lot more fun than childish sex, they are well on their way to maturity. The real goal is for the dumb brother on the beach to get smart and realize that the girl looks better naked than in a bathing suit.

Chapter 11

PROSTITUTION

When did prostitution begin?

In one form or another, prostitution has been around a long time. "Harlots" are mentioned forty-four times in the Bible, "Whores" and "Whoremongers" are featured fifty-three times, and "Committing Whoredoms" is mentioned eight times. Obviously Love for Money was well established by 2000 B.C. From its origin until relatively recently, prostitution has been a more or less respectable profession.

How can that be?

The Ancient Hebrews were the first to condemn whores. Most of their complaints were directed against Hebrew women who took up the trade, however. Foreign prostitutes were relatively well tolerated among them. The New Testament began where the Old Testament left off and commenced a religious campaign against prostitution that took on all the attributes of a Crusade and which continues with its original fervor even today in certain countries (including the United States).

Things were not always that way. Among the Ancient Chinese, Greeks, and Syrians (to name only a few), prostitution was considered a noble calling and played a role in many religious ceremonies.

Nearly every temple had its official prostitutes; intercourse with them (for a small fee) was considered an acceptable form of worship. Many of these ladies were volunteers in the sense that they only worked for a year or so, donating all the proceeds of their labors to the temple. This was considered the equivalent of modern missionary work and brought with it great religious rewards. When their time was up, the part-time prostitutes returned home to their husbands and families with greatly enhanced prestige.

But isn't "prostitute" and "religion" a contradiction in terms?

Not necessarily. Remember that many of the early religions were closely tied in with the mysteries of fertility of crops and animals, with planting seeds and all the rest. Sexual intercourse played a magical role with them, and sex within a religious context was not the same as meeting a prostitute in a bar and paying her a hundred dollars for oral sex.

Even through the Middle Ages prostitution was accepted as a way of life and the more elegant whores moved freely in upper-class society. Under the euphemism of "courtesans," they consorted with royalty. Among the lower classes, the prostitute's life was harder, but not necessarily unrespectable.

What about in modern times?

Prostitution has remained a socially acceptable if somewhat expedient way of earning a living in many parts of the world right up to the present time. Suppression of ladies of the evening was instituted subsequently in France, Italy, Belgium, and Japan. However, "whore" is still not a nasty word in large parts of the world. Most of Asia recognizes legal prostitution as do many other parts of the world. Latin America, with certain exceptions, allows lawful prostitution. The closest neighbor to the United States, Mexico, has considered prostitutes legal for a long time.

Isn't prostitution a terrible thing?

A lot of people seem to think so, but the facts don't necessarily bear out their emotions. The major objections to professional prostitution usually fall into the following categories:

1. Prostitution increases sex crimes.
2. Prostitution corrupts young people.
3. Prostitution is morally degrading.
4. Prostitution spreads sexually transmitted diseases.

Let's take a look at these objections one by one.

Doesn't prostitution increase sex crimes?

It doesn't seem likely. In countries where the trade is legal, sex crimes are almost non-existent. If a few dollars buys a willing companion, raping a stranger doesn't make sense. Peeping, exhibitionism, child molestation, incest, all feed on undischarged sexual tensions. Is it better for a man to find sexual satisfaction with a prostitute or is it better to let him rape women at the bus stop?

How about the corruption of young people?

"Corruption" is a loaded word. If it means that prostitution encourages them to engage in sexual intercourse before society approves, then prostitution is not guilty. Sexual permissiveness and parental neglect push kids toward premature sex more than the existence of women who will have sex for money. Remember that most prostitutes charge more for one copulation than most teenagers see in a month.

Judging from the countries where prostitutes are freely available, the moral fiber of the nation doesn't seem to be adversely affected. In the United States, where the majority of college students regularly take drugs, prostitution might even be considered the lesser of two evils. If the choice is a night with a prostitute or a trip on drugs, most rational parents would reluctantly opt for the young lady—at least an evening in bed leaves the brain intact.

Making prostitution illegal doesn't keep girls from becoming prostitutes. As a matter of fact, by raising prices it makes the profession more profitable and therefore more attractive.

But isn't prostitution degrading?

Definitely. We make it that way. By looking down on those who sell their sexual favors, by making them criminals, by shutting them off from the rest of society, we succeed in alienating them completely. Some of the bitterness and contempt rubs off on the customers, who are more than willing to pass it on to the Lady of the Evening.

Prostitution is a fact of life. In itself it is neither good nor bad. Sexual intercourse for money goes against our moral grain because we have been indoctrinated that way. Instead of complaining bitterly about the result of the problem, it might make more sense to go to the source. Like the old saying, "If there wasn't the demand, there wouldn't be the supply."

What causes the "demand"?

Let one of the girls tell her theory. Bonnie is twenty-seven; she has been playing for pay since she was nineteen.

> *"The only thing that keeps us in business is the American wife, God bless her. Those overfed, overdressed, smug little bitches help me buy a new Mercedes every other year. If all the wives woke up at once and gave their husbands what they wanted, I'd have to go back to waiting on tables in a beer joint. But I'm not too worried—business gets better every month. As long as the average woman thinks she has a 'Golden Vagina' I'll be in good shape."*

Like every prostitute, Bonnie needs to justify her way of life, but she obviously has a point. Most of her customers, like those of every other prostitute, are married. Theoretically they have access to complete sexual gratification with their wives. But if they did, they wouldn't need Bonnie. A tabulation of the services customers demand from the girls is revealing.

What do they want?

The activity men most often seek from professional prostitutes is fellatio. At least 75 percent of the clients want to have their penises sucked. It's the ketchup campaign.

The ketchup campaign?

Some years ago one of the producers of ketchup decided to boost sales. They analyzed the market and discovered that women were complaining that they spent a lot of time in the kitchen cooking up fancy dishes and their husbands would come home and slosh ketchup over everything. The wives' rebellion was bad for sales so the company came up with what they thought was a brilliant ad campaign. The idea was to remind wives that their husbands enjoyed ketchup on their food and it wasn't considerate to deprive them of that pleasure.

The ad was a masterpiece. It featured a pretty waitress holding a large tray against her chest. On the tray were two plates with big juicy steaks and a prominent bottle of the company's ketchup. The waitress's ample breasts rested suggestively on the tray as she gazed down at two men waiting to be served lunch. The caption was

IF YOU DON'T GIVE IT TO HIM AT HOME, HE'LL GET IT DOWNTOWN!

Two weeks later the ad was withdrawn.

But men who don't get fellated at home *do* get it downtown. And that keeps thousands of prostitutes in business.

How do the girls feel about it?

They love it. Not because it's their idea of ecstasy (no prostitute is in the business just for sexual pleasure anyway), but because it's a lot more profitable than anything else. A blow job, or "B.J.," as it is known in the trade, is fast, easy, and clean. No linen to change, no washing up to do (except for a swish of antiseptic mouthwash), and if the girl is crafty, she doesn't even have to get undressed. As one lady who should know puts it:

"I could do B.J.s all day without working up a sweat."

And thanks to the AIDS epidemic, it's better than ever.

How come?

Hardly any prostitute will do a B.J. without a condom these days. That means there's no spillage, minimum risk, and no big mouthwash bills. The only hazard is the occasional broken condom and, of course, the client who brings his own lubricated condom. As any girl will tell you, they taste awful!

The next most popular activity with the gents is cunnilingus. The girls don't like that so well.

Laurie tells how it is:

"I always charge them extra if they want to work on me down there. It takes such a long time and then they want a regular trick too. In this line you got to please the customer, but a girl still has to make a living. I usually charge an extra seventy-five bucks for it at least—and they have to use a condom."

How does a man use a condom when he performs oral sex on a woman?

Like this: He holds the condom up to the light, cuts off the top and carefully slits it from base to tip. Then he puts it over her clitoris and vagina and licks her through the condom. That keeps her secretions out of his mouth and his secretions out of her vagina. And hopefully it will keep the AIDS virus out of their lives.

Plastic wrap from the kitchen will do in an emergency, as will a sandwich bag, but condoms are preferred. Condoms are everywhere these days and they are only part of the new routine for sex—especially with prostitutes.

What else has changed?

A lot of little things. For example, you should never brush your teeth within four hours of having sex with a prostitute.

Why not?

Every time you brush your teeth, you make little tiny cuts in your gums. Sometimes you see blood on your toothbrush, sometimes you don't—but it's there. The AIDS virus can be in every body fluid—urine, blood, vaginal secretions, human milk, saliva, tears, and all the rest. If you get any of those secretions in your mouth with cuts on your gums, you can get AIDS. And as they say, "Fun is fun, but AIDS is forever."

Do many prostitutes have AIDS?

It depends on where you go. In some parts of Africa, up to 70 percent of all prostitutes have the AIDS virus. In most Western European cities, about 3 percent of the girls are infected. In the United States the percentage is about the same—with one important exception.

What's that?

About 35 percent of the girls who use intravenous drugs—like heroin or cocaine—may have the AIDS virus, usually from contaminated needles and syringes. And it's not as easy as it once was to know who's who.

Before the AIDS epidemic, you could spot the needle tracks on a girl's arm or leg and know she was shooting up. But prostitutes who are drug users know that clients are terrified of AIDS. So, being limitlessly resourceful, they shoot the drugs between their fingers or toes.

Between their fingers or toes?

Right. Many of the girls are artists with hypodermic needles. As a sideline, they do body piercing on their clients and even temporary cosmetic surgery.

They do temporary cosmetic surgery?

Yes, that's right. Some male customers have unusual tastes—and are willing to pay to have them satisfied. It works like this:

Suppose one evening a man says to his wife:

"You know Ellen, our sex life has been kind of routine for the past year or so. Do you think we could do something to, you know, make it more exciting?"

The wife has read all those magazine articles about "Keeping Your Marriage Young," so she says:

"Certainly Roger Dear! What do you have in mind?"

Her husband smiles and says, "I'm glad you understand! Let me get undressed and then . . ."

Ellen feels a little tingle of anticipation.

Wide-eyed, Roger whispers hoarsely:

"And then I'll put on the dog's collar! And then I'll put on your push-up bra and your red silk panties! And then I'll lie across your knees! And then you can wallop my bare backside with the fly swatter while I play with myself! And then I'll . . ."

That loud screech you hear in the background is tires burning rubber on the driveway as the wife takes off for her mother's house—never to return.

But will prostitutes do that?

They love to do things like that. As a matter of fact, Roger's offer to his wife is exactly what a lot of men pay prostitutes for. Terry describes it:

> *"I have this movie actor who comes to see me once a month. He's a big action star in films but he likes my action better. The first thing I do is a 'boob job' on him. I get a sterile salt solution from the druggist and I inject it around each nipple in five spots. It gives him real boobs for about twelve hours. Then he gets dressed in my bra and panties—well, he thinks they're mine, anyhow. And then I whip him a little bit and then I give him a B.J. and he goes back and makes another tough guy movie. It takes an hour, I make nine hundred dollars, and I don't even get wet. And I'm getting acting lessons free!"*

Prostitutes are actresses?

Certainly. Some of the best performances in America aren't done on Broadway—they're done every night in hotel and motel rooms all over the country.

Listen to Terry again:

> *"Listen, Doctor, to be a good hooker, all you have to learn is five lines. Here they are:*
>
> * *'Oh, it's so big! I've never seen one that big!'*
> * *'Oh, put it in me, put it in me! I can't wait!'*
> * *'Oh! Oh! Shove it in all the way!'*
> * *'Uhhh! Don't stop! I'm coming!'*
> * *'You were terrific!'*
>
> *"But remember, you have to say them in the right order."*

What does "trick" mean?

Prostitutes have their own private language. It gives them a feeling of togetherness and helps keep the customers in the dark (even more in the dark than they already are). Some of the trade lingo is original with the girls, some is from carnivals, the underworld, and drug dealers. Since some prostitutes served an apprenticeship in these fields, they come by the slang naturally.

This form of expression is fluid and constantly changing—these examples can only be considered representative.

- **Around the World**: to perform fellatio, anilingus, (licking of the anus), and regular intercourse with a customer in addition to licking his body from head to toe.
- **B.J.**: fellatio or blow job.
- **Balling**: the same as Turning a Trick.
- **Dyke Whore**: a prostitute who is a lesbian with masculine characteristics.
- **Fast Ten-Oh**: a fast trick, without extras, charged at the current basic rate: one hundred dollars.
- **Freak**: a customer with bizarre tastes. (Prostitutes worry about these johns, and with good reason—many of them are sadists, and bruises are bad for business. Some are murderers—murder is worse for business.)
- **Get Burned**: perform intercourse without getting paid; prostitutes hate this.
- **Girl**: a prostitute, sometimes specifically a call girl.
- **Go Down On**: perform active fellatio.
- **Half-and-Half**: fellatio and regular sex.
- **Halfway Around the World**: fellatio, anilingus, and copulation without the licking.
- **Hooker**: any kind of female prostitute.
- **In the Life**: working as a prostitute.
- **Jane**: a lesbian customer.
- **John**: the same as a Trick.
- **KU'd**: knocked-up or made pregnant by a customer; prostitutes hate this even worse than getting burned.

- **Lot Lizard**: a prostitute who works the big trucks in the parking lot of a truck stop.
- **Slam-Bam-Thank-Ya-Ma'am**: a very fast ten-oh, usually at the customer's request.
- **The Game**: working as a prostitute.
- **The Racket**: working as a prostitute.
- **Three-Way Girl**: a prostitute who is equally at home with vaginal and anal intercourse and cunnilingus; she commands extra fees but ranks low on the social scale.
- **Trick**: a male customer.
- **Turn a Trick**: perform sexual intercourse with a John.
- **Turned Out**: to be mistreated by a Freak; one of the many occupational hazards of prostitution.
- **Whore**: disparaging term used by a prostitute; means a low-class prostitute although it sometimes has a reverse meaning. Some women use it as a general descriptive term.

How does a girl get started as a prostitute?

Fortunately the terrifying tales of "White Slavery" exist mostly in grade-B films.

> *"HELPLESS YOUNG VIRGINS FORCED INTO
> DEGRADING SUBMISSION AGAINST THEIR WILL!"*

went over big at the Saturday matinee, but real-life prostitution is a different story.

Most girls become prostitutes because they deliberately decide to do it. The transition from a "straight" girl to a straight "girl" is usually a gradual one. It can start with run-of-the-mill promiscuity, maybe a divorce or two, then a job in a cocktail lounge as a waitress or barmaid. Freelance sex with customers for gifts plus association with full-time professional hustlers who hang around the club often prompt a girl to put the pieces together and get "in the life."

Rhonda tells how she got started:

> *"First of all, don't think I'm making excuses. I know what I'm doing and I like it—I could quit anytime. I started screwing when I was fourteen. In the crummy hick*

*town where I grew up there wasn't anything else to do.
By the time I was seventeen I'd laid every jerk in the
county. I wasn't a hustler then—I mean I'd let 'em take
me out to dinner and all that, but I just did it for kicks. I
got married when I was eighteen and we moved to the
city—boy, what a jerk he was! After six months, I left him
and got a job in a bar.*

*"There wasn't much to do so I started screwing around
again. We had a couple of hookers working the bar and I got
friendly with them. One day they said to me:*

*"'Jesus, what're you giving it away for? You want to put
us out of business?'*

*"After closing time that night we went out for a few
drinks together and they laid it out for me. I tried it a couple
of times with guys they sent over and it wasn't so bad. I
mean, I get paid for what I was giving away before and the
johns get what they want, so everybody's happy."*

Unfortunately Rhonda missed one point: in prostitution,
nobody's happy.

Almost every man who has pay-sex with a prostitute would
trade it in a moment for real sex with a loving woman. And almost
every prostitute would prefer a happy home with a husband and
children who love her fondly instead of absorbing the ejaculations
of thousands of strangers year after year after year.

But all prostitutes are not the same. Just as there is a difference
between the drunk who scrapes out fiddle tunes on the street corner
and the concert violinist, there is a difference between the prostitute
at the bottom of the sex-for-pay roster and the one at the top.

The lowest ranking prostitutes are the "street whores."

What's a "street whore"?

Usually an overage hustler, an alcoholic hooker, or one that's on
drugs. Many of them are mentally retarded or schizophrenic. They
have become so dilapidated that they are willing to trade the use of
their vagina for the price of their next drink or rock of crack. These
are the ones that most commonly fall into the hands of the police.
These young—and not-so-young—women are truly victims and
deserve rehabilitation rather than persecution.

The next step up from the street whore is the "outcall girl."

What's an outcall girl?

An outcall girl is a prostitute who makes most of her arrangements with customers over the telephone. She can work independently or has an "agency" make her dates. Daphne is "independent"—this is how she works:

She is twenty-six and operates in Southern California; she has been in the "racket" about six years. As she sits in the coffee shop, she looks like a young actress or a fashion model—actually she has worked as both. Tall, slender, with long blond hair and bright blue eyes, she has the look of a well-scrubbed teenager.

> *"Well, Doctor, my line of work is not exactly ideal. Of course it's a lot better than trudging around to the casting offices all day. I had to put out all the time to get a job when I was in films anyway. The funny part of it is, I'm still putting out for the same crummy studio guys, but now they're paying for it. Anyhow I get up about noon and I'm ready for the first trick at two in the afternoon. That's when the 'Breakfast Club' starts checking in."*

The "Breakfast Club"?

That's right. Let Daphne continue.

> *"The 'Breakfast Club' is the guys who are so afraid of their wives they can't come up with an alibi for being out at night so they come over in the afternoon for a quick one. I don't mind them—it breaks up the day. But I always get some jerks who want a discount because it's still the afternoon. Sometimes I get mad and tell them off. Yesterday I said to one:*
>
> *"'Look man, what do you think this is, the kiddie matinee? Sure, you can come over for half price but you only get half a screwing!'*
>
> *"Between us, when business is slow I even take those jerks on for a fast one—it's better than nothing.*
>
> *"Anyhow, about six I get ready to go out—most nights I have tricks waiting. I'm usually pretty busy from then until about 2 A.M. Then things slow down unless there's a convention in town, and then it's wild. That's all those convention guys can think of—making it with a whore. You'd think they never got any at home!*

"When I finish up, sometimes I meet a few of the other girls and we have coffee and then it's home to bed after another thrilling night. What nobody understands, Doctor, is that it's hard work to hustle. Letting ten guys lay you every night is like digging ditches. Unless you're in top shape, it gets to you after a while. Sometimes I'm glad when my period comes on—at least I get to lie down without someone jumping on me."

Do girls call customers?

Yes. Prostitutes are in business, and when things are slow they have to promote, just like any other business. The old days of standing under the lamp post with a slit skirt are gone forever—except for the "street whores."

On a slow day (or night), Daphne calls around to see who wants a little action. Some girls carry the personal approach a little further—they may send Christmas cards and even birthday cards to valued customers. Some prostitutes even take credit cards.

Credit cards? Isn't that a little obvious?

It doesn't have to be. The credit card statement that reads

"Lulu La Belle—Professional Services"

won't get by the bookkeeper—or the wife.

But the one that reads:

"Paradise Builders: Erections and Demolitions"

is likely to pass unnoticed.

The relationship between Hooker and John sometimes gets closer than just anonymous sex. Sometimes men frequent the same prostitute once a week or so. When a good customer separates from his wife or gets divorced he may receive a sympathetic call from his favorite Hooker and sometimes even a trick on the house to console him for his loss.

Although they don't usually talk about it, prostitutes sometimes have closer relationships with certain Johns, especially if they are "regulars." It happens most often with celebrities—especially actors.

Actors have to pay for it?

It may sound strange but many "leading men" in Hollywood *want* to pay for sex. They deliberately select hookers over all those pretty young aspiring actresses so willing to trade sex for stardom. They feel much happier in long-term relationship with prostitutes. Steve is a good example.

At the outdoor café in Hollywood, Steve sits safely behind his top-brand-name sunglasses. His muscles are bursting through his tight black tee-shirt. He combs his long hair back as he speaks:

> *"I know it sounds strange, Doctor. I could have any girl in this town—almost. But I wouldn't survive. Those groupies are poison! The last one I had wanted to make a plaster cast of my penis! Sure, brilliant idea!*
>
> *"And they all end up selling the story of their one night of passion to some fan magazine. That's not the right career move for me! So I have two or three hookers that I've known for years. I see one of them about twice a week, and when I film on location I take one with me and we both stay out of trouble. It's expensive—I pay about five hundred a pop. But it's cool and clean and I avoid a lot of problems."*

Sometimes the relationship gets closer. Romance between Hustler and John can happen. Every so often an unfortunate man with fantasies of rescuing a girl from "the life" talks her into marrying him. Their chances for happiness are microscopic. The hookers themselves have a saying—"Once a Hooker, always a Hooker, and once a John, always a John." Sadly, that's usually the way it is.

Is doing outcalls safe?

More or less. The experience can range from OK to disastrous. But that's what prostitution is all about—two strangers are suddenly launched into a supercharged emotional relationship and no one can predict the consequences.

Most of the time nothing much goes wrong. Mechanical sex, ejaculation on schedule, and off to the next client. But sometimes there are surprises.

Some prostitutes will check a fellow's wallet when he's otherwise occupied. They may take any cash they find and also write down his credit card information. Sometimes they use that to charge a new stereo or a fur coat to his card. And sometimes they use it for "insurance."

Insurance?

Sure. The second worst nightmare of a prostitute is not getting paid. (The worst nightmare is getting killed or injured.) But if she has the john's home address—often in another city—she's protected. If he stiffs her, she can always give him a call when he gets back home. And if that doesn't scare him into paying, there's the deadly "Honest Maid" letter.

What's that?

A hooker who gets burned always has a few tricks up her sleeve. She knows that the john's wife was home taking care of the kids while he was enjoying half-and-half with her in his hotel room. She simply takes a pair of her panties—a worn pair is fine. She drips a little cooking oil in the crotch to make a nice stain. Then she sends the panties to the john's wife with this note:

Dear Mrs. Jones,

I am the maid in the Cosmos Hotel where you stayed with your husband in Room 347 last week. When you checked out, I found your underwear that you left behind in the room and I thought you would like to have it.

Sincerely,
Gladys, the Maid

Within minutes of the moment when Mr. Jones gets home from work and sees his wife standing on the front porch with the letter in her hand, he will wish a thousand times that he had paid that prostitute in full.

In many ways prostitution is just like any other business.

How is that?

The classier prostitutes have their own informal code of ethics. If it were ever written down, it might go something like this:

- Never recognize a customer in public unless he greets you first.
- Never reveal the identities of your customers in a way which might embarrass them.
- Never steal another girl's johns (she might do the same thing to you).
- Help a "sister" out if she is in trouble (if you don't risk anything by doing it).
- Never help the cops.

What's a "bar girl"?

If business is bad, a call girl (like Daphne) may work as a "bar girl." The neighborhood girls hang around cheap corner bars; the Club Girls make themselves available at selected nightspots. The more expensive hookers choose the more expensive cocktail lounges in the fashionable hotels and motels. Call girls don't like to cruise the bars—they consider it degrading, but as one of them said, with a wink, "A girl has to eat to live!"

At about the same level in the pecking order are the "Incall Girls." These are the ones who work the massage parlors and places like that. Generally they charge about fifty dollars for a massage. And every customer has to have a massage. After that, the "fun" starts as the client negotiates for "other services." In some places the list is fairly complicated and can go something like this:

1. Masturbation of client by girl—girl fully dressed (no touching by client).
2. Masturbation of client by girl—girl topless (no touching by client).
3. Masturbation of client by girl—girl topless and bottomless (no touching by client).
4. Any of the above with handling of breasts.
5. Any of the above with handling of buttocks.
6. Fellatio in any of the above categories.
7. Full sex.
8. Anal sex.

The first item on the list usually adds about fifty dollars to the price of the massage. If the customer picks number 8, it can add two hundred dollars to the total. Everything else is in between.

Some massage parlors are roach-infested joints. Others are spotlessly clean and well maintained. Some even have facilities for handicapped customers.

And almost without exception, the massage parlors follow the new trend in condoms.

What's the new trend?

Almost all prostitutes these days insist on condoms. One exception is the "street girls" who are sometimes too drugged or drunk to care. Another exception is the girls who charge extra for going "barefoot"—sucking a penis or having sex without a condom. They know that some men will pay as much as double for the feel of naked penis against naked vagina. The men sometimes also pay with their lives—and the girls run the same risk. AIDS is a one-way trip.

But the new trend is even more conservative. Most girls insist on a condom for fellatio, a split condom for men who want to perform oral sex on them, and two condoms for vaginal sex. From a professional point of view, it makes sense. In the old days, a broken condom—if they bothered to use it—might mean pregnancy and an abortion. Now it can mean death. And not just from AIDS.

Not just from AIDS? Isn't that the biggest danger?

Not really. Hepatitis can also be transmitted sexually, and worldwide, hepatitis kills more people every year than AIDS. There is no cure for hepatitis, and up to 35 percent of prostitutes carry the hepatitis virus. To make matters worse, syphilis and gonorrhea are still around and going strong.

When it comes to Sexually Transmitted Diseases (STDs), the United States is one of the most dangerous countries in the world.

There are about 12 million new cases of sexually transmitted diseases every year in the United States. That's the highest rate of any industrialized country on the planet. As a comparison, the incidence of gonorrhea in the United States is about fifty times greater than in Sweden. Maybe two condoms aren't enough!

Realistically, what are the chances of getting a sexually transmitted disease from a prostitute?

The chances are good. Here's the problem. Even if the rate of AIDS among prostitutes (or as some people like to call them, "CSW" or

"Commercial Sex Workers") is small, the law of probability works relentlessly against both the girls and the clients.

How come?

Condoms aren't perfect. Not every girl and not every customer uses a condom, and condoms sometimes slip off or break. As a result, every night the girls are being flooded with body secretions from their customers—orally, anally, and vaginally. Given an average of seven clients a night, a girl has about two hundred exposures a month or over two thousand a year. In spite of multiple condoms and every precaution, it only takes one accident to give them AIDS, hepatitis, syphilis, herpes, chlamydia, gonorrhea, or any of the other more exotic venereal diseases (or STD's). It's the massive multiple exposure that tilts the odds against the customer and the girl.

Look at it this way: if you take a water pistol and shoot at a target two thousand times a year, eventually you're bound to hit it.

How much do the girls make?

Prostitutes have high gross incomes while they are working, but their expenses eat up most of the profit. For the average high-class girl, the balance sheet might run something like this:

Nineteen working days per month with an average of seven customers per day at an average of $150 (including extras) per customer equals $19,950 per month gross income. The girls have to set aside an average of six days a month for menstruation. They can work "freaks" during their periods, but many don't like to do it.

They also take about four days off a month to relax—after all, they are performing manual labor and need some time off to recuperate.

Upper-bracket hustlers must have a place to take customers from time to time, and even small nice apartments cost money. Including maintenance and linen service (twenty sheets a day), it can easily run to $1,500 a month.

Clothes, shoes, cosmetics, hairdos, and other "front" expenses range up to $2,000 a month. Prostitutes usually pay more than others for their clothes, hairstyling, and everything else. Everyone they deal with knows they make a lot of money and charges them accordingly. The girls have all had to struggle and that makes them generous tippers. As long as the money comes in from the johns, the hookers are willing to pay.

A girl who is expensively dressed in the latest fashions with every aspect of her personal appearance at its best brings in the customers. No one wants to rent a dumpy-looking hustler.

What else do they have to pay for?

Probably the biggest item for the average big-time prostitute is payoffs and tips. Prostitutes are in a strange position. Their livelihood depends upon their availability to the greatest possible number of men. Yet in many places (especially the United States) their activities are illegal. If a girl succeeds in letting the johns know what she does, she invariably lets the cops in on her little secret. For a prostitute to work, the police have to look the other way—and some cops charge for this service.

In addition, the hustler has to pay for referrals—from cab drivers, bartenders, bellhops, and other contacts. The going rate is $10 to $20 per customer, which eats into profits fast. According to the girls, everyone else has a hand out, too. The elevator operator who brings the customers up to her apartment, the building manager, even her maid, all want their share. It can add up to about $2,000 a month.

Smart hookers spend a lot on doctors and drugs—infections are bad for business. Those at the top of the profession get a medical checkup every week and take antibiotics regularly. Their drug bill is about $500 a month and the four visits to the doctor run a total of $500 or more. This includes a thorough vaginal exam and bacterial cultures. (Doctors who specialize in treating prostitutes charge more too.)

Every top-drawer hooker has her own pager service and cellular phone. This makes life easier in many ways. First, it helps to insulate her from the police, cutting down but not eliminating one of the big risks of her trade. Second, it increases her availability to customers. Third, it saves time—when she finishes with one john, all she does is call in for the location and time of her next "appointment." A sophisticated communications service may cost $500 a month or more.

In these fast-moving days a girl needs transportation. If she drives, she can't pull up to the client's hotel or apartment in a jalopy. Girls who are just starting out lean to compact cars, but successful hookers like to go first class. They feel better in BMWs and Cadillacs, and some of the higher-priced ladies make the rounds in Mercedes and Corvettes. Car expenses or cab fares can run up to $1,000 a month or more.

Is there any other big expense?

Another major expense for hookers is what might be described as a contingency fund. In spite of payoffs and precautions, sometimes a girl gets arrested. The bail bondsman and attorney won't settle for taking it out in trade; they want cash and a lot of it. Legal fees for a simple arrest can reach from $3,000 to $5,000 easily. The girls are willing to pay; thirty days in jail can cost them up to $19,950 in lost gross income—and most of their expenses go on while they are serving time.

Another expense is abortion. Most hookers don't want to get pregnant and especially not by their customers. Even if a girl can tell for sure the exact week she got KU'd, the father could be any one of a hundred men. The biggest objection, of course, is being out of business for seven months or so. Although there are exceptions.

Exceptions during pregnancy?

Sure. There are some customers who are willing to pay double to have sex with a pregnant prostitute—especially during the last few months of her pregnancy. These are the "freaks"—the men who go in for kinky sex. Some girls like them a lot because often they are less demanding.

Anita has been a hooker for ten of her thirty-four years. She's studying psychology in her spare time—looking toward the time when her hooking days will be over. She's six months pregnant with her first child:

> *"There just isn't too much demand for pregnant hustlers, Doctor. So I take what I can get. I mean, even if I'm PG [pregnant] I still have to eat, and having a child is a big expense. So if I can get twice as much for each trick, that means I can work half as much. Besides, PG freaks are usually timid, gentle guys. They treat you like you were their mother."*
>
> *She paused a moment.*
>
> *"Hey, I never thought of it that way! I'm pregnant and they treat me like I was their mother! I'm going to ask about that in class tomorrow!"*

But most girls choose abortion. It's available and legal in most places, and motherhood puts a crimp in their professional pursuits.

Based on an eleven-month work schedule, the average upper-level hooker should gross about $220,000 a year if she services her full quota of customers. Expenses, calculated conservatively, run to about $60,000. Her take-home pay figures out to about $160,000 before subtracting the contingency fund.

With payoffs and legal fees, her net income runs about $100,000. For about two thousand assorted acts of sexual intercourse, she reaps about $50 a trick for herself.

But that's assuming that the girls work every day. Don't they take time off during their menstrual periods?

Some do and many don't. The girl who turns seven tricks a night at an average of only $150 a trick loses over $1,000 for every night she takes off.

Listen to Jennie's point of view. She's twenty-nine and she's been "In the Life" 6 years now.

She chuckles as she says it:

"Now I know why they call it 'The Curse,' Doctor! When I was a secretary I was delighted to sit around with my legs crossed for one week out of the month. Sometimes I'd even call in sick to work. You know: 'Ohh, these cramps are so bad!'

"But now this is how I make my living—there's no pension plan for ladies like us. So when my period starts, I get out these sponges that I sterilize carefully, and before I turn a trick, I push 'em right up there and they hold back the flood."

Jennie paused.

"Of course, I have a few regular johns who call me just when my period comes around. They keep track better than I do, and that's the only time they like to have sex. I stopped trying to figure men out a long time ago. If that's what gets them off, it's all the same to me."

Jennie shook her head quizzically, then continued:

"If it's too bad, I don't let them do oral on me, and sometimes I use a tight-fitting diaphragm. It works fine. I'm thinking about trying that Extractor that some of the girls use to keep from getting pregnant. They say it sucks it all right out and you don't miss a trick."

Is it true that most prostitutes only keep half their income?

It's even worse than that. Because prostitution is considered to be a "crime," prostitutes are not eligible for Workmen's Compensation, Unemployment Payments, Health Insurance, or Social Security. It is an occupation without fringe benefits.

But they don't have to pay taxes, do they?

According to the law, they should. The ever-present tax collector always has his eye on these charming last bastions of free enterprise. These chaps are ready to make professional calls on hustlers (their profession, not the girls') to collect the government's share of the take.

As one of the girls complained:

> *"So I told him, 'What the hell do you guys want me to do, stick a taxi-meter between my legs?'*
> *"He just shook his head and walked out."*

If prostitutes don't wind up with so much money, then why do they do it?

Most prostitutes are "in the life" because they want to be. Obviously some women who choose to rent their vagina to dozens of men a week have emotional problems. These are the ones who find prostitution glamorous, exciting, and strangely gratifying. One of the hustlers explains it this way:

> *"I know some people think it's terrible to be in the 'racket'—but they don't understand what it's really like. Always knowing that men are running after you, knowing that they leave their own wives just to make it with you, controlling them just with your sex—there's nothing else that can make a girl feel so powerful."*

Another hustler is more direct:

> *"I love to see them beg for it. They act just like babies, pleading for a B.J. or whatever they have to have. I get a kick out of taking their money. A hundred bucks for fifteen minutes work—I never had it so good!"*

Some prostitutes have another characteristic in common—they hate men.

Why is that?

The full answer is a complicated one related to the underlying emotional situation that drove them into "the game." Basically, prostitution is an ironic form of revenge against all men, acted out on the johns. An expensive hooker in Dallas summed it up this way:

"They think they're screwing me, but that's all wrong, Doctor. I'm the one who screws them. Oh, I put on a big show, but take it from me, I never feel a thing. None of these 'great lovers' ever made a dent in me."

To be honest, prostitutes don't exactly see men at their best.

How come?

Prostitution is a hard life. The average call girl turns about six to twelve tricks a night. Some nights the fast ten-ohs are few and far between. And an evening full of freaks can be mighty hard on a young lady.

Some men have original ideas. It is not unusual for a man to pay a girl to watch while he masturbates in front of her slowly and deliberately. Sometimes he keeps up a running conversation; sometimes he has the girl do the talking according to his script. Some men like to masturbate while the prostitute urinates on them. Some men pay just to watch a girl masturbate. Sadism can be time-consuming and risky—occasionally what started out as a friendly whipping ends with a trip to the hospital for the hooker—without Workman's Compensation. Masochistic males who like to be tied up and B.J.'d can also waste a lot of time on a busy night. A diversified girl has to be ready for anything.

Some men like (and are willing to pay for) two girls at once.

What can a man do with two girls at the same time?

Obviously most of the gratification is emotional—one penis can't be in two vaginas simultaneously. Some men seem to enjoy this form of conspicuous consumption—others are attracted by the allure of doing something forbidden. It usually amounts to variations on a theme.

Sometimes the man has regular intercourse with one of the girls while he performs cunnilingus on the other. He may also have the unoccupied girl titillate him anally while he is working on her partner.

Occasionally these little parties can get crowded. A prostitute may team up with a male assistant (usually a homosexual) for a special customer. The girl and her associate have sexual intercourse and variations thereof while the john watches. When he gets tired of watching he has his choice of further fun with either one—or both. The ultimate in this type of scene is the three-decker: the customer has vaginal intercourse with the prostitute while the other man has anal intercourse with the customer.

Sometimes the customer does it another way. He hires two girls and has sex with one the "regular" way. The other girl puts on a harness and a dildo and penetrates the man anally.

Sometimes it's the other way around. Three (or more) men hire a three-way girl. They have oral, anal, and vaginal intercourse with her simultaneously. It's great for the girl, who usually charges triple her usual fee plus as much more as she can get. Of course, three-way girls have to charge more—they wear out faster.

Why do people do these kinds of things?

Men who pay for these sorts of sexual capers often have emotional problems. Cunnilingus and fellatio are relatively routine these days, and if the johns could arrange it with their wives, the girls would probably lose the business. But the triple-decker, the three-way girl, and the two-gents-one-lady routine are pushing the limits of heterosexuality.

The chap who pays to see two ladies perform also has his problems, as do the father and son who patronize the same hustler. Whether she realizes it or not, the prostitute frequently functions as a sexual safety valve. The exhibitionist who masturbates in front of a hooker makes a better choice than if he masturbated in front of the ladies in the supermarket. It's probably preferable for a dedicated voyeur to pay a prostitute to masturbate in front of him instead of climbing over fences to look in the neighbors' windows.

Why don't prostitutes get pregnant all the time?

The risk of pregnancy is never as high as it seems. Many hustlers contract gonorrhea or chylamidia early in their careers and end up sterile from sealed fallopian tubes. And of course, some customers don't do things to a girl to make her pregnant, which is one reason fellatio and cunnilingus are fine with hookers.

Birth control pills have also changed everything. Nowadays it is rare for a hooker to get pregnant unless she wants to. Most of them aren't interested.

And AIDS has cut the risk of pregnancy even more. Since the "two condom" rule, accidents hardly ever happen. The sperm that gets through two condoms and past the birth control pills could probably get a girl pregnant through a brick wall. Prostitutes who get pregnant these days are either unbelievably careless or high on drugs.

If prostitutes have sexual intercourse as often as twenty times a day, doesn't it affect their sexual organs?

It doesn't seem to have much effect. The lining of the vagina is composed of mucous membrane almost identical with the lining of the mouth. If the girls are careful to use adequate lubrication (natural or artificial), friction is kept to a minimum and the amount of wear is insignificant.

Occasionally a problem does come up when a girl has had a great deal of stimulation in the course of an evening resulting in congestion of the clitoris and labia that tends to linger after working hours. An experienced hooker clears this up quickly with a masturbation-induced orgasm.

Since most of the girls are conscientious about attending to minor irritations and vaginal infections, their genitals are usually in better condition than those of the average woman.

Don't prostitutes enjoy sex?

Almost never with their customers. Only in the rarest situations does the hustler experience any sexual feeling, much less sexual gratification. The customer, however, insists that the girl have an orgasm—or a reasonable facsimile—and is willing to pay for it.

Do prostitutes ever have orgasms?

Certainly, but they are few and far between. On one occasion when a detective was questioning a girl who had just been arrested in a raid, more for his own curiosity than anything else, he asked her:

"Say, do you girls ever really make it with a customer?"

The girl gave him that look that hustlers reserve for cops and answered:

"Do you cops ever get parking tickets?"

Occasionally hookers begin to have regular orgasms with the johns—for them it is bad news.

How come?

Prostitutes know that orgasm means emotional involvement, and getting hung up with their customers is a sign of the beginning of the end. From their own experience, hookers know that orgasms at work are often the first sign of an impending nervous breakdown. Every hooker can tell a story about someone she knows who committed suicide or started on drugs shortly after letting the tricks make her come. When it starts happening, they take a long vacation until things cool off. If that doesn't help, sometimes they get worried enough to see a psychiatrist.

Why do men want the prostitute to have an orgasm?

A lot of wives never reach orgasm during sexual intercourse with their husbands and some of them complain about it. In some men this breeds the nagging fear that they may be inadequate sexually— that their wives don't reach a climax because the husbands aren't doing it right. Often the husband seeks out a prostitute to prove he can do it. He pays, the hooker plays the role of the passionate woman he never married, and everybody wins—or loses, depending on how you look at it.

Doesn't the customer realize that the girl is just pretending?

If the customer thinks too hard—if he really analyzes the situation, he would probably jump up, put on his clothes, and run home. In addition to leasing her anatomy, the good hooker also sells some fantasy; the grinding, moaning, and clutching that she substitutes for an orgasm are all part of the illusion that sexual intercourse is taking place.

But isn't it sexual intercourse?

Not in the real sense. Masturbation in a vagina is probably a more accurate description. Besides, the hooker and the john are really adversaries. He wants to make it last as long as possible to get his money's worth. She wants to speed it up so she can get another penis working for her. He wants her to feel something; she wants to protect herself against any emotional relationship with him. The outcome is usually a compromise. He looks down on her but needs the use of her vagina; she despises him but likes his money. Prostitution is a hard life—in many ways.

Are there male prostitutes?

Yes. In every large city there are dozens of tall, athletic young men whose sexual services are for rent. Urbane, sophisticated, well dressed, they can be had for an hour, an evening, or a month. They are skilled in every possible sexual nuance—they will engage in every type of sexual intercourse except one.

What type of intercourse won't they perform?

Intercourse with women. Most male prostitutes are homosexuals. Mirror images of their sisters in many ways, they cater to the small army of homosexual men who want a penis for hire. There are, however, certain important differences.

Almost every gay hustler is a four-way fellow: fellatio, active and passive, and anal intercourse, active and passive, and whatever else a customer can think of. In one way the gay hooker's life is easier. Since male homosexual customers rarely make a pretense of romance, there is no time wasted on counterfeit love. Every transaction is cash and carry and things go a lot faster. An enterprising gay guy can service twice the customers a female hooker can. Of course his capacity for orgasm is limited, but there are ingenious ways to overcome that.

Nickie, one of the busier hustlers in his part of town, tells how he does it:

"Well, I'm only twenty-two, so I can still go pretty good, but what's the use of throwing it away if I don't have to? For the first job in the afternoon I try to let the man go down on me.

It kind of gets me warmed up for the rest of the night. For the next five or six tricks I always schedule old guys—you know, senior citizens. They pay better—they have to—and they always want a blow job because they can't come any other way. What do I care?

"I work a few 'rips' (active anal intercourse) after that because I'm a little tender around the mouth by then. Just before dinner I look for the guys who like to 'brown' (passive anal intercourse). I don't have to do anything but lie there and groan like I'm feeling something big, if you know what I mean.

"After dinner the prices go up, and I have to do whatever the customer wants. But I'm not rough trade (coarse or tough homosexual prostitute) and I keep away from the S&Ms (Sadists and Masochists).

"I do mostly B.J.'s until midnight unless I'm working an orgy." (Homosexual orgies are similar to their heterosexual equivalents.) "Those damn orgies really wear a guy out and they don't pay that much. Those queens (effeminate male homosexual) want you to spend all night with them. They think they're doing you a favor—they don't realize that I'm in business. A guy's got to make a living."

Gay hustlers have a couple of other distinctions. The rate of AIDS among "trade" is much higher than among female prostitutes. Male hustlers have a lot more customers to catch things from, and strangely enough, some of them just don't seem to care. The big problem, of course, is that anal sex is the primary way to get—or give—AIDS.

Male homosexual prostitutes only have one real professional advantage over female prostitutes—so far no gay guy has ever gotten pregnant. But there are some prostitutes who don't fit into either category.

Who are they?

Those are castrated men who have had an artificial vagina constructed. These are "transgender" chaps and some of them end up as prostitutes catering to men. Some estimates calculate that in San Francisco, for example, 25 percent of the people working as "female prostitutes" are really men with an artificial vagina. When he realizes what he has been doing, that can give an unsuspecting john an unforgettable moment or two.

Are there any male prostitutes who cater to women?

In spite of the adolescent fantasies of being pursued by hordes of beautiful girls willing to pay for a night of passion, male hustlers have never really caught on with women. Few ladies have any trouble finding willing partners at the corner cocktail lounge—if they are so inclined. Most women recognize intuitively the basic absurdity of sex for hire and insist on at least the illusion of emotional involvement in their sexual encounters. Even the enterprising young gigolo who is hired on a long-term basis by his middle-aged mistress has to go through the motions of love. If he allows his true feelings to peek through, he finds himself looking for a new matron to make up to. The middle-aged lady and her handsome young companion are about the closest thing to male heterosexual prostitution in our society.

What about female homosexual prostitutes?

Among the hookers this is not a recognized specialty. Most hustlers will take on anyone, women included. Since some prostitutes are female homosexuals in their private lives anyway, making it with another girl is like a busman's holiday.

Isn't a pimp a man who finds customers for a prostitute?

In popular slang, that's what he's called, but in the lingo of the hustlers a pimp is the man who lives with and from a hooker. These days most girls have their established clientele expanded by referrals from cab drivers, bartenders, and other key people. Besides, most modern johns know what they want and where to find it—pimping, as a trade, has been made obsolete by updated communications, improved merchandising, and greater consumer sophistication.

But no one can replace the pimp. He is the only man a girl can really talk to. When she comes home in the wee hours of the morning after drawing three freaks in a row, after being "burned," and in general having a bad night, it's her pimp who understands. If she feels like sex (she doesn't really consider her professional activities *sex*), the pimp is ready to oblige. If she is arrested, he is there with bail and a lawyer and sympathy. Her pimp is her own private boyfriend who provides her with what little emotional warmth he is capable of.

What does the pimp get out of it?

For his services he takes a big cut of the girl's earnings. Out of the average hooker's $100,000 net, the pimp may cut himself in for $60,000 or more. In spite of his promises, if a girl falls on hard times, her pimp may simply find himself another hooker who is doing better. In a grim form of poetic justice, the hustler hustles the john and the pimp hustles the hustler. (Another hustler inevitably hustles the pimp and everything comes out even.)

Most hustlers have a hard time making the transition from john to pimp. Their professional frigidity carries over into their personal lives; few prostitutes achieve orgasm even in the privacy of their own bedrooms.

What happens to prostitutes when they get old?

That's when things get tough for the girls. Some of the lucky ones have managed to save enough out of their earnings to go into a small business. One of the favorite lines is a ladies' ready-to-wear shop supplying fashionable clothes and fancy underwear to other hookers. A few hustlers retire into the straight world by getting married. They usually marry men who are unaware of their previous line of work; the girls are in no hurry to confess their past. As one of them said:

> *"How do you think my husband would like it if he knew I was screwed by 25,000 other men before he came along?"*

Less often they marry johns, and even more uncommon is a wedding between hooker and pimp; as they say:

> *"We know too much about 'the life' to ever trust each other."*

Contrary to popular folklore, ex-hookers do not make ideal wives. Their underlying—and understandable—bitterness toward men almost always breaks through and makes trouble for both partners. Some of them just can't resist the temptation to turn a few tricks on the side. Alice is one of those; her explanation summarizes the basic problem that hustlers run into when they try to settle down and live like the squares:

> *"Well, after putting in fifteen years on my back, I thought it was time to live a nice respectable life—you know, work in the kitchen instead of the bedroom. Was I wrong! After six months I thought I'd go out of my mind! And talk about dull—the biggest thing in the crummy straight world was what band was playing at the Country Club that weekend! Remember, I used to go out every night with guys who thought spending five hundred bucks was just warming up! So I got bored, and just for something to do, I turned a few tricks—just a couple of fast ten-ohs, and when my husband found out about it, that was that. I got mad and told him what he could do about it and here I am back in business again. Married life was lousy anyhow."*

How about the girls who don't get married?

They may try to get along with occasional jobs—acting in pornographic movies, posing for pornographic photos, and taking whatever else comes along. The most common solution is the one chosen by Tina. She describes it:

> *"Well, I'm forty-two now and I've put on about thirty pounds—there's not exactly a big demand for overweight hookers. I tried some of the other angles but it was too much of a comedown. I used to be right up there when I was in the racket, and I can't see turning twenty-five-dollar tricks. So I figured I got started waiting on tables and I might as well go back there. It's regular hours, I'm building up Social Security credits—which is one thing I never got in the racket. So I work standing up instead of lying down, so what? For me it's the best way out."*

A lot of other girls finish their careers by coming full circle—they go back to work as barmaids, hostesses, and waitresses. They manage to come out of "the life" with their minds and bodies intact. They are the lucky ones.

Chapter 12
BIRTH CONTROL

Important Note: Nothing in this chapter should be taken as medical advice. It is authoritative information of a general nature. For specific medical advice, see your doctor. After all, that's what we doctors are for.

What is birth control?

Birth control refers to the hundreds of methods that have been employed to separate the Art of Copulation from the Act of Reproduction. Since the earliest stages of civilization men have sought ways to deliver sperm into the vagina—and not one inch farther. Regrettably these little creatures have a compulsion to swim upstream and unite with an expectant egg; they stubbornly resist any effort to impede their progress.

The specter of unwanted pregnancy has always cast its shadow over sexual enjoyment. The prospect that each act of intercourse might result in a new addition to the family has dulled the sexual appetites of untold billions of husbands and wives. The possibility that sexual intercourse might start a family has also ruined the fun of a lot of people who aren't married. Some of the saddest lines ever spoken during sex are these:

- "Don't stop, Roger! Ooooh! Don't stop! Oh, this is the wrong time of the month! Stop! Stoooooop! Don't Stop!"

- "Don't worry, Alice, your period is sure to start tomorrow—isn't it?"

- "I was just thinking, Milt. What will my husband do if I get pregnant while he's away?"

and the all-too-common:

- "We might as well go ahead; I'm three weeks late already."

But now things have changed—in many ways.

Why is that?

Birth control has entered the Space Age. Based on modern knowledge of human physiology, there is a whole new arsenal of defenses against that unrelenting army of sperm.

Think of it this way. Every act of copulation is a sexual "Game of Tag." The 100 million Sperm that the man launches with each ejaculation are "It." The single and exclusive mission they have in their very short lives is to tag that helpless little Egg. The job of contraception is to keep the Egg from getting tagged by the Sperm.

Every time a blast of Sperm hits the vagina, the game starts all over again. Sometimes the Egg has the advantage.

How come?

Well, the Sperm only has so long to do its job. On the average, a little sperm only has seventy-two hours to live—although a few Super-Sperm can hold out for seven long days and nights. On the other hand, the Egg has a mere twenty-four hours of existence each month. If a Sperm doesn't tag her in that time frame, there is virtually no chance of pregnancy.

That means a woman can only get pregnant one day a month?

Many people who believed that are now pushing baby carriages. Actually a woman can be fertilized for *at least* seven days each month and maybe more.

Say, for example, her husband delivers Sperm into her vagina on a Monday night. Some of them immediately enter the cervix and start their migration upward toward the fallopian tubes.

Then the woman ovulates a week later. There may still be some surviving Sperm somewhere between the cervix and the fallopian tubes—and it only takes one to tag that Egg. That's why the simplest and oldest form of birth control seems the most logical.

Which one is that?

It involves putting some kind of impenetrable wall between the Sperm and the Egg so the sperm can't get through. It's the sexual equivalent of a "Catcher's Mitt." The most common "Catcher's Mitt" is the condom.

How well does the condom work?

Fair. It has a tough assignment. Sex is all feeling, and for a man that feeling is in the penis—especially in the head of the organ. But the head is also where all those Sperm come shooting out. So cover the head of the penis with something thick and you zap the feeling. Cover it with something thin, and you might let a few million sperm trickle out. That's why the early condoms were called:

> *"Armor Plate against Pleasure and a Cobweb against Disease."*

It's not that bad these days, but that's why so many different kinds of material have been used to make condoms.

The best material for feeling is what used to be called "skins." These were made from the intestines of lambs and allowed pretty good sensation. But they also allow bad viruses like AIDS to get through and that isn't good news for anyone.

The most common type of condom is made of latex rubber. That keeps the Sperm where they should be—most of the time—but the feeling isn't that great. It's really like having sex with your penis encased in one finger of a rubber glove. Making that glove thinner and thinner helps, but when you get to the point where you can really feel everything, you're in real danger of spilling a few million little wigglers all over the vagina. And of course there's the "desperation condom."

The "Desperation Condom"? What's that?

That's the one you use when you can't find a regular condom. It happened to Charlie:

> *"Last December I drove to my cousin's wedding in Cincinnati. I met this really nice girl there and we drank a lot of champagne and we found ourselves back in her room at the hotel about 2 a.m. Just as we were about to get down to it—you know—I realized that my condoms were in the trunk of the car in the parking lot. It was two degrees above zero and snowing."*
> *Charlie shrugged.*
> *"What was I going to do? Do it without a condom? With a girl I just met? I was half out of my mind anyway when I spied a green balloon from the party on the bedside table. I grabbed it, cut it open, pushed it over my penis, and had sex. It wasn't exactly great but I suppose it was better than nothing. And I'll tell you one thing, Doctor. Anyone who does it with a party balloon will never ever complain about lack of feeling with a condom!"*

Other people—in similar desperate situations—have resorted to plastic food wrap or plastic sandwich bags. It's not a brilliant idea, but a desperate man resorts to desperate measures. Perhaps that's what the old saying means when it says:

> *"When a man's Little Head wakes up, his Big Head goes to sleep."*

Strangely enough, plastic wrap for the penis has now become "Respectable."

Plastic wrap for the penis?

That's right. But it's not a sandwich bag anymore. It's a polyurethane condom. That means it's strong and can be made very thin. The sensation is good, but the old problem comes back to haunt us. The thinner it gets, the more "tearable" it gets and some reports say that the polyurethane condoms break almost seven times as often as the latex versions. They also seem to slip off six times more frequently than rubber condoms.

But users confirmed that when it came to sensation, "less is more." They liked the plastic condoms because they allowed a better "feel."

It's a tough equation. You can gain protection and lose sensation or you can gain sensation and lose protection. Wouldn't it be wonderful if a man could use a condom without having to wear one?

Is there a way to do that?

Sure. It's called the "female condom." The concept is brilliant. Take what looks like a little plastic sandwich bag, put a flexible plastic ring at each end to keep it steady, and push it carefully up into the vagina. The vagina is then lined with the plastic bag. During intercourse, the penis slides against the plastic, the ejaculation is in the "bag," and nobody gets pregnant.

Does it work?

Sort of. One problem with the *male* condom is that it interferes with the building excitement of sex. At the most crucial instant, the woman has to stop playing with the penis and the man has to stop caressing the clitoris and fingering the vagina. He tears open the foil pack, pulls out the condom, and the magic of the moment slowly evaporates.

Some women try to keep up the feeling by putting the condom on their partner's penis. (A few talented professional ladies go one step further. They have mastered the art of applying a condom without using their hands. It involves complex coordination of lips and tongue.)

But if putting on the male condom is a distraction, installing the female version is a major enterprise. Everything has to stop while it is inserted carefully and with precision. It has been suggested— very optimistically—that the manipulation be "made part of the exciting ritual of foreplay." It would seem to me that for most people, stuffing a plastic bag into the vagina is not exactly a turn-on:

> *"Now get ready for something really exciting, Dear. I'm unfolding this plastic bag and guess what I'm going to do with it!"*

In all fairness, the female condom helps prevent disease, although it hasn't been around long enough to compare its protection precisely with the male condom. But it's reasonable to assume that its failure rate in protecting against HIV will be about the same as its failure rate in protecting against pregnancy (we'll see that in a moment). If a man just won't use a condom, a woman can protect herself to some extent by using the female version. But that brings up an interesting question that proponents of the female condom need to consider:

What woman in her right mind would think of having sex with a man who refused to take the responsibility for protecting her from whatever disease he might have?

How are condoms as far as birth control is concerned?

Surprisingly good. There are all kinds of statistics about the effectiveness of birth control methods, depending on whom you talk to. In general, condoms are about 97 percent effective in preventing pregnancy—with an "IF."

That "if" depends on whether you use it perfectly each time. "Perfectly" means putting it on carefully with proper lubrication, grabbing the base of the penis to hold it on after ejaculation when the penis shrinks, so it won't leak or slip off, and in general being "perfect." In real life, the condom does its job about 88 percent of the time. That's not bad considering that it is cheap, fast to apply, and doesn't involve hormones that can affect the entire body.

It also has other advantages. Women can have one handy for impulsive moments, it comes in assorted colors, and some of them even have little faces painted on them for festive occasions. In addition, some condoms are treated with nonoxynol-9.

What is nonoxynol-9?

Nonoxynol-9 is a very effective spermicide—the primary ingredient of most contraceptive creams and foams. Some condoms are impregnated with N-9 (as it is known for short) in the hope that it will increase their contraceptive effectiveness. It probably can't do much, since it isn't in contact with sperm very long—but it may possibly cause irritation to a sensitive penis or vagina. (We'll see more about N-9 later on.)

How effective are the female condoms?

So-so. Their failure rate depends on whom you talk to. The most quoted figure is a failure rate of about 21 percent for real-world use. Add to that the fact that they are much more expensive than male condoms—plus one other little detail. Even after they are carefully and correctly installed, about an inch of the plastic bag dangles outside the vagina. Maybe that's what led one man to say:

"If my wife doesn't get home on time, maybe I'll just make love to the baggie!"

What about condoms and anal sex?

They just don't work that well. The typical male condom is about seven hundredths of a millimeter thick—much too thin to resist the friction of anal rubbing. Some companies have made extra-thick condoms for homosexuals to use in anal sex, but it's the old problem again. A doubly thick condom begins to feel like a bicycle inner tube. Some ingenious—or desperate—women have managed to accomplish the feat of installing the female condom in their anus for anal sex. That's not what it was designed for and it's not the world's most brilliant idea.

What are some of the other methods of birth control?

In an effort to restore the sensation to copulation that the condom takes away, contraceptive designers have moved the "Catcher's Mitt" inward and upward. Quite a few years ago they came up with the "diaphragm" which by comparison with the condom is so big that it begins to look like a real "Catcher's Mitt."

Basically a dome-shaped piece of rubber with a rubber-covered spring-steel-ring rim, it is filled with contraceptive jelly, folded, and slid sideways up the vagina. Ideally, it rests just behind the pubic bone and covers the cervix so the Sperm can't play that irresistible game of Tag with the Egg. The diaphragm has the advantage that you can pop it in ahead of time so you don't have to call a halt to the proceedings to erect your defenses against the Sperm Scrimmage.

Since rubber is waterproof (and sperm-proof), a diaphragm should be 100-percent effective. It isn't. Unless it is put in place precisely and remains fixed there throughout the inner turmoil of copulation, it merely serves to guide millions of little surfers into the cervix. Even with the diaphragm properly in place, a pinhole in the membrane is like the Holland Tunnel to a Sperm. That's why in actual use the device has a failure rate of about 18 percent.

There is also a mini-diaphragm known as the "cervical cap" and that's exactly what it looks like. It's a miniature rubber bonnet that fits tightly over the cervix like a shower cap. Like a good shower cap, its job is to protect against that hot shower of sperm. Sometimes the cervical cap doesn't fit tightly enough and can be found at the mouth of the vagina the morning after. The failure rate is about 18 percent—the same as its bigger cousin, the diaphragm. But there's one important detail to remember.

What's that?

The cervix *after* pregnancy isn't the same as the cervix *before* pregnancy. After the baby comes, the cervix is much more irregular and it's almost impossible to get a good fit with the cervical cap. Actually the cervical cap is a little condom turned inside-out. Imagine trying to keep a condom on a fat two-inch-long penis during hot and heavy sex. That's why after childbirth the failure rate of the cervical cap goes up to about 36 percent—bad odds even in Las Vegas.

There's one other in-the-vagina method that's worth mentioning.

What's that?

Sperm-killer, or "spermicide." The most widely used chemical is called "Nonoxynol-9" (previously mentioned). It's actually a powerful detergent that kills sperm by zapping their delicate surfaces. It also kills the AIDS virus and some of the microorganisms that cause Sexually Transmitted Diseases—in the test tube. No one knows how effective it is against those diseases in the vagina. But it does kill Sperm. The basic idea is to get enough of the chemical into the vagina so it can slaughter those stubborn little sperm before they can penetrate the Egg.

You can pump it into the vagina as a cream or a foam; you can push a little sponge impregnated with N-9 up the vaginal canal; or you can push a little square of plastic film soaked in N-9 up the vagina and stick it against the cervix. Spermicide has certain advantages. You can apply it well in advance of sex so you don't have to stop the proceedings. It also helps to provide lubrication if you need it. But it also has its disadvantages.

Like what?

For one thing, it tastes awful. And if you're into oral sex, that's important. And if you don't need lubrication, it can make things much too slippery. That's when you learn "The Fastest Four-Handed Game in the World of Sports."

What's that?

When the penis slips out.

And there's another problem. Spermicide is only about 80-percent effective in real-world use—so you can't bet your future on it. The protection against AIDS and STDs (Sexually Transmitted Diseases) is only theoretical and that too has its downside. N-9 kills bacteria and it kills good bacteria as well as bad bacteria. One example of "good" bacteria is the "Lactobacillus" found in the vagina. That protects women against certain vaginal infections and you don't want to do anything to harm it.

Another problem is that N-9 sometimes causes irritation of the skin as well as the vagina and penis in susceptible people. Theoretically that can make them more vulnerable to AIDS and STDs by reducing their natural skin defenses. It's nothing to lose sleep over but it is something to be aware of.

However there is one method of birth control that could be absolutely 100-percent effective—if it weren't for one little detail.

What method is that?

The "Rhythm Method" and all its variations. It depends on the physiological fact that fertilization is more likely to occur if intercourse occurs a few days before or a day after ovulation. A couple that uses the Rhythm Method assumes that ovulation takes place about the midpoint of the menstrual cycle and they simply avoid intercourse during this time. Theoretically it works fine. In actual practice it is a Reproductive Shooting Gallery—and the Egg is the Sitting Duck.

The big problem is that ovulation generally occurs fourteen days *before* the first day of the next menstrual period. So in order to win, the woman has to predict with perfect accuracy what will happen two weeks in the future. Nice try. If she can predict future events like that, she should be able to pick the winner of the Florida Lottery.

There is one other little detail. In reality, ovulation can actually occur on any day of the menstrual cycle, even during menstruation itself. Rhythm? That mischievous little Egg doesn't have any rhythm. And the proof is that the Rhythm Method flops about one-quarter of the time. But there's another method that works outside the vagina and is amazingly effective.

What's that?

The IUD or "Intra-Uterine-Device." If there ever was a THEORET-ICALLY perfect birth control method, it's the IUD—"theoretically" is the key word.

Look at it this way. All you have to do is insert a little plastic widget into the uterus and for the next ten years you can have sex every day if you want to and your risk of pregnancy is only about 1 percent. No pills, no condoms, no diaphragms, no messy creams. And when you want to get pregnant, just slip it out, and you're as good as new. Pregnancy should follow in a few months without any problem. No risk, no side effects, no danger.

Where do you buy an IUD like that?

On the planet Mars—or maybe Saturn. Because there is no IUD like that on Earth. We do have IUDs here, and they work fairly well in certain cases, but it's a long way from being the perfect means of birth control. As a matter of fact, the IUD has been controversial right from the start.

In what way?

In the beginning it was a political football. Aside from the ancient technique of popping an apricot pit into the uterus of a camel to avoid pregnancy on long caravan voyages, the modern IUD is not really so modern. Back in 1900 German doctors placed rings of catgut wound with metal wire in the uteruses of women to prevent pregnancy. The Japanese improved on that by adding another little twist so the IUD wouldn't pop out. Then the changing world situation made an increased birth rate a national priority in some countries and the IUD was put aside. But after World War II, the world suddenly decided that there were too many new faces showing up too soon. The new priority was "Population Control" and the IUD seemed like the perfect answer.

Is it?

Not quite. As more and more women used the device and we doctors learned more about it, a few problems began to show up. First of all, women aren't camels. Their bodies are very delicate and their sexual equipment even more so. Some of the first IUDs caused bad pelvic infections and had to be taken off the market.

These days there are two types of IUDs currently in use in the United States. One contains metallic copper and the other is impregnated with a female sex hormone—progesterone.

How do they work?

The truth is that no one knows exactly how they work. Copper and the chemical products that copper produces are poisons. The copper probably zaps the sperm and may also flow upward enough to affect the Egg and keep it from accepting the sperm.

The progesterone-loaded IUD releases a little of the hormone every day and makes the inner lining of the uterus atrophy and shrink up.

Currently the copper IUD can be kept in place for up to ten years according to government regulations. The progesterone IUD that is commonly in use in the United States uses up the hormone every year and has to be replaced. The first-year pregnancy rate of the progesterone IUD is about twice that of the copper device—but it's still only about 1 percent.

In other countries you can get hormone-containing IUDs that last ten years and are about as effective as the copper ones. But there is still one nagging question with IUDs. It's one that bothers some people while others couldn't care less about it.

What's that?

There are those who are seriously against abortion—in any form. Some of them suspect that the IUD may actually perform mini-abortions within the uterus. If a fertilized egg is prevented from attaching to the lining of the uterus because of the IUD, is that an abortion?

Is it?

I have no opinion whatsoever because I don't know. But it is a matter of concern to a certain number of people and it is worth mentioning. As we learn more about how IUDs actually work, that whole area will become clarified and hopefully set minds at ease.

Are there any problems associated with the IUD?

Where do you want to start? From the moment of insertion, there are problems. While the IUD is being pushed into the uterus, the woman feels strong pain and cramping. Afterward, the cramping may continue and often requires pain medicine around the clock. That pain and cramping can last a few months.

There is the risk of serious infection during the first three weeks or so after the device is inserted—about 1 percent of women get infected. And a lot of those infections depend on lifestyle.

In what way?

Strangely enough, the IUD is the only form of birth control that passes moral judgment. And it does it in an interesting way.

The human vagina is a strange place—it has immense colonies of bacteria constantly renewing themselves, and at the same time it maintains a very special and stable environment. If anything disrupts that bacteriological tranquillity, bad things can happen.

If a woman has regular sexual relations with one man, the conditions inside her vagina adjust to that man. If she takes on a new partner, the whole inner economy of her vagina changes. That's when she becomes much more susceptible to a serious vaginal and pelvic infection. But that's not all.

What else?

Amazingly, the vagina is so sensitive that even if she only has one sexual partner, if he has sex with another woman and then has sex with her, the bacterial environment of her vagina changes. So women who are having sex with more than one man—or having sex with a man who is having sex with someone else—are at much greater risk for a bad pelvic infection with the IUD.

In practical terms that means that the IUD is only a good choice for women—and men—who walk the straight and narrow. For anyone who strays, the IUD can inflict harsh punishment.

It's an interesting point. When I explained it to a female patient, she indignantly raised an eyebrow and said:

"It doesn't seem fair! Why isn't there an IUD for men?"

Are there any other problems with the IUD?

Yes. If the woman gets a STD (Sexually Transmitted Disease), the IUD has to be pulled out right away. The risk of keeping it in and spreading the disease upward into her pelvis is too great.

Can a woman get pregnant with an IUD in place?

Sure. Remember that statistics are like bikini bathing suits. What they reveal is interesting but what they conceal is vital. The pregnancy rate for the IUD may be 1 percent—but for the woman who gets pregnant, the rate is 100 percent. Pregnancy with an IUD is treacherous. If she is using the copper-containing IUD, the pregnancy will be *ectopic* about 6 percent of the time.

An ectopic pregnancy is one where the baby grows outside the uterus, usually in the fallopian tube. The treatment is emergency surgery to prevent possibly rupture of the fallopian tubes and fatal complications for the mother as well as the fetus.

Are there any other pregnancy-type risks with the IUD?

Yes, there are. If a woman gets pregnant with an IUD in place, she has a 50-percent chance of aborting spontaneously. Realistically that may not bother her too much since she is using the IUD because she doesn't want a baby. But if she changes her mind, she can cut the risk of losing the baby almost in half by having the IUD pulled out.

Pulled out?

That's right. Inserting an IUD is an interesting experience. A little plastic tube like a soda straw is inserted into the vagina and up into the cervix—the part of the uterus that extends into the vagina. The IUD is pushed through it into the uterus—a little like inserting a vaginal tampon with its applicator. There are two little strings attached to the IUD that hang out of the cervix—the doctor trims them enough so they don't dangle out of the vagina.

In the beginning every woman who uses an IUD should put a finger up into her vagina to feel those strings after every sexual intercourse. After that, she should check about once a month to see that the strings haven't been pulled up into the uterus. If the doctor needs to take the device out, the easiest way is to just pull it out by those strings. About 15 percent of women with IUDs will decide have those strings pulled before the first year is over, usually because of pain and bleeding. But sometimes the doctor doesn't have to pull it out.

Why not?

It can fall out by itself. That's why the woman should check those little strings regularly, and she should also look through her tampons and menstrual pads to see if the IUD has fallen out. If the IUD has fallen out, her chances of pregnancy suddenly increase astronomically.

If she can't feel the strings, that can simply mean they have just pulled up into the uterus. But it can also mean the IUD has poked through the wall of the uterus and is now floating around somewhere in her abdominal cavity. That means an operation to get it out.

Is the IUD a good choice for birth control?

That depends. Like every other medical decision, it has to be made in consultation with your doctor. It's interesting to note that less than 1 percent of American women have chosen the IUD as their means of birth control. But there's something else a woman can have inserted into her uterus that goes one step beyond the IUD.

What's that?

It's the last thing in the world that most people would ever think of. It's a handful of anti-malaria tablets. Although it may sound at first like the wires got crossed somewhere, more than a million women around the world have used malaria pills as the ultimate form of birth control.

"The ultimate form of birth control"? What's that?

Sterilization. Some years ago, scientists discovered that quinacrine, a common and inexpensive drug used against malaria, could also sterilize women quickly and permanently. The procedure is amazingly simple. The technician simply inserts the tablets directly into the uterus. (Strange as it may seem, in most places where this method is used a technician does it—not a doctor.) The operator uses the same gadget doctors use to insert the copper IUD to pop seven tablets high up into the uterus. A month later he repeats the process and the woman takes birth control pills for the next three months while the pills are working.

How do the pills work?

The active ingredient in the pills seeps up into the fallopian tubes and seals them off. The idea is to irritate the lining of the tubes enough so they stick together and keep Sperm and Egg from ever meeting. The method is a lot cheaper than the traditional procedure of carefully tying off the fallopian tubes with surgical sutures. That usually costs between two and four thousand dollars including surgeon, anesthetist, medicines, and hospital stay. The quinacrine procedure costs about five dollars. It has been used in over 100,000 women without a single death from the procedure.

But then why don't they use it instead of the expensive surgery?

There seem to be a few problems. First of all, most countries in the world don't approve the insertion of those little tablets into the uterus. Some say that their safety hasn't been completely established. There are other problems too. Since it can be done by non-medical people, the technique comes pretty close to a do-it-yourself sterilization procedure. The "Menstrual Extraction Machine" and the "Morning-After Pill" (details in this chapter) have already given control of a big part of reproduction to the individual woman. A technique that can sterilize a woman permanently, costs next to nothing, and doesn't even require a physician is very controversial.

But if a woman doesn't want to get pregnant in the first place, there is always the "pill."

What about the pill?

"The pill" or the "oral contraceptive" (or "OC") is a stroke of genius. For centuries scientists had been looking for something a woman could take by mouth that would keep her from becoming pregnant. Finally, about fifty years ago, they asked themselves this question:

When is the one time when it is almost totally impossible for a woman to get pregnant?

The answer was staring them right in the face:

When she is already pregnant!

So all they had to do was come up with a pill that would make a woman's body think she was sort-of-kind-of-maybe-pregnant.

This is the way they did it.

At the moment she is born, a baby girl has about 300,000 immature eggs in her little ovaries. From the time she is about fourteen years old until she is about fifty years old, every month one of those eggs will mature under the influence of two hormones that don't come from the ovaries.

These two hormones are really the "Fairy Godmothers of Female Reproduction." They're not well-known or even famous but they make everything else possible. Produced by the pituitary gland at the base of the brain, they are called "FSH" or "Follicle Stimulating Hormone" and "LH" or "Luteinizing Hormone."

FSH controls the growth of a few eggs each month and encourages the production of the female sex hormone, estrogen, by the ovary. Later, when the eggs are getting mature, the other Fairy Godmother, LH, triggers the "Event of the Month": The Egg Launch. When that tender little Unmanned Vehicle blasts off into Inner Space, you can almost hear Houston Control shouting:

"We have Ovulation!"

The remnants of the egg-maturity process that stay behind in the ovary give rise to a yellowish structure called the "Corpus Luteum" or "yellow body." That makes the female sex hormone called "progesterone."

Now the four Key Hormones of Reproduction are in place and the woman is ready for pregnancy. Very ready. If the average woman has sexual intercourse at random during any month, her chances of getting pregnant are 8.5 out of 10. That means that under normal circumstances, unless she uses some kind of contraception, she will eventually get pregnant.

Under normal circumstances, the velvetlike lining of the uterus matures under the influence of estrogen until the middle of the cycle. Then ovulation occurs and progesterone makes the lining warm, juicy, and succulent—just waiting for that fertilized Egg to touch down. Of course, as estrogen and progesterone increase, the levels of LH and FSH. slack off.

That's where the OC's (Oral Contraceptives) do their job. Most birth control pills these days contain a combination of two female hormones—estrogen and progesterone. The pituitary gland senses the presence of these hormones in the blood—but it doesn't know if they come from the ovary or from a pill that the lady has just swallowed. The poor pituitary gland reacts to the estrogen and progesterone it is sensing and decides that the woman might be pregnant. It immediately shuts off the release of FH and LH and blocks release of an Egg. Houston Control is in the "All Systems Ready" condition but that month the message is:

"No Launch! Mission Aborted!"

"Mission Aborted"? Is that really an abortion?

We'll see about that in a moment. But for now, let's follow the trail of an innocent Sperm on his way to fertilize an Egg protected by Oral Contraceptives.

As the sperm is blasted out of the penis into the vagina, he starts swimming desperately to make his way into the cervix. That's where he has his first unpleasant surprise. The opening in the cervix, the neck of the uterus that projects into the vagina, is usually sealed with a plug of mucus. But under the influence of the "Pill," that mucus gets thick and tough and the poor sperm finds himself clawing his way through something like thick glue.

If he manages to get through that, he swims upward through the uterus into the fallopian tube, where much to his dismay, he finds that there is no Egg to hurl himself into! He cruises up and down the dark passageway only to find himself totally alone and abandoned. The "Pill" has blocked ovulation, and it's curtains for Mr. Sperm.

Does it always work that way?

No. And that's when it gets really interesting. About 3 percent of the time (more or less, since no statistics about conception are anywhere near exact) ovulation happens anyhow. Then Mr. Sperm meets the Egg in the dark Fallopian Chambers and zooms into her. His chromosomes unite with hers and:

"Houston! We Have Fertilization!"

Now it's not an Egg and a Sperm anymore. It's a "zygote" or fertilized egg.

Within a few days, the new organism finds its way back down to the uterus. But things there are not what it expected. Instead of a thick juicy lining full of blood vessels and nutrition just waiting for it to attach, it finds a virtual desert. Because of the influence of the birth control pills, the lining is skimpy and atrophied, inhospitable and forbidding. Most of the time the zygote just withers away and dies. Implantation is a flop and contraception is a success. And it's all over until next month.

But you said something about "Mission Aborted." What does that mean?

That's a delicate subject. Some people believe—and they certainly have all the right to feel that way—that human life begins at the moment when the egg is fertilized by the sperm. If that is true, then it is conceivable that a pill that makes it impossible for that fertilized egg to survive is a pill that produces an abortion. On the other hand, if you believe that life begins somewhat later on, then it shouldn't be a problem for you.

Are there different kinds of birth control pills?

Yes. While there are more than forty versions on the market, they break down into three main types, although new categories can come along any day. The original versions were combinations of estrogenic hormones and progesterone-type hormones in fairly high concentrations.

The most common OC these days is the "micropill." It's called "micro" because it has less than 50 micrograms of estrogenic hormone. In an attempt to fine-tune the "pill," manufacturers have devised many different formulations. There are three major types—the monophasic, the biphasic, and the triphasic pills.

The monophasic variety keeps the amount of estrogenic and progesterone-type hormones at the same level during the month; the biphasic increases the amount of progesterone toward the end of the month; and the triphasic tries to imitate the natural hormone secretion by varying the dose of hormones during the month. The final result is pretty much the same—very effective protection against pregnancy. But like everything else, that protection has its cost.

What do you mean?

Birth control pills aren't gumdrops. They are very powerful drugs that alter the entire reproductive system and affect the entire body. For example, women who are taking OC's don't have menstrual periods. They may bleed every month but it isn't normal menstruation—it is basically a type of "withdrawal bleeding" when the hormones are abruptly cut off at the end of the month. There are also some other risks, thought to be primarily due to the estrogenic component.

Particularly in women who smoke and/or are over the age of thirty-five, there is a risk of blood clots that can cause heart attacks, sudden blindness, strokes, and problems like that. If a woman on the pill suddenly experiences severe headaches, blurred vision, numbness in the arms or legs, coughing up blood, severe leg pain, or a crushing pain in the chest, she should see a doctor IMMEDIATELY. Although the risk may be statistically low, if it happens to you, it is 100 percent.

There are also a few surprising fringe benefits to taking birth control pills.

What are they?

They provide some protection against the following bad diseases:

- Cancer of the ovary
- Cancer of the lining of the uterus (endometrium)
- Pelvic inflammatory disease (some types)
- Ectopic pregnancy
- Iron deficiency anemia
- Ovarian cysts

While the protection isn't absolute, it's a nice fringe benefit. Since most of the side effects of the pill have been blamed on the estrogen it contains, a new formulation has appeared called the "mini-pill." The hope is that women who take mini-pills will have mini-problems.

Does it work out that way?

Let's see. The mini-pill doesn't have any estrogen at all—it is 100-percent progesterone-type hormone but has only about half the progesterone in regular birth control pills. It can't always stop ovulation but it does make the cervical mucus thicker and of course makes it harder for the fertilized egg to implant in the uterus. But since about 60 percent of the women who take it continue to ovulate, it offers more material for argument to the folks who believe that a pill that impedes implantation in the uterus is really producing an abortion. Those are matters of personal belief that should be respected—I cannot venture an opinion one way or another.

But it is true that the mini-pill does have some problems attached to it?

Since it depends on its action against the cervical mucus, it has to be taken at precisely the same time every day. Even a few hours difference can increase the risk of pregnancy. And it is only about half as reliable in preventing pregnancy as the combined pill. It's also a good idea to use another form of birth control for the first three months of the mini-pill just to allow it to take hold.

The mini-pill can also cause spotting—bleeding between monthly bleeding episodes—and sometimes it stops the bleeding entirely. That can be a problem since it's a good idea to stop the pill if a woman is pregnant. But if she stops bleeding, is it because of the mini-pill or is she pregnant? That means if she doesn't have monthly bleeding, she should see her doctor right away.

That's probably the biggest point to remember with birth control pills. It's not a do-it-yourself project—although you can buy the pills without a prescription in Thailand, Korea, and Bangladesh. A woman has to work very closely with her physician to avoid the risks and get all the benefits of the pill—no matter what form she uses. If she misses a dose, has symptoms, or just isn't sure, a quick phone call can save a lot of trouble.

There is just one more problem with birth control pills these days—and it's no fault of the pills.

What's that?

They don't protect against AIDS or STDs. Unless a woman is absolutely certain of her partner, she still has to insist that he use a condom. And that wipes out two of the biggest advantages of the pill—natural sensation of penis against vagina and non-stop sex from kiss to orgasm. But it's a small price to pay. It only takes a moment to put on a condom—but AIDS is forever.

There are other ways to take progesterone-type hormones and they don't depend on a pill.

What are they?

The first one is a simple injection of a progesterone compound that lasts and lasts and lasts. All it takes is one injection every three months of medroxyprogesterone, a form of progesterone. The contraceptive effects last longer than three months—up to a year—but to be safe the shot is given every twelve weeks.

The injection acts the same way as the mini-pill and has about the same potential side effects. About 40 percent of users stop ovulating and don't have monthly bleeding. The protection against pregnancy is very good, with a theoretical failure rate of less than 1 percent. But like everything else, there is a price to pay.

Like what?

Well, every time you get a shot, you're committed for at least three months of infertility—maybe longer. With repeated injections, infertility can last a year. And whatever side effects you're going to suffer are pretty much going to last at least three months. The progesterone shot also has a tendency to cause weight gain—maybe two pounds or so a year. It can also produce spotting and later on, lack of any monthly bleeding at all.

But there are other major advantages. Women who suffer from certain kinds of epilepsy or sickle cell anemia may actually be helped by progesterone injections. Most important of all, there are some women who must avoid pregnancy for serious health reasons. For example, if a woman has to take medicine for a serious disease and that medicine can cause serious birth defects, what does she do? If she wants to be as sure as possible that she won't get pregnant, these injections might just be the answer.

But there's something that lasts even longer.

What's that?

Levonogestrel implants. This is a gee-whiz approach to medicine that gives reliable birth control for up to five years with a single application. Six little sticks of silicone rubber are inserted just under the skin of the inside of the upper arm above the elbow. They are about 1 1/3 inches long and about 1/10 of an inch wide—like little matchsticks. They are impregnated with a long-acting progesterone-type drug and they produce one of the most dependable forms of birth control available. The failure rate is probably less than two-tenths of a percent.

It has another advantage: it works almost immediately if it is inserted during the first seven days of a menstrual cycle. But there is also an unusual aspect—they are most effective in women who weigh less than 154 pounds. They can cause weight gain—but less than the progesterone injection—usually about a pound a year. (That's what some ladies gain just eating chocolate—and chocolate doesn't keep you from getting pregnant.)

Of course it has a high first cost and it does require minor surgery and it has to be removed if you want to get pregnant. In any event it has to be removed every five years. But for women who want or need very reliable long-term protection, they might fill the bill. Of course, every woman who wants to avoid pregnancy has to observe the Dr. Reuben's First Law of Contraception.

What's that?

See your doctor first and follow his advice! Every form of birth control has its advantages and its risks. Not only is every woman different, but the same woman changes from month to month and from year to year. Some methods can conflict with certain medications and some methods can cause avoidable side effects. These days, contraception is not a do-it-yourself affair. That's especially true when it comes to "Retroactive Birth Control."

What's "Retroactive Birth Control"?

It's a kind of modern medical magic. Let's say the condom breaks, the diaphragm slips out, you remembered too late that you forgot to take your birth control pills for more than two days. You're not married or you can't have another child right now or any one of a dozen other reasons that a pregnancy now would ruin your life. What do you do?

You sweat. You suffer. You count the days until your next period—or your wife's next period. It doesn't come and you start thinking about an abortion. The problems multiply as the days go by. It's Nightmare Number Nine and it won't go away.

But for thirty years there has been a simple and available solution—although except for research scientists and some doctors, few people knew about it.

Actually the solution was obvious all the time. If birth control pills interfere with implantation of the fertilized egg into the lining of the uterus, why not increase the dose and try to head off the zygote (fertilized egg) as it descends the fallopian tube on its way to the uterus? And that's what the "Morning-After Pill" is.

The routine is simple. The woman takes two double doses (or more) of certain common birth control tablets at twelve-hour intervals within seventy-two hours of unprotected sex. After that she should have only about a 2-percent chance of getting pregnant. Of course, there are some side effects. Nausea and vomiting are very common and sometimes the woman throws up the pills and has to take them again. But a bout of vomiting is easier to take than an unwanted pregnancy. The "Morning-After Pill" works very well but you have to take it in time.

So if a woman waits too long, there's no hope?

In medicine, there's always hope. There's another method of retroactive birth control that a woman can use up to seven full days after a contraceptive catastrophe. It's the copper IUD. If she has one inserted up to 14 days after the fact, she is almost sure to avoid pregnancy.

Of course, there are problems with that method as well. Having the IUD inserted brings all the typical problems of the IUD, and if the woman has a tendency to pelvic infections, that may be an additional complication. But like every other medical decision, that's a decision she has to make with the help of her doctor.

But can the "morning-after" techniques take the place of ordinary contraception?

That wouldn't be a brilliant idea—except of course if a woman wanted to use the copper IUD as her main form of birth control. But the high doses of oral contraceptives have their obvious drawbacks. The traditional methods of contraception are still the best.

However "morning-after" contraception fulfills a very particular need. Take the case of a sixteen-year-old girl who is raped by three drug addicts. Or a woman who is taking chemotherapy for cancer and forgets to take her pills for three days. She will almost certainly have a terribly deformed child if she gets pregnant. Those cases—and hundreds more—cry out for help. Those are the ideal patients for "morning-after" relief. For most other women who choose "retroactive birth control" it's an individual and very personal decision.

To get pregnant or not, when to get pregnant, how many children to have—these are the most delicate and personal of all human decisions. There are few choices in life that have a greater potential for happiness or the lack of it. That's why they deserve careful thought, up-to-the-minute information, and professional guidance. If you do it that way, you have the greatest chance of doing it right.

Chapter 13
ABORTION

Important Note: This chapter is neither in favor of abortion nor against abortion. It is simply a medical and scientific explanation of abortion—how it is performed and under what circumstances.

What is abortion?

Abortion is simply the interruption of a pregnancy at any stage before delivery. There is no doubt that abortion is an emotionally charged word, particularly when one realizes that it comes from the Latin word *aboriri,* which means "to disappear." The inescapable truth is that in an abortion the embryo, the fetus, the products of conception, or whatever we may call it, disappears. (Incidentally an embryo is what we call a developing baby from two weeks to two months after fertilization. It's called a fetus from the third month until it is born.)

There are two kinds of abortions—the accidental and the deliberate. The accidental ones occur when a pregnancy terminates itself. For some reason, the mother cannot maintain the developing child and her body casts it off. In medical terminology, it's called a "spontaneous abortion," sometimes delicately referred to as a "miscarriage." A vast number of abortions are accidental or spontaneous. About one out of every four pregnancies ends in a spontaneous abortion.

What causes a spontaneous abortion?

This type of abortion is probably nature's way of saying "no." About half of these result from product defects. The sperm or ovum is imperfect and produces an imperfect embryo. Such abortions, regretted as they are by the prospective parents, may be a blessing in disguise. The baby they have lost is actually being discarded by a vigilant reproductive defense mechanism. Virtually all such embryos are monstrosities. A twist of biological fate has rendered them unprepared for earthly life. Careful examination of the products of spontaneous abortion reveals a Lilliputian chamber of horrors. There are babies with no heads and those with two heads. Some have heads but no brains, other have gigantic hollow brains bursting through their skulls. There is no reason to regret the loss of these genetic mistakes.

What causes the other half of spontaneous abortions?

The remainder are determined in the brief moments of implantation when the fertilized egg is being attached to the lining of the uterus. Sometimes there is a lapse at the critical moment when the circulatory system of the mother is connected to the infant's blood supply. If this falters, the pregnancy must falter, either then or later.

When most abortions were illegal in most parts of the United States, any abortion that was done on purpose was called a "criminal" abortion. Now that abortion is legal in so many places, it's more accurate to call these events "deliberate "abortions.

Are deliberate abortions more common than spontaneous abortions?

Yes. Spontaneous abortions occur at the rate of about 1 million a year in the United States. For obvious reasons, it's hard to get exact figures for deliberate abortions, but probably about 30 percent of all the pregnancies in the United States are deliberately aborted—that would be more than 2 million cancelled pregnancies a year. (The "official" figures are somewhat less—the estimates are probably closer to reality.)

What about "therapeutic" abortions?

That term has a brand new meaning now. In the "old days," before legal abortion in the United States, every future physician was indoctrinated—from the very beginning—with the prohibition against performing an abortion except under rigid legal control. I remember that one of the first lectures we received in medical school was from the Dean of the Faculty of Medicine who informed us—in very somber terms:

> *"Gentlemen, if you are going to have honor and success in the practice of medicine, there are two things that you must never do. You must never begin a pregnancy or end a pregnancy in your office."*

These days we don't know for sure how many pregnancies are begun in a doctor's office but we do know that millions of them are ended there.

"Therapeutic" abortion had a kind of double meaning. It meant— as it does now—an abortion performed to protect the life of the mother or to end a pregnancy when it was obvious that the fetus was going to be terribly and incurably deformed. For example, therapeutic abortion was often allowed when the fetus had two heads—or no head—or the mother had a disease that would horribly deform the unborn child— like German measles. The concept was to prevent the birth of a hopeless, helpless being or to prevent the fetus from killing the mother.

But the idea of a "therapeutic" abortion was also flexible enough to allow some women to get abortions that perhaps weren't as urgent as they might seem. But that's all ancient history.

As things stand now, almost any woman in the United States can get an abortion with a minimum of delay—at least during the early part of her pregnancy. The specific laws vary from state to state but it's not too difficult to find a place that will allow her to do pretty much what she wants to do if she looks around hard enough.

But these days she doesn't even have to look around if she doesn't want to.

How come?

Abortion has now become pretty nearly a do-it-yourself project. And that's literally true. A woman can now find detailed instructions—including diagrams—on how to build her own "Abortion Machine." It's called a "Menstrual Extraction Device." Supposedly the purpose of the instrument is to suck out the menstrual blood at the time of the woman's period. But in addition to that, it has something in common with a sewing machine.

A sewing machine?

Yes. After World War I, Germany was strictly forbidden by International Treaties from building weapons of war. In the 1930s, a young German factory worker was working in a sewing machine factory and his wife was constantly nagging him to buy her a sewing machine. He didn't have the money to buy the machine so he decided to steal one by smuggling it out piece by piece and then assembling the pieces at home.

After three months of carefully sneaking out tiny pieces, he spent a whole weekend putting them together. To his surprise, he found he had a machine gun!

In the same way, the basic purpose of the "Menstrual Extraction Device" seems to be to produce an abortion. But if you read the description, it sounds like something completely different. It is offered to end users in a way that doesn't seem to make a lot of sense. Supposedly it helps a woman, "Avoid the inconvenience of a menstrual period on your honeymoon."

Terrific! That means a woman would use the device about once (or twice) in her lifetime. And if you really want to, "Avoid the inconvenience of a menstrual period on your honeymoon," you can buy a hand-held calculator or reschedule your trip. Figuring out when your period should come doesn't seem to be an overwhelming task.

If you analyze the machine carefully, you just might be able to use it for something else. A suspicious person might believe that it can also offer you a do-it-yourself early abortion in the privacy of your own home.

How does it work?

Like this. A big plastic syringe is attached to a long flexible tip that can be inserted into the uterus through the cervix. The woman—or a friend—inserts the tip into the vagina, then into the cervix, and then into the uterus. It goes without saying that everything should be hospital-sterile before starting—although it isn't always that way. Women who are worried about terminating a pregnancy are often scared, nervous, and anxious to get it over with.

It's very important to see to one little detail. There should be a one-way valve—a "check-valve"—in the system to prevent air from getting into the uterus. Otherwise "menstrual extraction" might also "extract" the mother to the cemetery.

Why is that?

During pregnancy the veins that supply the uterine lining are dilated and close to the surface, especially near the embryo. If air is accidentally injected into the uterus under pressure from the "Menstrual Extraction Device" it may enter these veins. It then travels to the brain where it causes coagulation of blood within the brain's small blood vessels. Death occurs quickly.

Anyone who even thinks of using this method should consult her physician first. One thing is being pregnant—another thing is being dead.

What happens then?

If everything is ready, then the "menstrual blood" is sucked out of the uterus. If there happens to be a fertilized embryo along with it, it also gets sucked out. That's in line with the promise of the device:

> *"Avoid the inconvenience of a menstrual period on your honeymoon."*

Fertilized embryos can also be inconvenient during your honeymoon.

It's also good to have a sealed glass jar in the system to catch whatever is drawn out of the uterus. That avoids the messiness when you have to rake through what you have sucked out to look for the dead embryo. Doing a pregnancy test after menstrual extraction isn't as reliable as actually seeing the embryo right there in front of you. Unless you can see it among the blood and tissue, you don't really know if the abortion was successful.

The Extractor is fairly effective up to about four weeks after fertilization, and since do-it-yourself pregnancy tests can be read after eight days or so, this system seems attractive to some women.

Is it a good idea?

I don't recommend it but some women will be attracted to it. You're poking a foreign body into the uterus and playing around with air bubbles—although the check-valve offers some protection. You may not be able to suck out the embryo the first time and have to go back again and hope to pull it out on the second try. And of course the woman has to sort through the bloody liquid to make sure the sucked-out embryo is there.

A woman who wants an abortion sometimes feels desperate and is eager to turn to this device. But it's more realistic to see it for what it is, a home abortion machine and not a handy-dandy way of timing your period to "avoid inconvenience."

Couldn't it just be considered a means of birth control?

Abortion, in a philosophical sense, is retroactive birth control. You're controlling the birth by making the embryo or fetus or "products of conception" disappear. That's the maximum in "control." But these days there are somewhat more elegant and graceful ways to prevent pregnancy than poking a plastic tube into your uterus every month and sucking the contents out with a big syringe.

You sound like you're against it?

I'm not against it and I'm not for it. Abortion is not something that anyone takes lightly. Ask any woman who has had one. And ask the doctors who have done them. It's a procedure that takes a certain emotional toll on everyone involved, and it's really a method of last resort. Anyone who had the choice would rather turn the clock back to that night when they had too much to drink or forgot to take the pill. If they could only do it over again, they would do it right and avoid that pregnancy. But where it's legal, woman can have abortions and doctors can do them.

What technique do doctors use?

Some use "Menstrual Extraction" but with precisely sterile methods and in a clinical environment. That's obviously the best way to use it. But there is another way. Especially later in the pregnancy—say after about seven weeks—doctors tend to favor the traditional "D&C"—short for "Dilatation and Curettage." The procedure is identical to the one done routinely in hospitals all over the country on nonpregnant women. Part of the operation uses a procedure that is more than five thousand years old.

What's that?

Let's start at the beginning. Here's how it's done:

The pubic hair is shaved and the entire vaginal area is washed with a germicidal solution. An instrument called a speculum is inserted into the vagina to distend the walls and provide access to the cervix. The cervix, or the neck of the uterus, is a tight solid tube like a section of sausage less than 2 inches or so in diameter. It has a lot of muscle and a tiny canal less than ¼-inch wide that connects the vagina with the uterus. If the doctor is going to get at that embryo clinging to the inside of the uterus, he has to dilate that opening in the cervix. He can do it by pushing bigger and bigger steel rods through the hole and stretching it. That's a tedious job and has some risk attached.

What many doctors do is exactly what their predecessors did thousands of years ago. They take a rod made of dried rolled-up seaweed and slide it into the cervical canal. Within several hours the seaweed absorbs moisture from the vagina, swells up, and forces the canal to widen. (The seaweed is then removed.) That's when a curved loop-shaped knife on the end of a stainless steel rod is inserted deep into the uterus and the lining of the uterus is systematically scraped to pull off the uterine lining and the one-inch-long embryo that is attached to the lining. That's a relatively routine procedure—the hard part comes later.

What's that?

Sorting out what the doctor has scraped out of the pregnant uterus. The combination of tissue, blood, and the remains of the embryo has to be raked through to make sure that everything has been removed. One of the serious complications of a D&C type of abortion is leaving part of the membranes that go along with the embryo in the uterus. That can cause bleeding, infection, and other problems.

If the operation is done under sterile conditions, the risk of complications is less than 1 percent. With good anesthesia and suitable drugs for pain, there is little subsequent discomfort. The woman is back to household activities in a few days, back to sexual intercourse in a few weeks.

But if the pregnancy is farther along, the D&C won't work.

Why not?

Well, after the first 12 weeks of pregnancy, the baby is getting pretty big and it's tough to scrape it out. The risk of complications also increases. So the doctors move on to another type of abortion called:

"Dilatation and Evacuation" or "D&E."

The technique is about the same as the "D&C" until the cervix is dilated. This time the doctor has to use several seaweed stems since the opening has to be wider, for one important reason. That's because the doctor has to cut the fetus up into little pieces and pull them out one by one through the dilated cervix. Then the doctor pushes a tube about ½ inch in diameter up into the uterus and sucks out the amniotic fluid surrounding the baby, the tiny placenta, and the odds and ends of the cut-up fetus that still remain. As usual, someone has to try to put all the pieces of the fetus together to make sure that the doctor sucked everything out. Any little arms or legs or pieces of head that might be left behind can cause an infection and serious complications for the former mother-to-be.

But you make it sound so horrible! Is it really that bad?

All the descriptions are taken from current medical textbooks—that's just the way it is. If a woman is going to have an abortion, it's only fair that she knows exactly what is going to happen to her body and to the body of the fetus or embryo inside her. To talk about "products of conception" and "menstrual extraction" is really avoiding reality.

Why is it so important to face such an unpleasant reality?

For one very important reason. One of the most common complications of abortion is depression and serious emotional problems in the woman who is operated on. That's compounding the already physical stress of the operation. A woman who faces—right from the start—the harsh facts of abortion has a much better chance of coming through it emotionally intact. An abortion usually takes an hour or so. But the mental suffering can go on for years. It's not fair for a woman to suffer because she hasn't been properly prepared emotionally. And there are some other problems with the "D&E" procedure.

What are they?

Well, the pregnant uterus is pretty soft, like a ripe pear—and it's easy to poke a sharp instrument right through it while you're cutting up the fetus. Perforation is a surgical emergency and sometimes requires a hysterectomy—removing the uterus once and for all. You can also puncture the nearby intestine, and that's a very serious problem when the intestinal contents spill out everywhere. That causes peritonitis and can be fatal.

That's why doctors like to use a different kind of abortion procedure after about the twentieth week of pregnancy. Since the fetus is getting to be pretty big and the uterus is so enlarged that it reaches the woman's belly button, another approach is indicated. It's called "Medical Induction."

In this method of abortion, the doctor takes a long needle, inserts it through the pregnant woman's abdomen into the uterus itself, and pokes through the amniotic sac. He takes out up to six ounces of the amniotic fluid and discards it. Then he pumps in about six ounces of a very strong salt solution. That usually puts the woman into labor in about twenty-four hours, and the fetus and placenta are expelled about twelve hours later. Sometimes other drugs are used like oxytocin, a hormone, or a prostaglandin.

What happens to the baby?

It's not called a "baby," remember? It's a "fetus." That is supposed to make it less emotional. In any event, the concentrated salt solution goes into the amniotic fluid and the fetus swallows it. It kills him. But isn't that the idea of an abortion?

Unfortunately, the salt solution can also kill the woman. Sometimes she absorbs the salt solution herself and joins her fetus. It's rare but it's tragic when it happens. And there are other dramatic moments that can occur in abortion.

Like what?

Like this. Another way to bring on labor is by giving the woman a type of drug called "prostaglandin." If the woman inserts a prostaglandin vaginal suppository or takes an injection of another kind of prostaglandin, she will go into labor even faster than with the saline injection method. But that can lead to a gruesome little problem.

What's that?

The fetus may come out alive. Because the prostaglandin simply starts the muscular contractions that expel the fetus, the fetus may survive. It can have a heartbeat and be breathing.

Then what?

Remember what the word "abortion" means? It means "disappear." If you are going to have an abortion, the fetus has to disappear. Period.

That's the point. Embryos, fetuses, and "products of conception" don't just go away to a "Special Land" where they live happily forever. They have to be disappeared and if they manage to get to the outside alive . . . well, you know what happens.

That doesn't mean a woman should or shouldn't have an abortion. It just means that there is one undeniable fact: aborted fetuses don't live. And everyone should be aware of it.

And there are other things we have to face as well.

Like what?

Like deliberate "termination" of the fetus, known by the disarming term "feticide." Lately a new concept called "multiple birth reduction" has become common. When a woman is going to have triplets or quadruplets or more, her doctor may decide that her chances are better if the "births" are "reduced." In plain old English, that means some of the fetuses have to get dead.

Since you can't take a gun to them under those circumstances, the usual method is to inject potassium chloride into their little hearts. By a strange coincidence, that's exactly the drug that is used to execute murderers in most states these days. But there are other ways. Some doctors have worked out a system of microsurgery where they can reach into the uterus, tie off the fetal umbilical cord, and the fetus suffocates as the oxygen-carrying blood supply is cut off.

But aren't there some important reasons for doing an abortion—like danger to the mother or to the child?

It's possible. If continuing the pregnancy is going to kill the mother or put her life in serious danger, you can make a case for aborting the fetus, curing the mother, and then trying again to have another baby—if that's what she wants. And there are some horrendous cases where a girl is raped by her father or a close relative—that makes for some difficult decisions.

Rape is one of the toughest areas in relation to abortion. If it's really rape—and not the "second-thought-morning-after-I-didn't-really-think-he'd-put-it-all-the-way-in" variety, then abortion has to be considered. The fifteen-year-old girl who is gang-raped by four drug addicts in their twenties doesn't look forward to bringing up their child. And the mother of three who is raped by a paranoid serial killer who just escaped from a mental hospital doesn't have much to look forward to. But for them there might be a better solution.

What's that?

The morning-after pill and the copper Intra-Uterine Device or IUD (the details are in the chapter on Birth Control). It's worth knowing that up to seventy-two hours after a rape occurs the pills can prevent nearly 100 percent of pregnancies. The copper IUD can work up to two weeks after the tragic event. That might well spare the victim the added trauma of an abortion, and with the sensitive modern pregnancy tests, the effectiveness of the after-the-fact birth control techniques can be carefully monitored.

But aren't a lot of abortions done just for that reason?

Strangely enough, no. For obvious reasons, exact figures are hard to come by, but probably no more than 3 percent of all abortions are done because of rape or incest. A serious threat to the mother's life or health accounts for about 7 percent of abortions. Danger to the mother's mental health is the reason for another 7 percent of abortions. Really bad deformity of the fetus is used to justify about 3 percent of abortions.

But how can you tell if the baby is going to be deformed?

There are some very sophisticated genetic tests that you can use these days. Amniocentesis is one of them. The procedure is relatively simple.

It's usually done about the fourteenth week of pregnancy, and although it doesn't sound like much fun, it's a fairly innocuous procedure. (However, complications are possible, including infection, poking the fetus with the needle, and triggering immune reactions in the mother.) After checking the location of the fetus with ultrasound, the doctor inserts a long needle through the abdomen of the mother directly into the amniotic sac, draws out some of the amniotic fluid, and sends it to be tested. That's it.

But can't that test itself bring on a spontaneous abortion?

Unfortunately it can, but the chances are slight. About 1 out of every 200 women will lose their babies as a result of the test. That risk may be justified in some cases by the information amniocentesis can offer.

For example, if the test detects Down's syndrome in the fetus, the parents might decide that an abortion is worth it. Down's syndrome used to be called "mongolism" or more crudely, "mongolian idiot." Children born with this condition are mentally defective—some very severely—and almost all of them die prematurely. The risk is a real one in women over the age of forty-five, about 5 percent of whose babies are victims of the condition.

Does that justify an abortion?

That's an individual decision—and a tough one. No one wants to have a mentally defective child and yet no one wants to dispose of a baby if it can be avoided. But there are worse kinds of birth defects—the "neural tube" defects, for example.

What are those like?

They are very bad. Babies with "neural tube" defects can be born without a brain or with their spinal cord bulging through their skin and with a hydrocephalic skull the size of a watermelon. The chances of that are about 2 in a thousand or two-tenths of one percent. But if it's your baby that has it, the chances suddenly become 100 percent. Brainless babies don't have any future, so aborting them isn't such a tough decision. If the amniotic fluid the doctor draws out shows alpha-fetoprotein (AFP), the baby probably has a neural tube defect and will be born with very serious deformities.

There's a whole range of genetic defects that can be detected with amniocentesis, and some of them require a lot of careful thinking to resolve. The decision is never easy. Abortion itself is a very complex question and every case is different.

Here are a couple of examples:

"Listen, Doctor, I'm desperate. I just can't have this baby! Even if it's going to be a perfectly normal baby! I just can't have it!"

The woman who was speaking was about thirty-one, dressed in a smart powder-blue wool suit with a pale yellow silk scarf around her neck.

"Doctor, this is an impossible situation! My husband is the President of the bank and we already have one child! And I'll die if I have to have this baby! Just think! It would be born right in the middle of Ladies Garden Club Annual Lily Show! What would everyone think?"

The next patient was a young girl, about seventeen, obviously depressed. Although she had taken off her cap, it was obvious that she was still wearing her waitress's uniform. She looked tired, and strands of pale blond hair were in her eyes. She brushed them away as she spoke:

"I just don't know what to do, Doctor. I live alone now—my father's gone and my mother's in a nursing home. I work nights, so I could take care of the baby in the daytime, but I just came from the clinic and they tell me there's something wrong with his spine."
"Did they say, 'spina bifida'?"
She nodded.
"I think so. Something like that. They said he would have a very big head and maybe couldn't walk—ever. But I'd like to have him even if I'm not married—they said it's a boy and I always wanted a boy. What should I do?"

Under current United States laws, both women are entitled to an abortion. But from a human point of view they are worlds apart.

What can a woman do if she waits until later on in the pregnancy to have an abortion?

If she has waited as long as twenty weeks from the time the pregnancy began she can have a procedure known as "Dilatation And Extraction" or "D&X." It is also known as a "Partial Birth Abortion." It is not for the faint-hearted.

Since the mother is so far along, the baby can weigh about a pound and measure 8 inches or longer. With a baby that size or bigger, the cervix has to be dilated much more; it can take several days of using the seaweed stems to open it enough. Then, under general anesthesia, the doctor reaches into the uterus and turns the baby around so that the feet will come out first. Then he grabs one of the baby's legs with forceps. He pulls the baby out until the head jams against the narrowest part of the uterus—the inside of the cervix. At that point the baby is stuck. His little head is just too big to get through the narrow opening in the cervix. So the doctor has to take the next step. He pokes a pair of scissors into the baby's skull, makes a hole, inserts a tube, and sucks out the baby's brains. Then he collapses the skull and pulls out the rest of the body. He removes the placenta and the abortion is over.

Do they do this kind of abortion very often?

No. For obvious reasons, it is fairly rare. Probably no more than three thousand a year are done in the United States, although it could be more or less. No one knows for sure. There is a lot of legal, social, political, and emotional discussion about this procedure, and no one can predict whether it will continue or be stopped or regulated. The outcome will probably be found on the front page of your local newspaper sometime in the future.

Isn't there a gentler form of abortion?

There are a couple of methods that are not quite so dramatic, although when you're talking about abortion, "gentle" is a relative word.

For example, there is the now famous RU 486. So much has been written about the controversial "abortion pill" that it's time to put it all in perspective. RU 486 is a chemical called mifepristone and it has an unusual characteristic: it occupies the places in the body where an important hormone called "progesterone" would like to land. It's as if you're going to the theater and when you arrive you find some big tough guy got there before you and is sitting in your seat. Unless you want trouble, you should probably just get your hat and go home.

If a woman has been fertilized and the embryo is starting to grow in the wall of her uterus, it needs progesterone—and plenty of it—to thrive. If she takes RU 486, the ovaries still secrete progesterone but when those progesterone molecules arrive at the uterus, they find their seat has been taken by big tough molecules of RU 486. The embryo can't survive without a constant supply of progesterone and it just dies.

Then the woman can just go to the drugstore, get her pills, take them, and that's the end of the pregnancy?

Not quite. First she needs a doctor's prescription. Then she should have a pregnancy test to make sure that she's really pregnant. RU 486 is not exactly a jellybean and it has some potentially serious side effects. You have to have a very good reason to take it.

Then she needs to have an ultrasound test to make sure the pregnancy is in the uterus. In some rare cases, an embryo can lodge in the fallopian tubes. That's called a "tubal pregnancy" and it's generally a surgical emergency. If the baby continues to grow there, it will rupture the narrow fallopian tube and cause havoc inside the mother. Once the doctor is sure the baby is in the uterus, the woman can have the go-ahead to take the pills. Except if . . .

Except if what?

Except if she's more than 7 weeks pregnant. And except if she is a smoker and except if she is over 35 years old. There is a much higher risk of side effects if she falls into any of these categories. But assuming she doesn't, she takes the pill and then it starts.

What starts?

The reaction. She may have nausea, vomiting, headache, weakness, or diarrhea. Then a day or two later she takes a dose of prostaglandin that starts powerful uterine contractions. She may have painful cramping and, of course, some bleeding. That's when the embryo is usually expelled. She should come back to the doctor's office in a couple of weeks for a checkup to avoid an unpleasant surprise.

What kind of surprise is that?

If RU 486 doesn't do away with the embryo, it can cause very bad birth defects. So if the embryo has survived, the woman is a candidate for an old-fashioned surgical abortion. About 5 percent of the time, RU 486 doesn't do the job.

As a means of abortion, RU 486 seems like the first TV sets or the first refrigerators. It works, but not the way you wish it would. The ideal abortion pill would terminate the pregnancy about fifteen minutes after you take it with no side effects, no bleeding, and no risk. It may take a long time for that kind of pill to appear.

Isn't there something else?

Yes, there is. It's an interesting and ingenious combination of drugs with an ironic twist. Doctors have discovered that a drug called "methotrexate" combined with a drug called "misoprostol" can bring on an abortion. It's an fascinating set of circumstances.

Methotrexate is a killer drug that saves lives. That sounds like a contradiction, but medical science is full of apparent contradictions. For more than forty years we've been using the drug to save women from a deadly form of cancer of the uterus called "choriocarcinoma." It has also been used in cancer of the breast, ovary, and cervix.

The drug is what we call a "folic acid antagonist." It works against cancer by stopping the growth and reproduction of malignant cells and kills them by disrupting the metabolism of a substance called "folic acid." That's another strange paradox.

Why?

Folic acid is essential to human nutrition. Pregnant women who don't get enough folic acid—a common ingredient in multiple vitamin pills—can give birth to seriously deformed babies. So pregnant women need to consume enough folic acid.

But there's another deadly problem lurking in the amazingly complex world of the female reproductive system. Sometimes a baby grows in the wrong place. Instead of the wide-open spaces of the uterus, the fertilized ovum can get trapped in the tiny macaroni-like conduit of the fallopian tubes. As the baby grows it inevitably ruptures the tube and can kill the mother. Doctors discovered that methotrexate could kill embryos in the fallopian tubes before they could grow big enough to threaten the mother's life. The drug can destroy a life—and save a life at the same time—by aborting an embryo that could kill its mother.

But methotrexate can also kill embryos that are where they should be—clinging to the lining of their mother's uterus. In a strange and contradictory way, the drug treats the developing baby as if it were a cancer and kills the newly growing cells—and the embryo that contains them. But that's only half the battle.

What's the other half?

You can't leave the dead embryo there. So it's back to our trusty prostaglandins. That's what "misoprostol" is. It triggers powerful contractions of the uterus and pushes out the dead embryo. The whole procedure is something like this:

Before the ninth week of her pregnancy, the woman gets an injection of methotrexate. From that moment on, her fate is sealed. She must have an abortion one way or another because if it doesn't kill the embryo, methotrexate will produce a horrendously deformed baby. There are the usual possible side effects: nausea, diarrhea, cramps, hot flashes, and sores in the mouth. The woman can also have vomiting, headache, dizziness, and even vaginal bleeding.

Then she waits a week. During that time she has to be careful not to take any vitamin pills containing folic acid since that will counteract the effect of the methotrexate. After the week is up, she inserts four tablets into her vagina—that's the prostaglandin. That should bring on powerful uterine contractions and expel the deceased embryo. If the contractions don't start after two days have gone by, she inserts another four tablets into her vagina. That should bring on strong cramps and bleeding as the embryo and placenta are expelled. But it isn't always that fast.

How come?

No one knows exactly why, but the process can drag on for a month. If she hasn't aborted in thirty days, she must have a surgical abortion. This combination of drugs—a kind of abortion cocktail—is about 90-percent effective and of course has the usual risk of uncontrolled bleeding, which can generally be handled by a D&C and perhaps a blood transfusion in serious cases.

Another little drawback is that the mother has to sort through the blood and tissues that she passes through the vagina to identify the dead embryo and the placenta. Otherwise no one knows if she really had the abortion or just had some vaginal bleeding from the drugs.

Raking through that combination of blood and tissue looking for a tiny embryo is not exactly the most exciting part of a formerly pregnant woman's day. But that's the reality of what has to be done if that's the choice she makes.

What if a pregnancy has really gone almost to the end?

About the only possibility there is an operation called a *hysterotomy*. (It's different from a hysterectomy where the entire uterus is removed.) It's really a cesarean section and it's a big operation. The doctor makes an incision in the pregnant uterus and pulls the baby out. What happens to the baby then is better left to the imagination—but remember what the word "abortion" means.

The death rate for the mother from this operation is much greater than just a simple D&C, done in the earliest stages of pregnancy.

All right, now answer the hard question. Is abortion good or bad?

I'm only a physician and surgeon and a psychiatrist, I don't know. But I do know this. Abortion is part of human existence. It's been with us since the beginning of the human race. In so-called primitive tribes, women poke an "abortion stick" up into the uterus to abort. Modern women suck out the uterine contents with a nice clean plastic syringe. It's still an abortion.

Most doctors can remember when abortion was illegal in the United States. We can remember the gaping mouths and the eyes filled with fear of the women who were dying from backstreet abortions. We all saw the women who pumped caustic chemicals into their vaginas to abort a baby—who desperately swallowed all kinds of poisons to terminate their pregnancies—and only terminated their lives.

As long as there are pregnant women who don't want to be pregnant, there will be abortions. Every doctor knows that.

The ideal solution is easy-to-use, absolutely reliable, inexpensive techniques of birth control that make abortion unnecessary. A society that effortlessly sends men into the vast reaches of Space should be able to find an equally effortless way to keep a tiny sperm from entering that very small space where a single ovum lies waiting. Let's all hope that day comes as quickly as possible so that the whole problem of abortion will only exist in old newspapers and dusty history books.

Chapter 14
SEXUALLY TRANSMITTED DISEASES

Venereal Disease

Why are syphilis and gonorrhea called venereal diseases?

Venereal refers to Venus, the Goddess of Love. This makes the term especially inappropriate. You don't give diseases like this to someone you love, and you certainly don't love someone who gives them to you—that is, once you realize what you've got.

Actually the expression has come to mean any disease transmitted by sexual contact.

That was the first question in the chapter on "Venereal Disease" in the Original Edition of this book. Quite a few things have changed since then—to put it mildly.

First of all we don't call them "Venereal Diseases" anymore. That was too romantic—invoking the name of the Goddess of Love. Now we call them "STDs" or "Sexually Transmitted Diseases."

Something else has changed too. "Venereal Disease" (or "VD" as we called it when we didn't want to say the whole shocking name) consisted of about five diseases: syphilis, gonorrhea, chancroid, lymphogranuloma venereum, and granuloma inguinale. Gonorrhea was the most common, followed by the few cases of syphilis that were still around. The other three were relatively rare diseases usually seen only in "VD Clinics" in big city public hospitals. Now there are more STDs than there are signs of the Zodiac.

How many are there?

It depends how you classify them but here's a partial list:

- HIV-AIDS
- Candidiasis
- Chancroid
- Chlamydia
- Pubic Lice
- Human Papilloma Virus (Condyloma Acuminata)
- Gonorrhea
- Granuloma Inguinale
- Hepatitis A
- Hepatitis B
- Hepatitis C
- Herpes Simplex Virus
- Lymphogranuloma Venereum
- Nongonococcal Urethritis
- Pelvic Inflammatory Disease
- Syphilis
- Trichomoniasis
- Bacterial Vaginosis

That's eighteen and there are new ones coming up every year or so. An estimated 10 to 12 million new cases of sexually transmitted diseases are reported to the Centers for Disease Control and Prevention every year.

New STDs are discovered every year or so?

Not necessarily "new" diseases but we are discovering that some old diseases can be transmitted sexually. One example is "Type C Hepatitis." Recently cases of this form of hepatitis were found to have been passed by sexual intercourse. Actually the list can get pretty exotic—perhaps that gave birth to the following story:

An auto worker from Detroit went to Miami on vacation and met a prostitute in a bar. She invited him up to her room and had sex with him. Two weeks later, back in Detroit, he came down with gonorrhea. The following year, on vacation in Miami again, he met the same prostitute in the same bar and she invited him up to her room again. He shook his head.

"Not a chance! Last year you gave me gonorrhea!"

She shook her head.

"That wasn't my fault. It was just a little bad luck. Give it a chance!"

He shrugged and followed her up the stairs.

Back in Detroit, it wasn't long before he developed syphilis. And a year later, again on vacation, he met the same girl in the same bar. She strolled up to him, threw an arm around his neck, and murmured:

"Hey, Big Boy, let's have some fun!"

He frowned at her:

"Whoa! What are you selling this year? Cancer?"

Can you get cancer from sex?

We'll see. It used to be that the worst thing you could get from sexual intercourse was a bacterial infection known as syphilis. Provided you got to the doctor in time, penicillin or some other antibiotic made short work of that disease. But now things are different. These days what used to be little insignificant maladies are suddenly targeting the sexual organs and causing a lot of problems. Who would have imagined that a pesky cold sore that popped out on our lip the night before the Senior Prom would come back to haunt us?

A cold sore can affect you sexually?

That's right. That annoying blister that no makeup can cover is caused by a virus known as Herpes Simplex. On the upper lip it's a nuisance—on the vaginal lip or the penis, it's something else. A variety of the virus called Herpes Simplex Virus Type 2 can infect the sexual organs of men and women and get in the way of a lot of good things.

It starts off like this:

One day you notice a little blister or two on the end of the penis or on the labia at the vaginal entrance. Your reaction might be:

"Hmmm, what's that?"

The next day the blisters break and begin to form little ulcers— and those ulcers hurt. They are a very big nuisance. In women they can make urination painful and difficult. In men they can be very painful when they rub against clothing or underwear. And they drag on and on—usually for several weeks.

What should a person do if they have an outbreak of HSV?

See their doctor right away. The treatment is simple—antiviral medicine to alleviate the symptoms as quickly as possible. And it usually works nicely—the pain and discomfort gradually go away and the ulcers heal. But that's not the end of it.

Sooner or later those little blisters show up again. The second attack is usually not as severe, and the same antiviral medicine usually helps. But as the blisters and ulcers go away there's one thing you can be almost sure of—they will be back. Then it's more medicine and wait until those yucky blisters clear up. Most patients have recurrences from time to time and it's something they have to live with. At this moment, there is no "cure" for genital herpes. All a person can do is try and pinpoint those things that might bring on a recurrence—and avoid them. Everyone is different but here's a partial list:

1. Stress—emotional or physical
2. Fatigue
3. Other infections
4. Marijuana
5. Very energetic sex with lots of friction
6. Menstruation
7. Ultraviolet light

8. Pregnancy

9. Problems with the immune system

What can you do about HSV?

The best thing you can do is avoid it. Some measures are obvious. Like don't let anyone perform oral sex on you if they have a blister on their lip. (Who would?) But it isn't that easy. Men or women without a blister on the lip or without any other symptoms can have the virus in their mouth tissues and spread it to your most tender parts.

Always use a condom. That keeps any virus that may be lurking around the vagina or on the penis from getting onto you and triggering an infection. Unfortunately it doesn't always work with Herpes because the virus may be on the skin around the sexual organs where a condom doesn't go. The only solution would be a condom like a pair of boxer shorts—and that has obvious disadvantages.

Choose your partner carefully. Although it sounds too clinical, these days it's sensible to check your new sexual friends for sores, ulcers, and spots on their sexual equipment. Perhaps you can do it discreetly—you don't have to take a flashlight to bed. But it's important. Herpes doesn't do anything for your sex life.

Don't be afraid to ask. You can be as subtle as you want. You could say something like:

"I was reading the other day that about 20 percent of people have Herpes these days . . ."

If your new friend glances quickly at their pubic area—keep asking.

Or you could be more direct:

"Listen, I like you a lot but I also like sex. If you have Herpes or any other disease that I could catch, please tell me now so I can keep on liking you!"

Of course it's a personal question. But your sexual happiness is also a very personal question.

Asking if someone has Herpes doesn't solve the problem, however. Even if they answer honestly, it may not help, because 75 percent of the people who have HSV don't know they have it! Beyond that, one out of five of all Americans over the age of thirteen is infected with the virus. The estimate is that 40 to 60 million Americans have the condition today—and more tomorrow.

The best solution of all is to find one sexual partner that you know is free of any STD and stick with them. And of course, make sure that they stick with you. Unfortunately the stakes get higher every day.

What do you mean?

You can guess. I mean HIV—Human Immunodeficiency Virus or the worst disease to strike the world since the Bubonic Plague in 1348. It's hard to find anything nice to say about this organism. It's a bad little virus that gets inside the victim's cells—instead of living on the outside where it's easy to get at. It mutates almost constantly, so the vaccine you make today probably won't work next week. It leads almost inevitably to a disease called AIDS—Auto Immune Deficiency Syndrome. That disease zaps your immune system so that any other disease that comes down the pike can gobble you up in one bite. And most grotesque of all, it makes the joke about the man from Detroit come true. Sexual intercourse can give you cancer if you get AIDS from it.

How does that happen?

There is a relatively rare kind of cancer (not rare in people with AIDS) called "Kaposi's Sarcoma." It is a skin cancer that later spreads throughout the body and eventually causes death—unless the patient with AIDS dies of another complication first. AIDS can also bring on another form of cancer called "lymphoma" which affects the lymphatic system and is also fatal.

(We make the distinction between "HIV" and "AIDS" for this reason. Technically, HIV is the condition where the virus is present in your blood without causing any other symptoms. When someone—almost inevitably—starts to have symptoms, they then have AIDS which is the "syndrome" or collection of symptoms that make up the actual disease. We doctors like to make things complicated sometimes—it exercises our minds.)

Realistically a full explanation of HIV-AIDS would take this entire chapter and this entire book and perhaps a set of encyclopedias as well. My goal here is to tell you the most important facts about HIV-AIDS that somehow or other didn't get to you: for example, the true facts about condoms and HIV-AIDS prevention.

Don't condoms prevent HIV-AIDS?

Yes, no, and maybe. The relentless—and vitally important—campaign promoting the use of condoms as a way of avoiding HIV-AIDS doesn't begin to tell you the whole story. It's a necessary oversimplification to encourage mass compliance. For example, in most antirabies campaigns you are exhorted to vaccinate your dog every year, although most rabies vaccines are effective for two years. But that's the way to make sure that the campaign reaches as many dog owners as possible.

HIV-AIDS is a bigger problem. The disease is easily transmitted by sexual intercourse, almost uniformly fatal, and there is no cure. What can we tell the billions of people out there who are having sex day after day? We tell them the only thing we can tell them: *Use Condoms*! The truth is, that will help to reduce the number of new cases. But the actual protection that it provides for a specific person in a specific sexual act is worth analyzing.

Let me pause a moment to say this:

What follows is a medical-scientific analysis based on current medical research. Please understand that I do not recommend having sex without a condom. If anyone says that I do, I will be rather annoyed. (Incidentally, "rather annoyed" is a polite way of saying that I will call in the lawyers.)

According to one careful analysis of research, condoms are effective in protecting against HIV-AIDS, on the average, about 69 percent of the time. Another research paper suggested that with what they call "consistent" use of a condom, the protection rate is between 90 and 95 percent. Another study found that in "typical use," which is the way people really tend to use them, condoms fail to protect against HIV-AIDS about 9.7 percent of the time. In still another research project, almost 8 percent of condoms broke during sex or while being withdrawn or they slipped off during sex. An additional 7 percent or so slipped off while being withdrawn. There is a very important message in those figures for everyone— a life-and-death-message.

What's that?

Condoms aren't perfect. After all, the typical condom is seven hundredths of a millimeter thick. That's mighty thin—and that's all that stands between you and a terrible fatal disease. At least one and a half percent of condoms bought at random burst on testing in a recent survey. To make matters worse, you can't safely test a condom yourself. If you unwrap it and blow it up you may weaken it and make it even more likely to fail at the critical moment.

So what can you do?

Analyze the situation carefully. Condoms aren't perfect. Let's take the very best possible statistic, the one that sounds almost too good to be true. Assume that a condom protects you against HIV-AIDS 95 percent of the time. That's about the same as putting a gun to your head and pulling the trigger, confident in the knowledge that you only have a 5-percent chance of blowing your brains out! That bullet can slam into your skull on the first trigger pull or on the ninety-sixth—but sooner or later it will happen.

But what about the scientific finding that says condoms only protect you 69 percent of the time? If that's the case, by the time you pull the trigger three times, you will probably kill yourself. In other words, even if you use a condom, on the average, one out of every three copulations with an infected person will expose you to HIV-AIDS.

As we have mentioned, statistics are wonderful but they are like a bikini bathing suit. What they reveal is interesting but what they conceal is vital. If you are the man or woman who gets HIV-AIDS in that 5-percent (or 31-percent) lapse of condom protection, as far as you're concerned it's exactly the same as if you never used a single condom in your entire life!

That's why some analytical observers have come up with the radical theory that THEORETICALLY you would have less risk of contracting HIV-AIDS if you didn't use a condom at all. (Remember what I said—I don't recommend not using a condom.)

Their reasoning is interesting. If you trust a condom to protect you, you will have sex with people you are not really sure of. Remember that guy you met in the singles bar with the tattoos?

Would you try it with him without a condom? How about that really sexy girl at the party who's wearing long sleeves on a hot night? Is she trying to cover up skinny arms or a few needle marks? Would you have intercourse with her without a condom?

If you believe that a condom offers 100-percent protection, you might risk it with them. But if you contemplate sex with them "barefoot"—without a condom—you probably wouldn't do it.

Now here's the lifesaving message that comes from all this: Don't ever have sex with anyone unless you are personally convinced that you would feel totally safe doing it without a condom.

THEN USE A CONDOM!

And ALWAYS use a condom!

ALWAYS!

Is there anything safer than using a condom?

Sure. Using two condoms. No, it's not a joke. You can cut the risk of condom breakage almost to zero by using two condoms. I know, what can you feel through two condoms? The answer is: you can feel safe.

Life is funny. Sometimes you get into a situation where you don't think you should have sex but it's hard to resist and, well, you know how it is. That's the time for double the protection. And so what if you only have half the fun? Remember, HIV-AIDS is forever.

But what about other kinds of sex—oral sex for example? How do you use a condom there?

Remember the story about the duck who stopped in at the drugstore and purchased a condom? The druggist dropped it on the counter and said:

> "Here it is! Shall I put it on your bill?"
> The bird frowned.
> "Put it on my bill? What do you think I am, some kind of perverted duck?"

Just as there are no condoms for ducks to put on their bills, there are no condoms to put on your tongue. But there are what they call "dental dams." These are little squares of latex rubber—the same that rubber condoms are made of. The idea is to place them over a lady's clitoris and vagina before performing cunnilingus on her. It may not sound like fun—unless latex is a turn-on for you—but it's better than HIV-AIDS or any of the other horrible STDs.

You can make it a little better by washing the latex first and then putting a water-soluble lubricant on one side and a flavored lubricant on the side you're going to lick. Then press it against the appropriate spots and it's all yours! But—if it drops off during the festivities, be sure you don't get it reversed and start licking the lady's side. That's precisely what you *don't* want to do.

There's also a do-it-yourself version that you can whip up on the spot. Just take a condom—unlubricated and without 9-nonoxynol (the spermicide that some condoms are impregnated with)—cut off the tip, slit it up the side, and apply your lubricants. But there's still one disadvantage.

What's that?

As you can see, it takes two hands to keep the latex in place, and that kind of cramps your style. But there's a solution to every problem. If the lady is wearing a garter belt, you can simply take the snaps on the garters and use them to clip the latex in place. That should leave your hands free. Of course, her stockings will fall down.

Protection while performing oral sex on a man is less complicated. Just slip on a nonlubricated and non-N-9 condom. (Those chemicals don't come in gourmet flavors.) Then you're ready to go. Although your chances of getting HIV-AIDS from oral sex are not as great as from regular intercourse, it can still happen. So be prepared. I know, licking latex isn't great—but it's better than pushing up daisies.

Except by regular sex and oral sex, how else can you get HIV-AIDS?

Anal sex is by far the biggest risk. The anus is not designed for a hard elongated penis, and the trauma that occurs leaves blood vessels open. That's why the majority of cases of HIV-AIDS are male homosexuals, and that's where women can run a big risk as well.

It's not surprising that women run a bigger risk than men in vaginal intercourse. Some estimates say than a woman has four times greater chance of getting HIV-AIDS from regular sex than a man has: That's because of the volume of infected semen that she takes on as well as the greater surface area and vulnerability to trauma of the lining of the vagina. If she has sex during her period, the risk is increased even further.

Any body-fluid contact is a risk for HIV-AIDS, of course. The virus has been found in blood, human milk, sweat, tears, and urine. It may also be present in feces and vomit. Sharing razors, or straws for sniffing cocaine, or intravenous needles can also transmit the disease. Hospital workers can be infected by needle sticks or blood from an infected patient spurting into their nose or eyes. (Just one more thing we doctors have to worry about.)

But there's one more possible mode of transmission that no one wants to talk very much about.

What's that?

Insects. Here's the question: A mosquito bites someone with HIV-AIDS and sucks up their blood. Then it flies across the street and bites you. Can it give you HIV-AIDS?

It's a logical question and needs to be answered. Insect bites draw blood, and blood is where the bad virus is. The *official* explanation goes something like this.

You can't get HIV-AIDS from an insect because:

- People who have HIV-AIDS don't constantly have high concentrations of the virus in their blood.
- Insects don't retain a lot of blood on their mouth structures.
- Insects don't normally travel from one person to another immediately after biting.

It's understandable that Public Health people are always afraid of causing something called "panic" in the population. But HIV-AIDS is such a terrible disease that I think everyone has a right to know the truth so they can protect themselves. Here is the truth:

- People who have HIV-AIDS might possibly have a high concentration of the virus in their blood at just the moment when an insect bites them (Murphy's Law).
- How much HIV-AIDS-infected blood do you want in and on your skin?

- Maybe insects don't "normally travel from one person to another immediately after biting," but they just might do it the evening you're sitting out on in your backyard (Murphy's Law).

Scientific studies have shown that the HIV virus can bind to the following insects:

1. Mosquitoes
2. Fruit flies
3. Mediterranean flies
4. Stable flies
5. Bedbugs
6. Ticks

It has also been shown that the virus lives eight days in bedbugs and ten days in ticks. According to several studies in the scientific literature, there is agreement that insects could possibly be a source of the AIDS virus.

Does that mean that insects can transmit HIV-AIDS?

Not necessarily. But it doesn't mean that they can't. Here are the three links in a possible chain:

- HIV-AIDS lives for a week or more in common blood-sucking insects.
- HIV-AIDS-infected blood can get on their mouth-parts or in their bodies.
- When they bite people they draw blood and sometimes regurgitate on them. (Polite way to say the insects vomit on your skin.)

I think you have to know this because medical science isn't perfect. (Is that really a surprise?) Researchers sometimes make mistakes and sometimes they make new discoveries that are the opposite of what they thought before. I'm telling you this because I don't want to pick up a scientific journal one day and read this:

"Oh, by the way, we just discovered that insects do transmit HIV-AIDS! Sorry 'bout that!"

The best advice is to play it safe. Avoid insect bites whenever you can. When biting insects are around, wear long sleeves and long trousers, use insect repellent, and even stay inside. If you do everything else to avoid HIV-AIDS, with all the sacrifice it entails, you don't want to be done in by a mosquito or a stable fly.

Will condoms protect you from all the STDs?

Regrettably, no. As we've seen, it isn't completely effective against Herpes.

It works very well against gonorrhea because the bacteria of gonorrhea infect the urinary tract. In males the bacteria are pumped out through the urethra to infect sexual partners and enter through the urethra to infect the man. (As you recall, the urethra runs through the center of the penis.) If you put a condom on the penis, you hold back the flood of gonorrhea. Besides, gonorrhea is usually not thought of as a lethal disease, as in this story:

> *Marlene and Melanie were talking one day at the beauty parlor. Marlene turned to Melanie and said:*
> *"Say, what ever happened to Emily?"*
> *"Oh, Emily. Well, she died."*
> *"She died? I thought she was going out with Two-Ton Charlie! What did she die of?"*
> *"Uh, she died of gonorrhea."*
> *Marlene wrinkled her brow:*
> *"The gonorrhea? Nobody dies of gonorrhea!"*
> *Melanie shrugged:*
> *"You do if you give it to Two-Ton Charlie!"*

But if gonorrhea doesn't kill anybody, why is it worth worrying about?

Because Marlene was wrong. Gonorrhea *does* kill people. It doesn't happen very often but people have died from it. Besides that there are three very important reasons to worry about gonorrhea.

First of all, it looks as if gonorrhea is just about to escape from our control. When antibiotics first came out, penicillin zapped gonorrhea in a flash. Now new strains have developed that are immune to virtually every common antibiotic available. These days it takes a specially powerful and expensive drug to defend against the disease.

Secondly, it's a very common disease and most people don't take it seriously enough. In big cities, it's really a serious problem. For example, Newark, New Jersey, recently had the distinction of being the Gonorrhea Capital (per capita) of the United States, with 942.5 reported cases of the disease per 100,000 residents. There are about 1 million new cases of gonorrhea reported each year in the United States, but the real figure is easily twice that and maybe more since many cases don't get reported.

The third reason to take gonorrhea seriously is that although it rarely kills anybody, it can cause sterility and prevent millions of people from being born. Gonorrhea is one of the major causes of PID. or "Pelvic Inflammatory Disease." PID is bad news—it happens when an infection of the vagina and cervix spreads upward into the uterus, fallopian tubes, and ovaries. It can even extend all the way to the abdominal cavity, and that's when it can kill.

But is Pelvic Inflammatory Disease very common?

There are millions of cases per year in the United States. No one knows how many, since most doctors don't report every case of PID to the Health Department. Most of the infections are caused by gonorrhea or another bad actor known as "chylamidia." (We'll get to that problem shortly.)

As with any disease, the more you are exposed, the more likely you are to get infected. Women who have sex with more than one man are almost 500-percent more likely to get PID. Not surprisingly, women who use IUDs for birth control have a 350-percent greater risk for PID. The problem, apparently, is the little string that's attached to the IUD and hangs down into the vagina from the uterus. It's easy for a vaginal infection to climb up that string into the uterus and creep upward from there.

There's another interesting aspect to PID caused by gonorrhea. About 70 percent of the women who have PID from gonorrhea get infected in the first week after their period. That impressive infection rate might be the fault of hitchhiking.

Hitchhiking?

That's right. If a woman has sex during her period, the gonorrhea germs may go piggyback with the sperm to form a sort of "sperm-germ" team. That can spread the infection to the uterus, fallopian tubes, and ovaries.

PID is really bad news. Even if the infection is cured, about 12 percent of women are permanently sterile. After the second infection, even if that one is cured too, almost one-quarter of the victims will never have children again. Three infections with PID leave more than half the women permanently unable to become pregnant. But even if the woman can still become pregnant, the risk of ectopic pregnancy—pregnancy outside the uterus—increases about 1000 percent. That's because the scarring that occurs in the fallopian tubes makes it more likely for the fertilized egg to attach somewhere besides the lining of the uterus.

What's the treatment?

Before we get to that, the best advice is: "Don't get infected!" Use a condom—for whatever limited protection it offers. Don't do anything dumb. Choose your partner wisely. Remember the story about the prostitute who was performing oral sex on a regular customer?
While she was working on him, he said:

> *"Listen, I'm a little short of cash this week. Is it OK if I pay you just this once with a coupon for a dozen dinners at that new barbecue restaurant around the corner?"*

She paused in her endeavors and looked up at him.

> *"I guess it's OK just this once—but are you sure the restaurant is a clean place?"*

That's the point. Too many people pick their sexual partners with less care than they pick the place where they are going to eat lunch.

The symptoms of PID are pain in the lower abdomen, a vaginal discharge that looks like pus, and fever. See your doctor right away if those symptoms occur—especially in the first week after your period. The treatment is carefully chosen antibiotics. If the condition doesn't clear up quickly, it may mean a stay in the hospital. An ovarian abscess can form (that's a pus-filled sac involving the ovary) and sometimes emergency surgery is the only way out. Gonorrhea can also cause intestinal obstruction or sepsis (the common name is "blood poisoning"). Those are the kinds of complications that can prove Marlene wrong—and confirm that gonorrhea can kill.

One other little point to consider: infection with gonorrhea and most other STDs makes you much more vulnerable to HIV-AIDS. That's not exciting.

You mentioned chlamydia. What's that?

Chlamydia is a strange bacteria dating back to Ancient Egypt and it exists in many forms—some of them rather surprising. One of these is called "chlamydia trachomatis" and it causes a disease called "trachoma." Currently about 500 million people around the world are infected and about 7 million are blind from the infection.

But the same bacteria can also infect the sexual organs, and although it can't cause blindness there, it can do other things. Chlamydia seems to be everywhere these days. Chlamydia affecting the sexual organs is the most common bacterial STD in the United States today; 90 percent of all the PID in the United States is caused by either chlamydia or gonorrhea.

It's also a very contagious disease. Every year there are about 90 million new cases in the world, and 4 million of those are in the United States. Even worse, the infection sterilizes about 50,000 American women every year. And it's a weird disease. Birth control pills seem to make a woman more resistant to gonorrhea. (Be careful: "resistant" doesn't mean "immune.") But the same pills make her more vulnerable to chlamydia! STDs have certainly made the world more complicated.

Men can also have the sexual version of chlamydia but they usually don't have any symptoms. That's not especially good news because they can spread it to women without even knowing it. Women aren't much better off in that regard—about 60 percent of all chlamydia in women is undetected but can still cause PID and all the other problems. Besides that, children born to infected mothers can develop serious chlamydia eye infections.

The best solution is to get a simple chlamydia test from your doctor and take the antibiotics necessary to clear up the infection. That's that. But be sure to put it on your list of things to do before it can sneak up on you and cause trouble. Of course, the precautions are the same as for gonorrhea:

Don't have sex with anyone unless you would willingly use their toothbrush because if you have sex with them you're going to be using something else of theirs that can carry a lot worse things than their toothbrush.

Even better, find one person that you can trust and whom you love, and organize your sex life around them. That was always a good idea, but now it's even a better idea since it can save your life in the process.

Save your life? Are STDs really that bad?

You can decide for yourself. There's another one that's come to prominence relatively recently called "Human Papilloma Virus" or HPV for short. "Papilloma" comes from the Latin word, *papilla*, which means "nipple" and the Greek word, *oma*, which means "tumor." As someone once said,"Any word that is half Latin and half Greek can't be any good."

They were, of course, talking about the word "television" but it applies even more to HPV. It's really a disease that could have been invented by a mad scientist from Mars. "Papilloma" means a benign (not cancerous) skin tumor, and that's the way HPV looks—but don't be fooled.

Usually it takes the form of something that looks like a wart. But they are warts on the penis—at the entrance to the urethra, on the foreskin, or somewhere on the shaft. They can also occur around the anus or the vagina. Sometimes they are even *inside* the vagina or the anus. For years these were known as "condyloma acuminata"—and they still are. For years they were never really taken seriously. Now they are taken very seriously.

How come?

It turns out that those little tumors—which are not really the kind of warts we are used to seeing—are caused by a very special virus. Remember when we were kids we used to be afraid that we would get warts from handling toads? Well, you can't get HPV warts from handling toads but you can get them from handling other things—like a penis or a vagina.

The Human Papilloma Virus is quite contagious and can be spread by sexual intercourse. If you have a papilloma on your privates, you almost always have virus there that you can spread to someone else. And you will probably keep the virus in your body for the rest of your life. But even if you don't have any papillomas right now, if you've had them in the past, you can probably give the virus to your partner.

Will they get the papillomas too?

Probably. A lot depends on how good their immune system is, but they will most likely get infected. But there's good news too. Most of the time these papillomas go away by themselves in from three to six months. But, as we said, the virus will stay on. And from time to time the papilloma may come back without any warning. And there's one other problem.

What's that?

Human Papilloma Virus causes cancer—and that's not good. As one of my patients said,

> "What's this world coming to, Doctor? It's like you can't have any fun anymore! It used to be if you got it on with the wrong person you got the Clap [gonorrhea]. Now you get the Cancer! Or you get Dead!"

Strangely enough there's a lot of truth to that. It is now fairly clear that an infection with HPV can cause potentially fatal cancer of the cervix, the penis, the clitoris and labia and vestibule, the vagina, the urethra, or the anus. A particularly serious complication is cancer of the cervix, the short tubular neck of the uterus that extends into the vagina. Cancer of the cervix is the second most common cancer affecting women in the entire world. It's a bad cancer that has killed millions of women.

Fortunately not all the news is bad. There are about twenty different kinds of HPV that cause tumors on your sexual organs. The ones that cause those "warts" are usually types 6 and 11. They very rarely progress to cancer.

But there's something else. A man can have the virus lodged deep inside his urethra—the tube that carries semen and urine through the center of his penis. If that happens, he may be pumping virus into his partner's vagina every time he ejaculates. It's not an exciting prospect.

If HPV is so dangerous, how can you keep from getting infected?

It's not easy. Even if you use a condom, the condom doesn't cover everyplace the virus goes and that means that condoms are only from 10 to 50 percent effective in preventing HPV. That means that, at best, when you pull the trigger, the gun will go off at least every other time. At best, it goes off one time out of ten. Spermicides seem to help a bit but you can't put them everywhere, especially in some of the orifices where those warts grow. Since it's so hard to protect against, it's a good thing that HPV isn't HIV-AIDS— although it's bad enough on its own.

As always, the best solution is avoiding exposure. The truth is that the way things are these days, bungee jumping is safer than sex with someone you don't know.

Are there any other STDs to worry about?

Not necessarily to worry about but there are some you should know about. For example, there's a curious condition that affects the vagina—it's puzzling in every way. It's called "bacterial vaginosis" and even the name is strange. In medical lingo we usually use the ending "itis" to indicate an infection of an organ. For example, "tonsillitis" is an infection of the tonsils. But this condition is called "vaginosis" which means involving the vagina but not necessarily infecting it.

But it gets stranger. The disease has hardly any symptoms except for a moderate vaginal discharge. But women who have it run a much bigger risk of infected abortion, premature labor, and premature delivery. Even the diagnosis is unusual. The doctor takes a bit of the discharge from the vagina, puts it on a glass slide, treats it with a common chemical—and then turns the scientific clock back ten thousand years! He makes the diagnosis by smelling the specimen! If it smells fishy or musty, it's most likely bacterial vaginosis.

But the mystery goes beyond that. There is none of the usual evidence that indicates a man can transmit BV to a woman. But— and no one knows why—if a man uses a condom, the incidence of BV in his partners drops significantly!

The treatment is antibiotics administered by your doctor. The results are usually good.

Are there any other vaginal infections?

Yes, there are two more important ones. These two, along with bacterial vaginosis, are responsible for 90 percent of all vaginal infections—and the annoyance that goes with them.

Trichomonas is the name of the first disease and it's a very strange one. It isn't caused by a bacteria and it isn't caused by a virus. It's caused by an animal that lives inside the vagina. As you can imagine, it's a very small animal, about the size of an amoeba. It belongs to the same family as the "protozoa," the simplest type of one-celled animal. The full name of the animal is *Trichomonas vaginalis,* and by itself it causes about 25 percent of all cases of vaginitis.

Women don't like this disease because it causes a greenish-yellow bad-smelling frothy discharge which is messy. It also makes the area around the vagina tremendously itchy, which is sometimes hard to deal with at job interviews, first dates, and visits to your prospective mother-in-law. It's also a problem on the job for waitresses, airline stewardesses, and fashion models.

Men don't like it because it makes sex painful for women. That means it makes sex nonexistent for men. Trichomonas is a true STD and a Ping-Pong infection besides. The man gets the disease from the woman, Ping-Pongs it back to her, and she Ping-Pongs it back to him. That game can go on forever unless the doctor calls off the match. That means that he has to treat the woman—and the man—simultaneously to stamp out those millions of little wiggling animals once and for all.

There's another common and annoying vaginal infection that isn't caused by a bacteria or a virus—or even an animal.

What's it caused by?

It's hard to imagine but it's caused by a yeast. The name of the yeast is *Candida albicans* and usually it's very well behaved. About 30 percent of all women have this little yeast growing normally in their vagina without symptoms. But if a woman is taking birth control pills or oral antibiotics, the yeast may suddenly multiply out of control. It is vaguely similar to the way yeast grows to make bread rise. However, the results are somewhat different.

The woman has a thick white discharge that looks almost "curdled." She also has that awful itch, itch, itch. It's interesting that the vagina itself can't itch. It doesn't have the kind of nerve endings that can "feel" an itch. But when the disease spreads outside the vagina, the awful itch begins.

The treatment is simple and effective but the infection has an annoying way of coming back again and again. One of the culprits can be vaginal douching, which changes the ecology of the vagina.

There's no reason to squirt liquids into the vagina unless the doctor prescribes it. (The way things are these days with HPV and Herpes you probably should even think twice about squirting semen into the vagina—except when you want to have children.)

Another useful way to avoid recurrent yeast infections is to think in terms of making bread rise. The yeast in the cake reproduces fastest when it's in a warm, dark, and moist environment. That pretty much describes the vagina, doesn't it? But a woman can help prevent re-infection by cutting down on the moisture by not wearing underwear whenever possible. Just that little drying of the atmosphere puts the brakes on the yeast. For those occasions when underwear is indicated, loose-fitting cotton may not be glamorous but neither is an itch you can't politely scratch.

By the way, speaking of baking, there's a little-known hazard there for home bakers.

Not long ago a woman came down with a vaginal yeast infection from an uncommon type of yeast. The doctor was interested in identifying the exact organism that caused the infection and ordered a complex laboratory analysis. When all the results were in, it turned out that the yeast infection in her vagina was from a very specific type of yeast found in two places. One place was the pizza restaurant where her husband worked. The other place was on her husband's fingers. Moral to that story:

"It is always a good idea to wash your hands after baking."

Technically a *Candida* infection doesn't qualify as an STD, but it can happen. Just as in trichomonas, the woman can infect the head of the man's penis or, if the man isn't circumcised, the yeast can grow under the foreskin. That's when the man needs to be treated as well. Treatment is simple and effective—your doctor can do it easily.

What are some of the other STDs that are important?

Well, there are two infections that most people don't think of as sexually transmitted—but they can be. Odd as it may seem, there are at least three types of hepatitis—inflammation of the liver—that can be transmitted sexually. They are Hepatitis A, Hepatitis B and Hepatitis C, three serious types of liver infection. Hepatitis A is usually spread by anal sex—the other two can be transmitted by regular penis-vagina intercourse.

The good news is that condoms prevent all three types of hepatitis from being passed from one person to another—within the limitations of the effectiveness of condoms, of course. Remember the estimates—condoms are 69-percent effective at the least and 95-percent effective at the most. No matter how you figure, that doesn't add up to 100 percent. So don't take any chances.

Are there any other important STDs?

They're all important if you catch them. They can also be very deceptive. Take pubic lice, for example. These are tiny lice that inhabit the pubic hair and neighboring areas. They are annoying and embarrassing—and contagious. If you didn't have them before, you may well have gotten them from someone you had sex with. A normal impulse is to head for the drugstore and explain to the pharmacist:

> *"Look, my uncle just called me. He has these lice on his—you know. And I wonder if you have anything for him?"*

The pharmacist will find you a very effective lotion or cream that will get rid of the lice in a day or two. Easy, safe and—it may cost you your life!

How could that happen?

Think about it. It isn't your uncle—it's you. And you didn't get those bugs from watching TV. If the person you had a sexual experience with was so contaminated that they had lice on their privates, think of what else they may have had—like maybe HIV-AIDS? If you have any infection or condition on or near your sexual organs, don't even think about treating it from the drugstore. See your doctor right away and let him run all the tests he thinks are necessary. The lotion from the well-intentioned pharmacist will zap the lice—but it won't do a thing about HIV-AIDS.

There's another STD that is similar.

Which one is that?

It goes by two names and the abbreviations are "NSU" or "NGU." Don't let the initials fool you—these are not the names of universities, although you can catch them at some universities. They are

"Non-Specific Urethritis" or "Non-Gonoccocal Urethritis." (As usual we doctors have a solution for everything. In medical language "Non-Gonoccocal Urethritis" means, "It's not gonorrhea and we don't exactly know what the heck it is!")

This condition, by either name, is an inflammation of the urethra—the tubing that leads from the bladder to the outside in both men and women. We call it "non-specific" or "non-gonoccocal" because it's not clear exactly what causes it in every case. These STDs are usually worse in women than in men, cause discomfort on urination, sometimes produce a little discharge, and are a nuisance. Usually they respond to antibiotics and the doctor can almost always clear them up easily. But they have the same risk as pubic lice. You don't get NGU or NSU from playing solitaire. You almost always get it from sex—and if you get *that* from sex, you may well have also gotten something else much worse besides. Even if it seems to go away by itself, see your doctor!

How about the other STDs?

Here are some of the lesser-known or less common STDs. One of their biggest hazards is that many of them tend to make you more vulnerable to HIV-AIDS—and that's the end of the trail.

Take chancroid, for example. Chancroid is caused by bacteria that get into the skin of the genitals and form little pus-filled blisters. These rapidly break down into painful ulcers, which spread over the entire pubic and genital area. The ulcers are particularly vicious since they attack the victim in two ways. One type burrows deep into the skin; in men it may penetrate through the penis into the urethra so that urine leaks out uncontrollably. The other type of ulcer spreads rapidly over the skin surface to cover the stomach, groin, and thighs. Because the skin is open at the site of the ulcers, it makes the victims much more vulnerable to HIV-AIDS. Condoms don't help much because the ulcers are over the stomach and groin. You'd need a full-body condom to do any good.

Next on the list is granuloma inguinale. Like chancroid, it is caused by bacteria and often passed on by anal sex. Little bumps slowly break out over the surface of the genitals. Gradually they turn into raw, oozing masses of tissue and spread out over the penis, labia, clitoris, and anus. Soon a pungent overpowering stench develops. Once in a while the penis, clitoris, or scrotum become permanently and outlandishly enlarged. If the patient happens to develop a resistant case, the entire lower half of the body becomes ulcerated, and the patient rapidly loses weight and dies.

Two other aspects make granuloma inguinale dangerous. The early manifestations are painless, encouraging victims to postpone treatment until the condition is well advanced. In addition, three months may elapse between exposure and the first sign of infection. By then the original carrier of the disease may have infected scores of others. And of course, the open ulcers make the patient much more susceptible to HIV-AIDS. On the bright side, if the disease is treated early and if it responds to antibiotics, good results can be expected.

There's another unattractive STD called Lymphogranuloma Venereum or LGV for short. It's caused by the same bacteria that causes vaginal chlamydia, *Chlamydia trachomatis*. To make matters worse, it has a pronounced effect on the entire body. The sufferer usually feels sick. Fever, chills, and joint pain are common. Unfortunately they are nothing in comparison with what happens later on.

The most humiliating and disabling changes occur when the infection spreads from lymph glands in the groin to those around the anus. At that point anal stricture occurs, and scar tissue completely obstructs the anus. The only hope is constant dilatation of the rectum—for a lifetime. In a desperate attempt to keep the vital passage open, the sufferer pays a weekly visit to his doctor, who inserts a gloved and lubricated finger into the rectum and vigorously stretches the opening. Although it affects heterosexuals and both men and women, more and more LGV is being spread from one homosexual to another via anal intercourse.

Another problem of LGV results from swollen lymph nodes breaking through the skin at dozens of different points. This pus drains through the openings constantly, particularly in the area between the genitals and the anus—the perineum. Because the pus flows from a dozen or more tiny holes simultaneously, the patient is said to have a "sprinkling-can perineum." Unfortunately it is an accurate description.

While these aren't common diseases in the United States, they do exist and people get infected with them. Be careful.

What about syphilis?

The history of syphilis gives us a fascinating bit of insight into the evolution of STDs. Back in the days when it was called a "venereal disease," syphilis was big and bad. But now, with the abundance of antibiotics and with increased public awareness, it has sort of taken a backseat. There are an estimated 300,000 cases of syphilis a year in the United States, and although that's 300,000 sick people, it doesn't loom as immense as the millions and millions of cases of the "Four H Diseases": HIV-AIDS and HPV and Herpes and Hepatitis.

Two other developments have helped to cut syphilis down to size. First, there is a fast, reliable blood test that is almost routine these days. Second, the disease still responds well to antibiotics.

What's the solution to all these terrible STDs?

It's a matter of waking up and smelling the coffee. It's a matter of facing reality. There is a fascinating psychiatric concept known as "I^2" or "The Immunity of I." It's the feeling that all too many people have that no matter how great the risk is, they will somehow be immune. It is a fantasy that is fed by the movies and television where the hero or heroine always manages to squeak by, no matter what. But real life isn't like that. If you're careless and impulsive about sex, those bad microorganisms are waiting for you. They never watched a sitcom. They don't know anything about happy endings. They know you're not immune. They'll just grow and grow until they do some awful harm.

The world around us is now full of incurable STDs—including the "Four H Diseases." Maybe the best advice is what my wise old Professor of Internal Medicine once told his class:

"As you go through life, you will face many challenges. Sometimes you will succeed and sometimes you will fail. Sometimes you will be wise. Sometimes you will be foolish. But at the very least, try not to get any incurable diseases. . . ."

Chapter 15
MENOPAUSE

What is the menopause?

Technically, the menopause is that time in a woman's sexual development when her menstrual periods stop. With that in mind, it should really be called "meno-stop." Because that's it—no more bleeding, no more cramps, no more pads! "The Curse of Womanhood" is finally a thing of the past! Good-bye to birth control, good-bye to fears of getting pregnant, good-bye to PMS! It should be a time for rejoicing and celebration.

But for all too many women, it doesn't quite work out that way. The menopause is also known as the "Change of Life," presumably so we don't have to say the word that scares men, "menstruation." The "Change of Life" might bring a lot of "changes" with it, and not all of them are welcome.

That includes annoying things like hot flashes, osteoporosis (thinning of the bones), depression, loss of interest in sex, increased risk of heart attacks, vaginal and urinary disorders, and half a dozen other problems.

What causes the menopause anyway?

It's a little defect in the design of human beings. About a million years ago, people were constructed with economy in mind. The real life expectancy was forty years or so and most human organs were designed to last about that long. (Vital parts such as the heart and brain were built a little better.) Then modern medicine entered the picture and made folks live much longer than they had ever been intended to. Once upon a time a woman expired before her hormones did. Today her body lives on for forty or more years after the ovaries have died.

Do the ovaries actually die?

From the standpoint of function, they do. As the fortieth year approaches, the blood supply to those small egg-shaped glands gradually decreases. Cell by cell, the organ withers away and is gradually replaced by scar tissue. Before the menopause, normal ovaries can produce as much as 300 micrograms of estrogen a day. By the time the menopause is well advanced, the ovaries have lost almost all of their function.

Does it make any difference if the ovaries stop working?

Only if you are a woman and only if they happen to be *your* ovaries. The entire basis for femininity is estrogen, the hormone produced by the ovaries. It is also produced to a lesser extent by the adrenal glands and surprisingly enough, by body fat!

This is the stuff that makes girls different from boys. Secreted into the bloodstream drop by drop, this liquid is continuously distributed throughout the entire body where it affects every organ. At the time of puberty it causes the breasts to develop, lays down deposits of subcutaneous fat at the hips, thighs, and buttocks, and keeps the complexion soft and relatively hairless. It also triggers development of the labia and clitoris as well as the uterus and vagina. It works under the direct supervision of the pituitary gland, which regulates the ovary by its own hormone, gonadotropin.

Estrogen is also responsible for that strange mystical phenomenon, the feminine state of mind. It makes girls think like girls. It makes girls act like girls, especially when it comes to sex. Estrogen rules women sexually—the word itself comes from the Greek word *oistros*, or "mad desire." It is the ebb and flow of estrogenic hormone during the menstrual cycle that strongly affects the variations in female sexual desire. Once the production of estrogen stops, the very essence of being a woman stops.

Estrogen is responsible for all the physical female sexual functions. It brings on sexual development, menstruation, ovulation, and plays an important role in pregnancy. It also affects the way women think sexually. Normal men and normal women both have a mature and realistic approach to sex. However, they arrive at it from different points of view. During the menstrual cycle, the amount of estrogen in the body tends to rise and fall. When there is more estrogen available, women tend to feel contented and confident. As the estrogen declines, they may become tense and restless.

One of the important reasons why women tend to be more sensitive than men is that about every thirty days their estrogen level goes from near zero to a very high level and suddenly back to zero again. Most women tolerate this admirably. If men had their sex hormones taken away and given back twice each month, they probably would have made a worse mess of this world than they have with their hormones intact.

How does it happen?

Let a woman describe it.

Irene is forty-eight. She manages a small dress shop to keep busy since her children married and moved away. Her periods stopped two years ago.

> *"Doctor, if I didn't know better, I would think I was being turned into a man. At first when my periods stopped, I thought, 'Thank goodness that's over. No more pains, no more nuisance.'*
>
> *"Now I'm not so sure. At least when I was having periods, I felt like a woman."*
>
> *"What changes have you noticed?"*
>
> *"The first thing I noticed was that my body was changing. It was as if everything were falling down. My breasts began to sag, the upper part of my body got thinner and all the fat went to my hips, abdomen, and legs. I'm not very happy about that.*
>
> *"Then my skin and hair got terribly dry and I began to wrinkle up. I feel like I've gotten ten years older in the past two years! If that wasn't enough, everything I eat seems to go to fat. Gaining 15 pounds in six months just isn't like me. And those hot flashes—when they hit me, I feel like I'm standing in front of an oven!"*

What's a hot flash?

An unbearable sensation of heat that menopausal women experience. It is probably the most common symptom of "The Change." Caused by sudden dilatation of blood vessels at the surface of the skin, most women describe it in dramatic terms:

> *"I'm sitting there watching TV with my husband and all of a sudden my living room turns into a blast furnace and I'm in the hottest part of it! Now I know what the sinners must feel in Hell!"*
>
> *"It can happen anytime. Sometimes I wake up at 2 A.M. on fire—I want to go out and roll in the snow!"*

These thermal reactions can occur as often as every ten minutes, day and night. The usual quota, fortunately, is about four a day.

Do all women have these changes at the menopause?

Almost all women have these kinds of changes to a greater or lesser degree. (Interestingly, women who are really overweight seem to suffer less from menopausal symptoms since their body fat produces a certain amount of estrogen on its own.)

In Irene's case, she was noticing the general effects of estrogen starvation. Weight gain, shifting of fat deposits, increased wrinkling of the skin, and dryness of the hair are annoying. Worse things might happen. Let her continue:

> *"But this is the reason I'm here, doctor. In the last few months I've started to grow hair on my face. And my voice is getting deeper. But that's not all . . ."*
>
> *Irene began to sound embarrassed.*
>
> *"I can't even have relations with my husband anymore."*
>
> *"Why is that? What seems to be the trouble?"*
>
> *"I don't know. I can't seem to describe it. My—my—it just isn't—he can't even—"*

She was gritting her teeth.

A few moments of patient questioning revealed what Irene was trying to say: her vagina was shrinking. The atrophy had progressed to the point where her husband couldn't even push past the entrance to the vagina. Her own interest in sex had evaporated more than a year before and intercourse was a monthly event. On the most recent occasion, it actually seemed to her as if her vagina had vanished. Combined with the other body changes, this dramatic event caused a panicky reaction.

Her description was accurate. Without estrogen, the quality of being female gradually disappears. The vagina begins to shrivel, the uterus gets smaller, the breasts atrophy, sexual desire often disappears, and the woman becomes completely desexualized. Actually it is a little worse than that.

What could be worse?

Although her supply of estrogen is being shut off, her adrenal glands continue, as they always have, to produce testosterone, the male sex hormone. That gradually tends to masculinize a woman. She develops more and more male characteristics.

Increased facial hair, deepened voice, obesity, and the decline of breasts and female genitalia all contribute to a masculine appearance. Coarsened features, enlargement of the clitoris, and gradual baldness complete the tragic picture. It's no fun.

Although she will obviously never really be a man, she has lost a lot of her feminine attributes and she is progressively being masculinized. To make it worse, at this stage emotional problems tend to weigh on women too. Their children have departed, their relationships with their husbands may have declined, and very often sex no longer interests them. Sometimes the husband suffers as keenly. This is how one of them, Harry, tells it:

> *"It's like some kind of bad dream, doc! Up until last year Peggy was a perfect wife."*
>
> *"A perfect wife?"*
>
> *"Well, we've had our little disagreements but nothing like this. Now it's crazy! No sex, no fun, nothing! Every time I turn around she's complaining about something else:*
>
> - *'Why don't we go out more?'*
> - *'Why don't I pay more attention to her?'*
> - *'How come I'm not like other husbands?'*

"Then if I don't get down on my knees and apologize, she blows up, starts crying, and won't talk to me for a couple of days. If this doesn't stop pretty soon, I'm going to be completely nutty!"

Unfortunately, Harry's situation is typical. In addition to physical changes the menopause can bring a lot of mental alterations too. Depression, irritability, and insomnia become the order of the day.

Are the mental changes from lack of estrogen too?

It's hard to say. When a woman sees her womanly attributes fading before her very eyes, she is bound to get a little depressed and irritable. This reaction, superimposed on an estrogen deficiency, can make plenty of trouble. At this stage the divorce rate takes a big leap, and the unhappiness rate (which is hard to measure precisely) goes through the roof.

To many women the menopause marks the end of their useful life. They see it as the onset of old age, the beginning of the end. Having outlived their ovaries, they think they may have outlived their usefulness as human beings. They may fear that the remaining years will just be marking time until they follow their glands into oblivion. But it doesn't have to be that way.

Repeat: It doesn't have to be that way!

Why not?

Many years ago, when I was studying Human Anatomy in Medical School, our Professor of Anatomy showed up one Monday morning somewhat the worse for wear. It was obvious that he'd had a difficult weekend; either too much work or perhaps too much liquid refreshment. His topic that morning was a bone in the skull called the "Ethmoid Bone." It's worth mentioning that the Ethmoid Bone (which sits at about the bridge of the nose) is the most complicated and frustrating bone in the human body to describe and understand. It is a veritable jigsaw puzzle of edges and surfaces.

That morning our professor began his lecture:

"The topic today, Gentlemen, is the Ethmoid Bone."

With bleary eyes and a furrowed brow he stared down at the bone before him, looked back at us, and said:

"Gentlemen, I have only one thing to say this morning regarding the Ethmoid Bone. To Hell with the Ethmoid Bone!"

And I have only one thing to say regarding the menopause:

TO HELL WITH THE MENOPAUSE!

There is no reason in the world for a modern woman to surrender her happiness, her peace of mind, and her sexual satisfaction to the twist of fate that has given her a longer life expectancy than her ovaries. Because two little glands have been shortchanged by Father Time is no reason for her to give up the battle. Remember this: the average life expectancy of a woman in the United States is approaching eighty years. If she starts the menopause at the age of forty, she is going to spend half her life in the menopause.

She might as well take control of her life as quickly and as firmly as she can. She has a full arsenal of weapons at her disposal, if she will only use them. If she is determined and if her doctor is skillful, together they can virtually turn back the clock and restore everything the menopause wants to take away.

How can she do that?

The easiest and most effective way is to simply replace the lost hormone. No one can bring back the ovaries, but the substance they once produced in abundance can be replaced. Most of the undesirable changes that come from lack of estrogen can be virtually reversed by the precise administration of replacement hormones.

For a woman who has suffered the discomforts of the menopause, the transformation can be astounding. The first thing she notices, within a week or so of replacing hormones, is a sudden feeling of well-being. After months or years of depression and discouragement, it's as if a light was snapped on in a dark room.

Evelyn describes it: She is in her fifties and stopped menstruating three years ago. Since then she just stood by and watched as her hormones drained away. Finally things got so bad she decided to see her doctor six months ago.

"I don't believe it! Even though it's happening to me, I don't believe it! When I went to the doctor I was so desperate I was even thinking about killing myself. I hated to get up in the morning. Now I feel like I'm sixteen again. It's even a little embarrassing. My breasts are getting bigger and I find myself thinking more about sex."

Other nice things began to happen. Her voice went up an octave, her facial hair diminished and got downier, and her breasts became firmer. (That's because the elastic fibers of the skin regain some of their strength.) At the same time, some of the unwelcome wrinkles may recede. The skin and hair got back their old consistency and sheen. With the help of a diet, the extra pounds she had gained came off quickly and her feminine figure began to return. The only word that describes the transformation is: "exciting."

The effect on the genitals is exciting too. As Evelyn said, it is almost like puberty. The uterus enlarges, the vagina lengthens, the vaginal lining becomes moist and receptive, the clitoris reverts to a more feminine size, and everything "feels right" again.

What about women like Irene whose vagina has really atrophied? Can they be helped too?

Almost always. The vagina is a fascinating structure in many ways. It has a very special lining made up of squamous cells, the same kinds of cells that line the mouth. But in the normal adult vagina, there are many layers of those cells and the lining is thick and durable.

As the estrogens dwindle, the vaginal lining gets thinner and thinner until it is only a few layers thick. That's bad news, because when the penis gets going, it makes a lot of commotion inside the vagina and bangs those cells pretty hard. If the layer is thin, it gets scraped away and that can hurt!

But there's good news. Direct application of estrogen to the vagina rebuilds the lining quickly and efficiently and helps restore function to normal. Irene's doctor would probably advise her to administer estrogen directly into the vagina in the form of a cream. After a few weeks of this treatment the vaginal tissues would stretch and soften enough to admit the penis. Although estrogen replacement helps in the healing, the real responsibility rests with Irene and her husband.

What would they have to do?

Engage in regular and frequent sexual intercourse. Any structure that isn't used regularly and vigorously withers away—and the vagina is no exception. Some medical textbooks recommend using a very special instrument to dilate the vagina. But Irene's husband has a very special instrument that does an even better job—and a lot more efficiently and enjoyably.

They should use it gently and carefully at first, but they should use it. If he can only insert his penis just at the entrance to the vagina and ejaculate there, the stimulation and increased blood flow to the vaginal tissues will be helpful. As time goes by he should be able to enter a little bit farther. It shouldn't take too long to get the vagina functioning normally again, and then the pleasant assignment is to keep it working.

There is also something very specific that Irene can do to help herself restore and rehabilitate her vagina and the related structures.

What's that?

She can apply the estrogen cream in a very effective way. If she uses the cream as a lubricant to masturbate twice a week or so for two or three weeks, she will help to bring things back to normal fast. It helps in two ways. Rubbing the cream over the clitoris and urethral opening brings the hormone into direct contact with the areas that need it badly. Inserting a finger or two into the vagina and massaging the cream directly into the vaginal lining will also help. This kind of thorough and direct massage is much more effective than just squirting some cream in the vagina and forgetting about it.

But there's more. The increase in blood supply that comes with the swelling of the tissues brought on by masturbation helps the hormone to be absorbed that much faster. And when she finally has an orgasm, the extra flooding of blood is even more helpful in getting the cream where it will do the most good.

But what if she doesn't feel comfortable masturbating?

In this case, it's not masturbation for fun, it's masturbation for therapy—to deal with a medical problem. But if she still doesn't feel right, that's what husbands are for. He can do the same thing for her. As he rubs and strokes her vagina and clitoris with the warm and slippery cream, everyone will feel better. They can also use the cream as a lubricant for sex—without exceeding the dose, of course (the husband should use a condom, he doesn't need estrogen on his penis). And they should have sex as frequently as they can without discomfort— keeping in mind that it takes a few weeks for the lining of the vagina to regain its normal thickness. Just go slowly and let the estrogen cream do its job. A combination of replacement hormone and conscientious copulation will preserve the genitals better than anything else.

What kind of hormone is used to replace the estrogen produced by the ovaries?

Many different kinds of estrogens have been tried. In the last century many of the "Tonics for Women" were really alcoholic extracts of plants that contained vegetable estrogens. Another common source of estrogen is extracted from the urine of pregnant female horses. These days a lot of the estrogen that is prescribed is synthetic estrogen, made in the laboratory.

The method of administration doesn't seem to make much difference either—with certain exceptions. Many women take their hormones by mouth, in tablet form. Many others receive it by injection. (At one time it was even given by implanting little pellets under the skin.) These days a skin patch to deliver estrogen is also available.

For direct application to the vagina, there is the estrogen cream and also a ring like a small doughnut that sits in the vagina and gradually releases estrogen into that structure. What matters is that it enters the bloodstream and is distributed throughout the body.

But why should a woman take hormones? The menopause isn't really a disease, is it?

Let's check the dictionary:

> *"Disease: From the Latin* dis = *'away from' and the French* aise = *'ease.'"*

That sounds like it, doesn't it? The menopause certainly has kept hundreds of millions of women "away from ease." And there's another aspect:

The things that a lack of estrogen causes—like osteoporosis, atrophy of the vagina, and depression, certainly *are* diseases.

But that's part of a kind of reasoning that has kept so many women from finding relief. The argument goes:

If the menopause is not a disease, why take medicine for it?

That sounds logical, doesn't it?

It sounds logical, but it isn't. People don't consider a headache a disease, yet they take medicine—acetylsalicylic acid, known as aspirin—for it. They don't consider an upset stomach a disease yet they take an antacid—aluminum hydroxide gel—for it.

Beyond that, estrogen isn't a "medicine" in the narrowest sense. It's a hormone that one takes to replace a deficiency. Women take thyroid unflinchingly for thyroid deficiency although a lazy thyroid gland can cause them far less trouble in the long run than an estrogen deficiency. And most important of all, estrogen does more than get rid of those hot flashes. It saves lives.

How does estrogen save lives?

By protecting women from the disease that kill more females than any other disease known to Modern Medicine. Half of all the women in America who die, die from heart attacks or strokes. It has been proven again and again that carefully prescribed hormone replacement therapy can cut a woman's risk of dying from a heart attack by as much as 50 percent! And a woman who takes estrogenic hormones cuts her risk of dying from a stroke by almost 70 percent! That's not a misprint. Women who take estrogens in the menopause can cut their risk of dying—from the diseases that kill more women than any others—by 50 percent or more.

Don't these hormones cause cancer?

There is no reliable evidence that estrogens cause cancer. Researchers have been interested in that question for years and have conducted many thousands of careful experiments. What they have found is fascinating. It is possible that women who take estrogen during the menopause will have a slightly greater chance of developing breast cancer. Researchers can't agree on the actual risk. Some studies say there is no significant risk of breast cancer with estrogen replacement; others put the figure around 20 percent.

But that has to be weighed carefully against the risks of *not* taking estrogen. The woman who doesn't take estrogen has doubled her chances of dying from a heart attack and almost quadrupled her chances of dying from a stroke. Besides that, the breasts are not exactly secret organs. They are right out there where the doctor can examine them and where they can be mammogrammed as often as is indicated. Any abnormalities should be able to be identified promptly.

At the same time, a careful look at the figures is very revealing. Each year, about 233,000 American women die from heart disease and 65,000 die from a hip fracture (a condition that estrogens help prevent), compared with 43,000 from breast cancer. That means a woman in the menopause has a 700-percent greater chance of dying from the diseases that estrogen prevents than dying from the disease that estrogen might possibly encourage. It shouldn't be a hard decision to make.

There is also a theoretical possibility that estrogens alone can increase the chances of developing cancer of the lining of the uterus—the "endometrium." But if the estrogen is combined with a small dose of progesterone, the other ovarian hormone, the risk is virtually eliminated.

What if a woman has had cancer of the breast or the uterus? Can she still take estrogens?

That's a question for her doctor to answer. A lot depends on the type of tumor, where it was located, how long ago it was treated, the family history of the woman—and other factors that only her personal physician can evaluate.

Is there any other advantage to taking estrogens during the menopause?

There certainly is. Hot flashes and depression are one thing. They're no fun—being roasted and toasted on a random schedule can make a woman miserable. Depression can take all the pleasure out of life. The amazing protection against heart attacks and strokes that estrogen provides is like a gift from Heaven, but you can't touch it or feel it. It just happens as the years go by and your friends who don't take estrogen disappear and you continue to enjoy a healthy life.

But there's one very special benefit that estrogen gives—a benefit that you can see and feel and experience every day of your life.

What's that?

Relief from the "Terrible Shrinking Disease," otherwise known as "Osteoporosis." (From the Greek words *ostion*, meaning "bone," and *poros*, meaning "passage" or "opening.") Osteoporosis is a strange and mysterious disease that strikes nearly every woman during the menopause. As of this moment at least 20 million American women are its victims.

As her estrogens diminish a woman gradually urinates away the calcium that makes her bones strong and hard. During the first five years of the menopause nearly every woman loses as much as 10 percent of her total bone mass. Later on she may continue to lose bone density at about the rate of 1 percent per year. Osteoporosis does bad things to a woman.

It starts off as ordinary aches and pains—in the back and in the joints. Most women don't pay much attention to it—they dismiss it as part of the menopause. Then one day the back pain may be a little worse and the woman decides to go to the doctor. He takes an X-ray—and then tries to find a tactful way to tell her that she has broken her back.

Broken her back?

That's right. Among all the other things it does, estrogen controls the very complex metabolism of calcium and phosphorus in the bones. Strange as it may sound, human bones are basically soft—something like a stiff gelatin. If you take an animal thigh bone and soak it in a weak acid for a few weeks to dissolve the calcium compounds, you will be able to take the bone and literally tie it in a knot! What makes the bone hard is the calcium and phosphorus that is deposited in all the tiny pores in that bone. (Those calcium compounds are something like what you find in the shell of a clam.)

If a woman is starved for estrogen, the calcium and phosphorus gradually drain from her bones (in the urine) and don't get replaced normally. At the same time, the protein or gelatin-like part of the bone starts dissolving too. A lot of the damage affects the spinal vertebrae, which carry the full weight of the body as they sit on top of each other like little square concrete blocks.

As the osteoporosis progresses the vertebrae may disintegrate, one after the other, like dominoes. The process is silent and insidious and relatively painless at first—the patient may complain of a little back pain. As the vertebrae slowly collapse, the woman actually loses height, sometimes at the rate of a half-inch or more per year. That's why osteoporosis might well be called the "Terrible Shrinking Disease." But it doesn't stop there.

What else happens?

At any time, without any warning, a woman with osteoporosis might have a minor fall or bump that results in a sudden fracture. The most vulnerable areas are the wrist or spine or worst of all, the hip. These are called "pathological fractures" because it hardly takes any force at all to break the brittle bones.

It's a real danger: the United States has the highest rate of fractures from osteoporosis in the entire world. And tens of millions of American women are at risk.

In their lifetime, almost half of all the fifty-year-old white women living in the United States will have a fracture of the spine, the hip, or the wrist caused by osteoporosis.

To put it another way, every year osteoporosis causes more than half a million fractures of the spine, 300,000 fractures of the hip, 200,000 broken wrists, and 300,000 other fractures in the United States. The direct cost of those fractures is more than ten billion dollars.

A broken wrist is disabling, a broken back is worse, but a fractured hip is really bad. A great number of older people who fracture their hips never lead a normal life again and at least 20 percent of them ultimately die of complications of their condition.

Caucasian women in their late fifties are more vulnerable, as are smokers and female athletes who have exercised to the point of stopping their menstrual periods.

What can a woman do about it?

Remember the professor and the Ethmoid Bone?

A woman can also say:

TO HELL WITH OSTEOPOROSIS!

All it takes is awareness, determination, and an understanding doctor. One of the basic problems is that calcium isn't being deposited in the bones. Some people, apparently well intentioned, tell menopausal women that all they have to do is eat more calcium.

But that's not the problem. Human bones are constantly being "remodeled." Old calcium is taken out and new calcium is put in. In the menopause, the woman can have plenty of calcium in her diet, but it just isn't getting deposited where it should go.

The solution is to take estrogen. Estrogen turns back the clock in relation to the bones. It takes over as a traffic cop again and runs the calcium traffic the way it should go. In a menopausal woman, replacing missing estrogens can cut the risk of osteoporosis fractures by 50 percent.

Once a woman is replacing the estrogen, of course, it's important for her to get enough calcium. She can take calcium pills, but they are expensive, and too much calcium—more than 2,000 milligrams a day—can cause kidney stones. Who needs that on top of everything else?

The cheapest, easiest, and tastiest way to get enough calcium is to eat it in your diet. Dietary calcium is abundant, and it's sometimes found where you'd least expect it. You can find it in milk products, but you can also get it from green vegetables.

For example, the beet greens that they often throw away in the supermarkets have nearly as much calcium ounce for ounce as milk. Spinach, collard greens, kale, broccoli, mustard greens, turnip greens, and similar leafy green vegetables are rich in calcium. Tofu, or soybean curd, also equals milk in calcium content. If you like Mexican food, corn tortillas are a good source of calcium. Maybe you're not used to eating spinach and broccoli, but it's better and cheaper than popping calcium pills. A calcium pill just gives you calcium, but a serving of greens gives you plenty of nutrition.

Exercise also helps fight osteoporosis since the more bones are used, the stronger they get. But don't overdo it. Too much exercise in a woman can deplete estrogens and worsen the calcium loss. Smoking is not a good idea either if you want to avoid bone density loss.

So to fight osteoporosis every step of the way, use a combination of estrogen replacement, natural calcium intake, and mild weight-bearing exercise such as walking, baseball, basketball, soccer, tennis, weight-lifting, aerobics, and dancing.

What about the new medicines for osteoporosis?

They're interesting but they have one basic problem. While they may help osteoporosis, they don't do much for the other problems of the menopause. Not only does estrogen fight osteoporosis, it also

protects against a myriad of other diseases in women including cancer of the colon. A woman who takes estrogens has only half the
chance of getting colon cancer. She cuts her risk of crippling
osteoarthritis of the knees by two-thirds.

She even protects her brain. Women who were taking estrogen
replacement had almost 300-percent less chance of contracting that
degenerative brain disease, Alzheimer's, than menopausal women
who didn't replace their hormones. As if that weren't enough reason to take hormones, estrogens also offer protection against age-
related cataracts of the eye. For an extra bonus, they reduce skin
dryness and wrinkling by at least 25 percent.

As one of my patients said when she heard the news:

"Where's the estrogen? Let me at it!"

Of course it makes sense. The decision to replace the most
important hormone in a woman's life should be made on unemo-
tional scientific grounds. In all sincerity, it isn't a job for well-
meaning amateurs who really want to help but haven't invested the
decades of study that are needed to really understand the
menopause. After treating 10,000 or so patients in the menopause,
one begins to understand why there is no substitute for estrogens.

The last word on the subject was written by a very special group
of women who are *better qualified to judge the situation than any
other group of women in the world.* If they say "yes," one can have
complete confidence in their decision.

What group can know so much about estrogens and the menopause?

Think of it this way. The overwhelming majority of male doctors are
in favor of replacing estrogen in the menopause. Yet only about 25
percent of women in the menopause take the estrogen they need. But
the most qualified group of people to evaluate the safety and effectiveness of estrogens must be women doctors in the menopause. What
decision do they make—as doctors and as women? Are they willing to
take a medication that could in any way put themselves at risk?

Here is the answer, according to a careful survey of one thousand four hundred and sixty-six lady doctors:

Almost 60 percent of these female MDs (59.8 percent exactly)
between the ages of forty and forty-nine—including a large num-

ber of female gynecologists—prescribe estrogen replacement for themselves!

That says it all.

Isn't it true that some women don't need hormones? Don't they just "get over" the menopause?

Women can't "get over" the menopause because they can't "get over" the permanent deficiency of a vital hormone. It's not as if a woman's periods stop and then after a few years, she "gets over it" and her estrogen starts again, her periods return, and everything is like it was before.

The idea that a woman "gets over" the menopause is like the farmer who bragged to his neighbor that he was teaching his mule to get along without eating.

"Sounds great, Clem! How'd it work out?"

Clem paused a moment to scratch his head.

"Dunno. I got to where I almost had him convinced and then he up and died!"

It is true that a small group of people believe that the menopause is something women go through and eventually get over. They never give hormones or much of anything else except manly advice like:

"Just get hold of yourself!"
"Don't pay attention to those hot flashes!"

This group is composed exclusively of men; men who have never had a hot flash, never watched their breasts shrivel up, never had their spinal column collapse.

There are also other points of view. Some physicians believe that menopausal women should get estrogen and, at the same time, a little supplement of the male hormone, testosterone.

Is it good to give male sex hormones to women?

They've been getting them all their lives. The adrenal glands, the small organs that sit atop the kidneys, produce testosterone throughout a woman's lifetime. That's one of the reasons a lack of estrogen results in masculinization. Unopposed male hormone brings on things like clitoral enlargement, extra hair growth, and a deepened voice. As the woman grows older the secretion of testosterone begins to decline as well. But women need testosterone too—although in much smaller amounts than men. One of the most important effects of testosterone is to maintain sexual interest and drive during the menopause. A very small supplement of testosterone seems to help eliminate the hot flashes. It also improves the texture of the vaginal lining. Most important of all, it can perk up a woman's interest in sex, which very quickly helps everything else improve.

Do women lose their sexual desire in the change of life?

Many of them do. With depression, hot flashes, aches and pains, osteoporosis, and all the rest, a lot of women couldn't care less about sex. Restoration of estrogens with a little testosterone added does wonders for this problem. The beneficial effects of orgasm with the oxytocin that it adds can be most welcome at this stage. Among other benefits, oxytocin is a powerful anti-depressant. (See Chapter 16.)

On the other hand, some women have a tremendous increase in sexual drive after menstruation stops. No more menstruation, no more birth control, no more anxiety about pregnancy—now they can concentrate on the pure enjoyment of sex and sexuality. This resurgence of sexual drive may bring on two other problems.

What are they?

The first one concerns the husband. At the time when his sexual interest and ability may be slipping, his wife is suddenly rejuvenated. Her demands may be more than he can handle. The second problem is pregnancy. It is possible to become pregnant during the Change of Life. Menstruation may stop but ovulation occasionally goes on. Unless she plans on it, a Change of Life Baby can be quite a surprise.

How long is birth control necessary for a woman?

To be reasonably safe, she should continue contraception for at least one year after the last menstrual period. If another period shows up after eleven months, she needs to wait another year.

That's usually long enough, but human physiology is notoriously unpredictable—more than one woman in her fifties has started buying baby diapers again. If she has any doubt, it's better to stick with birth control a while longer.

Do women who start the menopause early because of surgery—having their ovaries and/or uterus removed—need hormones too?

Women who enter the menopause surgically need estrogens just as much or more than those whose ovaries give out gradually. The sudden withdrawal of hormone support requires prompt and energetic action on the part of both patient and doctor to minimize the discomfort and damage. Even if a woman has simply had her uterus removed with the ovaries left behind, the blood supply to those ovaries may diminish and their hormone production may decline. The same applies to the small group of women who start the menopause prematurely, at the age of thirty or even earlier.

Estrogens don't prevent all the changes of the menopause, do they?

Not all of them, but they keep those changes to a minimum. And it goes far beyond that. Many of the menopausal changes that women experience, such as the lack of energy, the weight gain, the loss of interest in daily life, and all the rest are similar to the effects of "aging." If a woman succeeds in eliminating the worst menopausal symptoms, for all practical purposes she is eliminating the worst effects of aging. That's good news!

But she doesn't have to sit around waiting for the effects of hormone deficiency to strike. Remember, even though a woman may spend half her life in the menopause, she has a right to enjoy every moment.

Is there such a thing as the male menopause?

There might be—if men menstruated. Remember that "menopause" means the end of menstruation and men can't have a "menopause." But just like women, they do get older and as they get older their supply of the male sex hormone, testosterone, declines. Most people call this change the "Male Menopause" but it's not the same.

About the age of forty, the cells of the testicle that secrete the hormone begin to break down. They are slowly replaced by scar tissue, just as in the ovary. Very gradually the output of testosterone diminishes and male sexuality wanes. The secretion of the hormone drops off at the rate of about 1 percent a year from the age of forty or so on. Of course, everyone is different and some men maintain higher levels of the hormone than others—and you can often tell just by looking at them.

How can you tell?

Since men also produce estrogen in their adrenal glands, as the testosterone diminishes the estrogen begins to show itself. Gradually the beard becomes thinner, the voice gets higher, the men put on weight, and their muscles start to get flabbier. Sometimes male breasts even become slightly enlarged. If you had X-ray eyes, you would probably notice that the penis and testicles were starting to diminish in size as well. But there's an interesting paradox.

Although men who lose their testosterone have a relative increase in estrogen, it's not enough to keep them from getting osteoporosis. However, osteoporosis is much less frequent and severe in men. A fifty-year-old white male only has about a 14 percent chance of having an osteoporotic fracture.

But there are other more subtle effects of testosterone deficiency.

Like what?

Men may become more irritable, more lethargic, more depressed, and worry more. In many cases they suffer sexual problems as well. But there is also a complicating problem. Because of the heavy on-the-job stress that many men suffer, sometimes it's hard to tell whether these emotional symptoms come from the job or lack of the hormone.

Why not just give them hormone replacement therapy like in women?

That would be the ideal solution. Just a shot every once in a while or a few pills now and then should put everything back the way it was—or almost. And interestingly enough, it works exactly that way. Men who suffer testosterone deficiency get stronger, more aggressive, more interested in sex, and have better and more frequent erections with testosterone replacement. They also make progress against the osteoporosis which may affect them.

But there's one little problem, which can become a very big problem.

What's that?

It's called the prostate gland. Sitting astride the male urethra at the outlet of the bladder, the gland is very sensitive to testosterone. If a man gets too much of the hormone, the gland begins to grow and can block the flow of urine. No one ever appreciates urination until they can't do it.

You can try it for yourself. The next time you really have to urinate, make yourself wait ninety seconds by the clock. That's just a tiny hint of what a man with a really enlarged prostate has to go through. So we come up against a real dilemma. If we replace the hormone, maybe you won't be able to urinate. If we don't replace the hormone, you can urinate but maybe you can't do a lot of other things that are more fun than urinating.

Of course an enlarged prostate can be removed surgically, but it's obviously better to avoid it than to have to have an operation. But there's something even more important to think about. There's no actual proof that giving extra testosterone to a man causes cancer of the prostate. But it's very likely that testosterone supplements can cause an already small cancer to grow very big, very fast. Since prostate cancer is the number one killer cancer of men (after lung cancer), it's nothing to play around with.

There's something else. Some older men have cancer of the prostate that never spreads beyond the gland and doesn't cause them any trouble. It only turns up at autopsy as a curiosity. But if you pump them full of testosterone, you might ignite that tumor and spread it everywhere.

To make things even more complicated, extra testosterone just might increase a man's cholesterol level and increase his chances of a heart attack or a stroke.

So what is a man to do?

Some doctors give injections of testosterone or recommend a testosterone "patch" which passes the hormone through the skin. Other people feel it's not a great idea. There is serious and sincere medical thinking on both sides of the question. The truth is that no one knows the long-term results of testosterone replacement therapy in men. But there are alternative solutions.

Thanks to the most recent medical discoveries a man can deal with the most pressing problems of the decline in testosterone individually. For example, he can manage the problem of diminishing strength by moderate weight lifting. He can deal with any potency difficulty by using the techniques in the chapter on Impotence. He can manage the osteoporosis by adding additional calcium to his diet, engaging in weight-bearing exercise, and getting non-hormonal medications for osteoporosis from his physician.

Is there anything else he can do?

Yes. He can take a clue from Asian men and make a few tasty additions to his diet. It's a fascinating medical fact that cancer of the prostate is almost unknown in Asian males who follow their traditional diet. At the same time, they seem to suffer much less from "mid-life" emotional disturbances and potency problems. Of course some of the emotional stability is cultural and that has to be taken into consideration. But there is no doubt that certain foods in the Asian diet have important concentrations of sex hormones.

Sex hormones in food?

That's right. They include both male and female sex hormones and can make a big difference in the people who consume them. For example, many Japanese men have been found to have cancer of the prostate during postmortem examinations. But the condition never bothered them while they lived and they were never even aware of it. Enlarged prostates are also unusual in Asian men. So by adding a little Asian flavor to his diet, the average man might be able to do himself a great deal of good.

What can he eat?

The easiest and most useful addition is soybean products. Soy contains powerful compounds called "isoflavinoids" which can lower cholesterol and fight osteoporosis. A glass of soy milk once a day will provide plenty of soy hormone benefits. Besides, it has most of the taste of cow's milk without a drop of cholesterol.

Tofu, or soy cheese, is also a good choice and nowadays you can find it in a dozen forms in the supermarket. You can also find roasted soy beans which can be eaten like a snack—instead of high-fat potato chips. The more soy you can get into your diet—within reason—the more you should benefit.

The ideal intake is about 30 grams of useful soy a day—a glass of soy milk has about 8 grams, a cup of roasted soybeans about 18 grams, and 4 ounces of tofu has about 10 grams. But only eat what you enjoy.

Is replacing the hormones enough to take care of the problem?

Not quite. There is one other vital ingredient. Both men and women need a loving and understanding partner who is willing to help them over the rough spots that the menopause or the male equivalent can bring. A kind and patient wife and a gentle and considerate husband can go a long way to guarantee victory over the tensions and pressures that declining hormones can trigger.

The lack of hormones can't really do permanent harm unless a person allows it to happen. With courage and determination you can beat back all the threats of the menopause, but it's a battle that is better won by two people. Remember, the wife who helps her husband deal with his midlife problem today may need him to do the same thing for her a few years from now. The husband who sees his wife through the first shocks of the menopause may need her to reassure him when his hormones begin to decline.

How about homosexual men? Do they have a change of life too?

Homosexual men are no different physiologically from their heterosexual brothers. Their hormones give out too. Replacement therapy can help them as well, and a homosexual partner who understands their problem and is willing to help is part of the therapy.

How long do women in the menopause need to take hormones?

As long as they want to feel good. If they want to feel good for the rest of their lives, they need to take hormones for the rest of their lives. They can stop taking the hormones anytime, but all the symptoms will come creeping back. The menopause doesn't "go away." Nothing is ever going to bring those atrophied ovaries back to life again. Once they go, they are gone forever. But replacing their vital secretions can make things almost the same as they were before—or even better.

Many years ago people used to look upon the menopause as "The Beginning of the End." But with all the new and exciting treatments and constant encouraging research underway, nowadays the menopause is nothing more than "The End of the Beginning." If you keep that in mind it can actually be the Introduction to a new, more satisfying, and more fulfilling way of life.

Chapter 16
SEPTEMBER SEX

When does a person get too old for sex?

Never. Because of their amazing resilience, the sexual organs just don't wear out. Though most women lose the ability to reproduce after the age of fifty or so, and men rarely become fathers after the seventh decade, sexual intercourse is feasible (and desirable) virtually until the day one departs for a Better World. As a matter of fact, continued sexual interest and activity after the age of sixty is therapeutic—in every sense of the word.

How can sex at that age be therapeutic?

Sexual intercourse and all the events leading up to it are fascinating, stimulating, and exciting. They provide our daily life with much of its vitality and verve. Men and women who have given up most of their other stimulating activities, such as working and raising a family, need sex more—not less—than before.

An elderly man who waits out his last years on a shuffleboard court leads a dismal existence compared to the gent who spends his days scoring in a different sort of game. A crotchety older woman moving back and forth in her rocking chair might discover that life still had a lot to offer if she had a chance to do the same movement in a cozy bed with a willing partner.

This doesn't mean that older people should be turned into sex maniacs (Whatever that is!) constantly looking for a way to titillate their throbbing libidos. But much of the isolation and depression that accompanies old age can be avoided by the socializing effects of searching for suitable sexual partners. If they had more sex on their minds, senior citizens wouldn't have to be prodded to get out and meet people—the problem might be more like getting them to come back home at night.

But isn't it sort of indecent for old people to have sex?

It's hard to understand why. If it's decent for a couple to have sex when they are forty-five and indecent for the same people to do the same thing in the same way with the same organs when they are seventy-five, somebody's mixed up.

Part of the confusion is due to the misconception, handed down through the years, that sex without reproduction is "sinful." As they get older many individuals feel they no longer have a "reason" for sex. But who says they need one? Sexual intercourse is enough reason in itself. If reproduction is the only reason for sex, the human sexual equipment has been grossly overdesigned.

A man only requires, in his lifetime, at the very most enough sperm to father ten to twenty children. Actually, in one ejaculation he has about 250,000 times that amount. For reproduction purposes the human female only needs sufficient eggs to produce a family—but she has the capacity to produce over 200,000. So if sex were only for reproduction, then the sexual organs should be made like hair. When you get to the age of forty-five or so, they would just fall off. Fortunately it isn't that way—which confirms the fact that we should use them for the immense pleasure they can bring us. And that, of course, is one of the true secrets of sexuality.

What's that?

The fact that sex is a "renewable pleasure." As a matter of fact, sex is one of the only two renewable pleasures available to human beings. Each sexual experience can be just as enjoyable as the one before—the two-thousandth time can be as much fun as the second time—or more. The other renewable pleasure is eating; a man of sixty can enjoy it as much as he did when he was sixteen—maybe even more, since he has developed taste and discrimination. Just as there is no reason in the world to give up eating just because you hit the age of sixty or so, there is no reason to give up sex.

Then why do some people give it up?

It may be the easy way out for men and women who never felt right about sex anyway. When age fifty-five or sixty rolls around they are relieved to be excused from what they have considered a burden. Being too old is a socially acceptable excuse for backing away from something they never learned to enjoy.

Occasionally the impetus to relinquish sexual activity comes from the children. Particularly if one of the parents has died, a daughter and son-in-law may say:

"You're too old for that kind of nonsense anyhow, Pop. Why don't you just settle down and forget all about that sex stuff?"

How about another question? Why don't the all-too-considerate children follow their own advice and give up their sex life if it's such a good idea? (Unfortunately some of them probably have.)

Some older people give up sex voluntarily when their partners die. After the first shock of being alone has worn off, their sexual powers and interest may have disappeared permanently. Others interrupt copulation for a while when either husband or wife is ill. That frequently spells the end of all sex. Some couples just lose interest gradually; for others sex goes out the window when the man loses his potency.

Interestingly enough there are some striking differences in the way men and women finally retreat from sex.

What are they?

The statistics reflect what everyone has probably been suspecting all along. In this country, women maintain their interest in sex much longer than men do. Among the age group sixty to ninety years old, the overwhelming majority of women give up sexual intercourse only because their husbands are no longer willing or able to satisfy them. Of these, about half the women bring their own sexual lives to a close when their husbands die. Only about one-tenth of females voluntarily choose celibacy.

On the other hand, more than half the men in this age range ring down the curtain on sexual gratification because of illness, impotence, and lack of interest.

The most important thing to keep in mind is that—after the age of sixty—if sexual intercourse is interrupted for a period of time, it may never start again. This is probably the most important single point for older folks to keep in mind. As a practical matter, if a period of more than sixty days voluntarily elapses without sexual relations between husband and wife after the age of sixty (and sometimes even before), the odds are against ever taking up an active sexual relationship again. When it comes to sex, the magic words are "Use it or lose it!"

Henry had an experience like that and it was a harrowing one. Henry is sixty-eight and a retired accountant; he tells what happened:

"Well, I was never too interested in sex, but I wasn't ready to give it up—once in a while I really enjoyed it. I would say that my wife and I would have relations about every four weeks or so. About six months ago, back in January, Irene had a bad attack of arthritis and it made our married life pretty uncomfortable for her. So I just did without for that time. Last month she was feeling better and I tried to start again but I couldn't get sufficient strength in my organ."

What Henry means is that after six months of enforced chastity, he couldn't get an erection. At the age of sixty-eight erections don't come easily to most men, and like blackbirds, once erections fly away it's hard to get them back. But like most women, Irene was more practical about sexual matters than her husband. She tells what happened next:

"Well, I'm not exactly what you would call a sex fiend, but I knew something was wrong with my husband. He didn't eat right and he just sat around the house brooding—he didn't even go for his walks anymore like the doctor said he should. And every time he tried to have relations with me and failed he just got worse. So I went downtown and got your books on sex—I'd never done anything like that before, but times are changing and I guess I'd fallen a little behind.

"One of your books said that if the wife handled her husband's organ when they had sex, it made it easier for him to have an erection. I was always taught that no decent

*woman did that kind of thing, but I suppose things are dif-
ferent now. To tell the truth, I didn't really care. I love my
husband and I was willing to do anything to help him be a
man again. The next chance that came along I did just what
your book said, and it was like magic—his organ got harder
than it used to get thirty years ago. That's when I thought
maybe I should have been doing it all along!*

*"But even more important to me, Henry was a changed
man. He's much more cheerful and optimistic and he even
wants to look for a part-time job now. And I'm not afraid to
admit it—I enjoy our relations much more than I used to.
I'm even thinking of trying some of the other things I read
about in your book!"*

In general women tend to be more practical about sex.

There are many examples of the pleasures of sex after seventy
in the folklore of various nations. For example, in Scotland, there's
a well-known poem about a widow lady of seventy-five who married the village blacksmith, a strapping man of forty-seven. The
fourth day of her honeymoon, her daughter sent her a telegram:

*"Mother—How is your honeymoon? Are you feeling well or
is it too much for you?"*

There was no answer until two days later, when she received a
telegram with this short message:

*"Farewell, my Friends!
Farewell, my Foes!
Your Granny's off to Heaven
On a Pintle's Nose!"*

(*Note*: In the Scots language, a "Pintle" is a penis.)

At any age, sex is good for you, but by the time you pass the
sixth decade, it is medicinal.

Medicinal? You mean it's like medicine?

No, it isn't *like* medicine. It *is* medicine. And as with medicine,
there are many different forms in which to take your medicinal sex.

If there was no other choice, Henry could have gotten his medicine another way.

How?

By masturbation. If he was a widower, or if he didn't have a sexual partner, masturbation would be an important part of the solution. As far as the body is concerned, all reflexes are similar. Physiologically speaking, the sexual reflex patterns are very much like those controlling digestion. If Henry didn't eat any solid food for six months he would have a very hard time going back on a normal diet. Unless the sexual nerve patterns are constantly reinforced after the sixth decade, they may simply fade away.

The body doesn't care how this reinforcement takes place. Henry's minister may not like it if Henry brings on his own orgasms, but the minister surely can't suggest a better method of preserving sexual function either. (Besides, ministers masturbate too.) If an aging man can understand that regular masturbation may help keep his sexual equipment functioning until his usual sexual partner is again available, both husband and wife will be spared a tremendous amount of suffering.

You mean doctors recommend masturbation?

Masturbation is certainly not the ideal form of sexual activity. For obvious reasons although it can't compete with sexual intercourse for lasting satisfaction, it plays a significant role in everyone's sexual evolution. Just as sexual activity kicks off with masturbation in childhood, it can extend sexual satisfaction in old age. If a man or woman has to choose between permanent loss of sexual powers or temporary masturbation, masturbation should win hands down. If the husband dies, it makes sense for the wife to masturbate to keep her copulatory reflexes going until she can find another sexual partner.

In men it's even more urgent. It doesn't take much mechanically for a woman to prepare for sex. But before a man can have sex, he has to set some very complex machinery in motion. For an older man, an erection can be just that—a complicated construction project to erect a rigid piston that can enter a waiting cylinder. When it comes to erections, once again, it's literally a case of "Use It or Lose It!"

What if the spouses can't get together because of excess weight?

Because of the amazing versatility of the human sexual equipment, it's almost always possible to bring penis and vagina together in one way or another. One of the biggest obstacles to sex—sometimes literally—is obesity. As a couple grows older and puts on weight, their enlarging abdomens push the vagina farther and farther away from an eager phallus.

Unfortunately the penis cannot increase in length to keep one step ahead of the tummy, and the vagina ultimately gets out of range. The ideal solution would be for both partners to lose weight. That's not always possible. The practical solution is to find a way to have intercourse that detours around the protuberant abdomens. One of the most effective positions is the "T-square" technique. The woman lies in the usual position on her back with her legs spread wide apart. Her partner lies on his side facing her with his hips under the arch formed by her raised legs. With both abdomens safely out of the way, the penis can make an end run and score a touchdown at the vagina.

Another simple solution is the famous "Cowgirl" position where the man lies on his back and the lady straddles him and rides his penis like a wild horse. There's also the "Reverse Cowgirl" technique where she rides him the same way except she faces his feet instead of his head. Both these positions give the penis and vagina a clear shot at each other. And they have some excellent added attractions.

With the woman riding on top, the entire upper surface of the penis races back and forth on the "Orgasmic Highway"—that super-sensitive strip on the front wall of the vagina extending all the way up to the clitoris. But the woman is in control and she can twist and turn to get just the exact kind of penis massage that delivers her right into the hands of a tremendous orgasm. The "Reverse Cowgirl" has exactly the same benefits—plus this one. As the woman bounces up and down he can watch his penis pumping in and out of the vagina. That can be just the extra stimulus that makes sex even better for an older man.

What about people with arthritis?

As time passes, almost everyone develops occasional aches and pains in the bones and joints. Sometimes the discomfort gets to the point where a person is afraid that sexual intercourse and the associated movement might make it worse. That's not necessarily a bright idea. For most forms of arthritis, frequent mild exercise is beneficial. And what better way is there to exercise mildly than in bed with an eager and willing sexual partner?

But there is even a better reason than that. The experience of sexual intercourse is not as simple as it looks—it isn't just penis-into-vagina-in-and-out-and-in-and-out-pop-goes-the-weasel. A lot of other things happen that we are just beginning to be aware of.

In the human being, all the glands in the body are interconnected and ruled by the master gland, the pituitary. Since the testicles in the male and the ovaries in the female are powerfully affected by sexual activity, every time a person has an orgasm, an urgent message is relayed to the pituitary which sits at the base of the brain. The pituitary transmits the message to the thyroid and adrenal glands which start pumping hormones. The most amazing thing is that the adrenal glands produce—among many other hormones—a hormone called "cortisol." By a wonderful coincidence, cortisol works to relieve the symptoms of arthritis! So, if everything works the way it should, regular and frequent sexual intercourse should tend to alleviate the symptoms of arthritis.

You mean sex is good for arthritis?

In a sense, yes. For a long time doctors have known that there is much less arthritis among those who remain sexually active. They used to think that only those who somehow were spared the crippling effects of this disease were able to keep having intercourse. Now, hormone studies have proved that it is sexual activity itself which helps protect those beyond middle age from the degenerative changes of this condition. But it doesn't stop there. There is another powerful pituitary gland hormone that can be decisive in a person's sex life—and their entire relationship with their spouse as well.

How can a hormone affect their relationship with their husband or wife?

Like this. Almost by accident, researchers discovered that when a person has an orgasm, the concentration of a hormone called "oxytocin" suddenly zooms up to 362 percent of its normal value! The implication of that finding is the best news anyone over the age of sixty could have. Oxytocin is a type of chemical called a "neuropeptide" because it acts directly on the nervous system. Oxytocin increases a person's interest in sex, it makes them much more affectionate, and it is a powerful antidepressant. That's one of the reasons that almost everyone feels warm and tender after sex. And that warmness and tenderness tend to persist long after orgasm has passed. Even more important, the more orgasms a person has, the longer and deeper the affectionate phase is. So the more orgasms they have together, the closer and more devoted they tend to become. That's why oxytocin can help a husband and wife get along better in every area of their personal lives—in areas far beyond sex.

But it doesn't stop with oxytocin. There's another set of amazing chemicals that orgasm sets loose.

Which ones are they?

They are called "endorphins" and they are amazing substances. When someone gets a shot of morphine for pain, the drug goes to the nerve endings that sense pain and prevent the pain from being felt. At the same time the morphine also goes to the brain and gives the patient a feeling of happiness and well-being.

"Endorphins" are similar to morphine but they are produced by a person's own body. That's why when someone is injured seriously, at least for a while they aren't in unbearable pain.

One of the most effective ways to trigger your own endorphins is by orgasm. Every time you reach a sexual climax, your brain pours endorphins into your bloodstream and you get that wonderful "high" that makes you want to go back for more and more. And that's why—during the peak of orgasm—if someone stuck you with a pin, you would hardly notice it.

One of the things that older people need most is a feeling of well-being, and one of the safest and most reliable ways to get that feeling of well-being is as close as their bedroom. Sex makes their relationship better, and a better relationship makes their sex better. It's a wonderful situation where everyone wins—if they take advantage of the opportunities that sex offers them.

And there are some wonderful benefits of sex that we never even dreamed of!

For example?

For one thing, sex—including orgasm—is excellent for the brain. When a man or woman has an orgasm, suddenly one of the most vital parts of their brain is flooded with fresh oxygen-rich life-giving blood. The part of the brain that gets a massive flow of blood is known as the "pre-frontal cortex of the cerebrum."

That's fascinating because that's where human beings do all their highest level thinking—where they analyze what's going on in the world around them. But that's not all. That part of the brain handles the most important planning and decision-making. It's also the headquarters for sexual arousal, self-understanding, and new ideas and concepts. As if that were not enough, this is where insight, art awareness, music appreciation, and imagination also originate.

What's the significance of that?

Let's think about it for a moment. As people get older, it's just those particular areas that begin to suffer. Planning and decision-making begin to get a little fuzzy, they become less receptive to new ideas, their imagination starts to fade—you've seen it a hundred times in people you know. Now imagine the tremendous benefit of sending an invigorating shower of fresh and revitalizing blood to this vital area with every orgasm. That's why people who have regular and frequent sex seem so much brighter and more vigorous. And they also live longer and avoid premature death.

You're saying there's proof that frequent sex can actually help you to live longer?

That's exactly right. Men between the ages of forty-five and fifty-nine are the ones at greatest risk for fatal heart attacks. For a period of ten years, almost 1,000 men were carefully observed in regard to their sexual habits, their cause of death, and their age at death. The results were staggering: men who had infrequent orgasms had twice the chance of dying of a heart attack compared with men who had frequent orgasms.

To state it another way, men who had a lot of sex were protected from death by heart attacks. Simply by having regular and frequent sex, they cut their chances of dying prematurely in half.

The scientists, who were British, summed up their sensational findings with typical British understatement: "Sexual activity seems to have a protective effect on men's health."

But how much sex do you need to get the benefit?

The ideal number of orgasms per year to get the maximum benefit is about a hundred. That's a climax approximately every three days, or about two per week. Although it may interfere with the schedule of your bridge game or Monday Night Football, it's worth the sacrifice to keep your brain going and to save yourself from a heart attack. And once you get into it you may even find it more interesting then either football or bridge—who knows?

Is there anything else that people with arthritis can do to make their sexual lives more enjoyable?

Certainly. Very often simply changing positions can be helpful in relieving the pressure on painful joints. There is nothing in the U.S. Constitution that insists that the man has to be on top and the woman must lie on the bottom during copulation. Sensible experimentation is often indicated—any reasonable means of bringing the penis and vagina in closer proximity is worth considering. Some of the far-out techniques have their drawbacks, however. Leonard ought to know—he tried them:

> *"Well, you know how it is, Doctor. Grace and I aren't as young as we used to be. We're both in our fifties and when I saw one of those books advertised last week, Make Your Marriage Young Again, I just couldn't resist. It was the chapter on 'Thirty-Six Exquisite Sexual Positions' that really got to me. Since Grace was willing, we tried them— not all on the same night, of course.*
>
> *Positions one through nine weren't too bad. Neither of us noticed anything 'exquisite' about them but they were a change from everyday. The next ones, ten through seventeen, were just too much work and didn't seem worth it. Position eighteen was the one that did me in. It was called The Egyptian Grapevine, and had our arms and legs all twisted up together. It was supposed to bring on unbearable ecstasy.*
>
> *"Well, it didn't exactly work out that way. It took about five minutes for Grace and me to get ourselves into it but when we were ready to have intercourse, we found we couldn't even move. We both started laughing so hard that I wrenched my back. I couldn't go to work for two days and I could*

hardly have sex for the next two weeks. I gave the book to one of the salesmen at the office—he's a bachelor. Let's see how the Egyptian Grapevine works for him. I wish him luck!"

How does sex affect the heart?

No normal heart was ever harmed by sexual activity. Actually a vigorous, healthy interest in sex and an active sex life are probably the best form of protection against a heart attack.

How is that?

Heart specialists agree that three of the major precipitating factors in heart attacks are lack of exercise, overweight, and nervous tension. Frequent, vigorous sexual intercourse helps to control all of these dangers.

There are few forms of physical exercise that provide the benefits of copulation. The vigorous pelvic thrusts maintain the muscles and joints of the entire spine in good condition. The circulation of the whole body is improved and deep breathing is encouraged. If you think about it, as a form of exercise, sex beats jogging.

Look at it this way:

One of the major goals of jogging is to raise the heart rate over about 120 beats per minute and thereby increase cardiac reserve. During intercourse, the heart rate usually rises to about 160 beats per minute just before and during orgasm. In addition, the blood pressure increases, for a short time, as much as 50 percent—this is considered beneficial. It has been calculated that the average act of intercourse consumes about 150 calories, which makes it attractive to weight watchers.

A single act of intercourse is the exercise equivalent of about half an hour of jogging. For most people, four times around the park on a cold rainy morning can't compare with once around a nice warm bed. Any man who thinks about it is bound to trade forty minutes of pounding the pavement gasping for breath for an hour or so in the fragrant embrace of a willing female. The other drawback of regular exercise is forgetting to keep it up. Sex is a lot harder to forget, and your partner is there to remind you. And sex has one other big advantage over jogging: it doesn't require any special shoes.

An active sex life keeps the weight down in other ways too. While some folks like their mates to be pleasingly plump, everyone wants to look their best when they take their clothes off. To maintain their sexiness, most men and women have a good incentive to watch their weight.

One of the biggest burdens on the heart is our frantic society. The daily frustrations and anxieties that plague us can cause progressive and relentless damage to the heart and blood vessels. That's where the oxytocin and endorphins come in. There is nothing like a good orgasm—and the natural tranquilizers it liberates—to wash away all the stress and tension of our daily existence. The peace and well-being that a full, loving sexual relationship can bring is unobtainable anywhere else—at any price. There is an added bonus: as the richness of a gratifying sexual relationship calms and relaxes the individual, the sexual experience itself becomes even more satisfying. In its best form, sex can be the ideal antidote to our crazy mixed-up world.

Doesn't sex bring on a heart attacks?

Not really. If a person's cardiac status has deteriorated so tremendously over the years that a heart attack is just about to strike, copulation may conceivably be the final stress that cuts off the blood supply to the sagging heart. That doesn't mean that sex *causes* heart attacks. Watching an exciting movie on television or running to catch a bus the next morning can do the same thing. Giving up sex at that point won't forestall the inevitable more than a few hours at the most. And when you get right down to it, there are worse ways to leave this world than "Riding High in the Saddle."

Is sexual intercourse safe for those who have had heart attacks?

Except in unusually severe cases, the danger to the heart from sexual intercourse is insignificant. The rule of thumb that most doctors use is this:

If a person can walk one block or climb two flights of stairs without heart symptoms, they can have sex.

The strain on the heart of a brisk walk is probably more than that of a brisk orgasm. Copulation requires an energy consumption of about five calories a minute, which is well within the range of most of those who have recovered from heart attacks.

As a matter of fact, researchers have precisely measured what it takes to perform sexual intercourse. As you would expect, oral sex—cunnilingus and fellatio—don't make much demand on the heart. Intercourse with the wife on top is slightly less taxing for the man, and man-on-top at orgasm only brings the heart rate up to about 160 beats per minute—but only for a very short time.

Because a heart attack does cause some immediate damage to the heart muscle itself, it is sensible to wait until the first stage of healing is well under way. To be on the safe side, sexual activity should be postponed until about eight to ten weeks after the original attack. As in every medical condition, your personal physician is the one who can give you the best advice. Please consult your doctor for guidance in any medical condition.

No one can really say for sure what would happen if copulation were to begin before then. Occasionally heart patients are visited in the hospital by their husbands or wives and have sex in the hospital room as early as a week or two after the heart attack without any ill effects. While this demonstrates the durability of the heart muscles as well as the durability of the human sexual instinct, it's better to wait a little longer.

Couldn't somebody die that way?

As far as we know, the number of people who die from heart attacks during sexual intercourse is very small. Some estimates suggest that about six out of every thousand people with previous heart attacks finally succumb during intercourse. As an interesting sidelight, about 80 percent of those who cash in their chips during copulation are making it with someone other than their own husbands or wives. For those who've had a heart attack and want to continue with sex, honesty may well be the healthiest policy.

In any event, prompt resumption of sexual activities after a heart attack (as soon as it can be done safely) is very important.

Why is it so important?

Many of those who suffer heart attacks, both men and women, feel as if they have somehow been damaged irreparably. They often tend to think of themselves as semi-invalids. Once they see that they are still effective and desirable as sexual partners they improve immediately. The wife who wants to spare her husband the strain of sex is making a mistake. It would be much better if she would stimulate him instead—tactfully. Alice handled it well:

"Jim had his heart attack about three months ago and it really hit him hard. He almost lost his business—he wholesales appliances. He finally managed to get back to work slowly and got things under control. Just when I thought everything was fine, it turned out I was doing him in by trying to be considerate.

"I just didn't know better. I figured he was a sick man and sex would be bad for him. He really used to be sensational before his attack—I mean he could make me turn cartwheels when it came to sex! But when he got home from the hospital I ordered twin beds so he wouldn't get all worked up sleeping next to me. The poor man thought I did it because he was all washed up. He really started to go downhill then. Fortunately I caught on fast and put those twin beds up in the attic. It was just like magic! He's even better than before—he says he appreciates it more now. His heart attack certainly didn't seem to damage any of his other organs!"

Is sex helpful in any other way to those who have had heart attacks?

Yes. Aside from the feeling of relaxation that comes from successful copulation, there is a hormonal advantage as well.

Some cardiac patients have a symptom known as angina pectoris, a medical term for pain in the chest. On exertion, after a heavy meal, or because of mental strain, the individual may develop a sudden agonizing, crushing pain behind the breastbone. The exact cause of this symptom is unknown—it may be related to lack of blood supply to the heart muscle, but the explanation is far from clear. In any event, the pain of angina pectoris is excruciating and prevents the sufferer from doing anything—sex included.

As we've seen, orgasm liberates a whole array of beneficial chemicals and hormones in the body. Just as in arthritis, men with angina pectoris who are sexually active seem to have less frequent attacks of pain. Though angina pectoris is five times as common in men, those unfortunate women who are afflicted with it also seem to benefit from regular sexual intercourse. In cases where chest pain tends to interfere with sex, nitroglycerine tablets (a common remedy for angina) taken a few minutes before intercourse may prevent the pain from developing. But remember, check with your doctor before you do anything that might cause you a problem. It's better to ask than to have any surprises!

Is there anything men and women can do to keep their sexual power perking right along?

There certainly is. The first step is to decide to do it. What's the point of going to the gym every day or watching what you eat or taking vitamins if you're going to neglect the most important and most enjoyable function of your organism? If you want to keep enjoying sex, you have to pay attention to your sexual equipment and keep it in top shape.

As we have seen, the sexual organs—both in men and women—are basically hydraulic. They depend on pumping blood under pressure through tubes and pipes. The penis doesn't just get erect—it is very deliberately erected. The clitoris doesn't just pop up—valves open and close and blood is pumped in under pressure. Orgasm depends in great measure on the buildup of blood under tremendous pressure—and its sudden and explosive release. If the pressure doesn't get high enough—if the blood is stagnant—the orgasm is puny. It's just a dull thud, and it should be KA-BOOM! BOOM! BOOM!

Like any hydraulic system, your sexual hydraulics require care and maintenance. You can't neglect the cooling system in your car—a hydraulic system. You can't neglect the oil pressure—also hydraulic. In the same way you have to take care of the hydraulics of your sexual equipment.

How do you do that?

The hydraulic fluid of sex is blood and you have to maintain excellent blood circulation to the sexual organs. Think about it this way. If you sit all day at a desk with your legs hanging down, pretty soon you are going to have varicose veins from the stagnating blood. If a patient lies immobile in a hospital for days on end, he may end up with a blood clot in his lungs and probably die from it.

If you want good erections and good orgasms, you have to do your part. Consider this. Almost everyone agrees on the benefits of massage. There's nothing like massaging your feet when they are sore and weary from walking or standing too long. A back massage is wonderful for relaxing and getting relief from sore muscles.

Many women believe in facial massage and pay big money to have it done. But the sexual organs—far more important than the face or the back muscles or the feet—are left to fend for themselves. Are they just supposed to hang out there and hope that everything will be all right when their big moment comes?

Men and women—particularly those over the age of forty—should be willing to offer their sexual equipment the same care and attention they offer to their feet. The goal is to maintain and increase the blood supply to these vital structures. Just think for a moment how you feel. After standing or sitting all day there is that heavy feeling in the perineum—the area between the vagina or the scrotum and the anus. Vague pressures and tensions in the groin area are another symptom of inadequate circulation to the sexual structures.

What's the solution?

The same elementary attention you provide to your feet or a sore muscle. Massage those vital structures and the areas around them daily. Although you've been told all your life "Don't touch yourself down there!" the truth is that only good things can come from "touching yourself down there" if you do it right.

For a man, this is the recommended routine. Every morning in the shower, with adequate lubrication, take your penis between the palms of your hands and roll it back and forth very gently about 25 times. Remember that's where you want the blood to pour in when you have an erection and a daily massage to improve the circulation is ideal. At the same time, gently massage the root of the penis at the point where it leaves the body. You can also gently massage both groin areas about 25 times each as well as carefully kneading the skin of the scrotum the same number of times.

Then to finish, grip the shaft of the penis gently in one hand and massage the head of the organ with the other hand—as if you were polishing an apple. This will bring blood to the head of the penis and help to achieve a better erection and increased sensitivity. About twenty-five polishing strokes should be enough.

You will feel the effect almost immediately with a gentle glow spreading over the area and a feeling of better tone and circulation in the tissues. That's because you have improved the flow of the fluid—blood—that provides the power to these organs. After a week or so of daily massage, you should see a change in sexual functioning, with greater sensitivity and better results all around.

Can women do the same thing?

Certainly. With adequate lubrication place one finger on each side of the shaft of the clitoris and move the fingertips gently up and down. Twenty-five times should be enough. Then stroke the labia minora from top to bottom twenty-five times. Gentle massage of the entrance to the vagina is also helpful. And don't forget the groin massage on both sides. The best time and place is the morning shower—that warm glow and the increased tone are because of the improved circulation. The real results should begin to show up in a week, and you can expect continued improvement as you continue the daily routine.

But isn't that masturbation?

Not really—just like massaging your feet when they are tired isn't a foot fetish. But for men and women of advanced age, there is an important role for masturbation. When something happens that prevents either partner—or both—from being able to have sexual intercourse, what do they do? Is that an end to sex for both of them and an end to orgasm and all the wonderful physical and mental benefits that come with it? It doesn't have to be.

Obviously the ideal form of sex is sexual intercourse. But mutual masturbation and oral sex are the next best. The most important thing is to keep those orgasms coming—and get their benefits—no matter what.

In many cases oral sex and mutual masturbation will only be temporary measures until the problem that prevents full-scale intercourse is cleared up. For example, a woman who has a broken leg may find regular intercourse uncomfortable and awkward, but there is no reason for her and her husband to go weeks without any sex at all. She can still perform fellatio, and he may be able to perform cunnilingus on her.

Sometimes more serious chronic physical problems like a stroke or emphysema may make full intercourse difficult. But oral sex may still be a practical approach and mutual masturbation equally effective. The key is to be resourceful, inventive, and enthusiastic. Generous lubrication is always important—both to massage the penis to ejaculation and to caress the clitoris and stimulate the vagina. Just as in regular sex, the man should concentrate on the anterior wall of the vagina, slowly and carefully inserting first one and then two well-lubricated fingers. With those fingers working on the front wall of the vagina and the thumb on the clitoris, a satisfying orgasm should be just around the corner.

Why do you specify "two fingers" in the vagina?

That's the old maxim: "One finger isn't enough and three fingers are too much!" It's really only a rule of thumb. But for most women who have had at least one child, two fingers give the right amount of stimulation. But her partner should listen to her—she knows best what she wants.

The same applies to the man. Sometimes he wants a vigorous massage of his penis—even with both hands alternating. On other occasions he may prefer the most gentle of caresses until the very last moment. Remember, the only time you can't talk during sex is when your mouth is busy—and even then you can take a moment to describe what you want.

But is sex really that good for you?

Of course it is. Just look around you at your friends who are having regular and satisfying sex—and compare them with the ones who don't have sexual outlets. The difference is obvious and speaks for itself. And most important of all, the older you get, the more important sexual activity and the benefits of orgasm become.

When does someone actually get too old for sex?

Judge for yourself. One day a little girl asked her grandmother:

> *"Gee, Grandma, you're eighty-five. When do people stop liking sex?"*
> *Grandmother put down her book, smiled, and replied:*
> *"I don't know, Jennie. For an answer to that, you'll have to ask someone older than me!"*

That's really the way it is. And for those who are fortunate enough to have a good husband or wife, there is an old and very romantic adage that says:

> *"A good husband and a good wife are like rare wine—as the years go by they get better and better and better."*